Top 50 Dermatology Case

Danya Reich • Corinna Eleni Psomadakis
Bobby Buka

Top 50 Dermatology Case Studies for Primary Care

Dear Aunt Lila—
May you never have to
deal with anything in this
book!
See if you can figure out
which relative's skin is
pictured on page 11
& page 331.
♥ Danya
H

Springer

Danya Reich, MD
Assistant Professor
Department of Family Medicine
Mount Sinai School of Medicine
Attending Mount Sinai Doctors/Beth Israel
Medical Group-Williamsburg
Brooklyn, NY, USA

Bobby Buka, MD, JD
Medical Director
Bobby Buka Dermatology
Section Chief
Department of Dermatology
Mount Sinai School of Medicine
New York, NY, USA

Corinna Eleni Psomadakis, BA, MBBS (2018)
School of Medicine
Imperial College London
London, UK

ISBN 978-3-319-18626-9 ISBN 978-3-319-18627-6 (eBook)
DOI 10.1007/978-3-319-18627-6

Library of Congress Control Number: 2016955819

Printed on acid-free paper

This Springer imprint is published by Springer Nature
The registered company is Springer International Publishing AG
The registered company address is: Gewerbestrasse 11, 6330 Cham, Switzerland

To the patients in this book as well as those whose cases did not make it in, and to all our patients who have agreed to have their skin photographed by us for educational purposes. We are grateful for your willingness to participate and for the privilege of being able to learn from you.

Preface

The goal of this book is to help primary care doctors get better at dermatology diagnoses and treatment.

This book came about because I was looking at a different dermatology book—aimed at dermatologists—that was heavy on text, light on pictures, and I said to my colleague, "Family Medicine doctors need a lot more pictures!" The publisher of that book happened to overhear me, and this book was born.

Over the course of 2 years, I photographed over 300 cases that presented to my primary care office. Sometimes I knew what the skin condition was, sometimes I did not, sometimes I referred to dermatology, sometimes I treated myself, sometimes it was a combination. No matter what, I photographed. Bobby and I reviewed the cases and out of all of them, we chose 50 for this book to represent a cross section of common and unusual, acute and chronic, mild and life-threatening.

As a collaboration between primary care and dermatology, the idea for this book is to present these cases as a primary care doctor encounters them—opening the door to the exam room and not knowing what medical condition or body part will be presented, seeing a patient's skin lesion, describing it, and figuring out what to do next.

To that end, each case was written first from the primary care point of view and then dermatology weighed in with differential and favored diagnosis, overview and presentation, workup, treatment, and follow-up. Each case then concludes with a Q&A between primary care and dermatology. Lastly, the book is organized by body part as that is often the way we first think of any medical condition—by location.

Our desire is that—with all this information and with the primary care/dermatology collaborative perspective—this book would serve as a useful, informative resource for primary care providers.

Brooklyn, NY, USA Danya Reich

Preface

It is amazing how much this dermatologist does not remember about other parts of the human body. The more experienced I become in the practice of clinical dermatology, the less I recall about general medicine from my training. I am quite certain that as a medical student I was the most well versed in all aspects of medicine that I will ever be, and that it has been a steady decline ever since. Could I manage a hypertensive patient today, the most basic of internist duties? Not a chance.

It is precisely for this reason that I hold the utmost respect for the fields of family medicine and primary care. These doctors are charged with the unique challenge of staying up to date on a dizzying array of advances in contemporary medicine, not just in one field, but in *all* of them. Clinicians like Danya are oftentimes the first line of defense against illness *in any organ system*, that is, the first opportunity to render an accurate diagnosis, and treat appropriately.

Danya and I first met as colleagues, and it was not long before we realized the unfortunate disconnect between specialist and primary care. The specialist letters I sent back to her gave an assessment and plan, but were painfully incomplete when it came to helping her appreciate how and why a particular diagnosis was made. And so this text and its format were born.

Each case will take you from presentation to differential diagnosis to pathophysiology to care, just like patients arrive on our doorstep. And just like the doctor ordered, with lots and lots of pictures. We encourage you to enter each case cold, photos first, do not turn the page! See if your differential comports with our own. It need not overlap entirely but should get you in the right ballpark. This approach will ensure you get the most from this text, whether you are a new student just entering the world of cutaneous medicine or an old-timer freshening up. Have fun with it!

New York, NY, USA
June 2016

Bobby Buka

Morphology of Dermatological Lesions

Macule A circumscribed flat, nonpalpable area of <1 cm with altered skin color.
seen in: freckles, café-au-lait spots, melanotic macules

Patch A larger circumscribed flat, nonpalpable area >1 cm with altered skin color.
seen in: port wine stains, vitiligo

Papule A solid, small (<1 cm) elevated lesion. Papules may be described in terms of their shape (dome-shaped, umbilicated, verrucous, etc.).
seen in: molluscum contagiosum, juxtaclavicular beaded lines

Plaque A flat, palpable lesion that is >1 cm in size and is elevated or thickened relative to surrounding tissue, analogous to a geographical plateau.
seen in: psoriasis, pityriasis rosea

Nodule A firm, elevated lesion that is larger and deeper than a papule. Nodules are typically >1 cm and may extend to the dermis and subcutaneous tissue.
seen in: dermatofibroma, inflammatory acne

Pustule A small, elevated lesion with green, white, or yellow purulence. The contents of a pustule may be infected or sterile.
seen in: folliculitis, pustular psoriasis, acne vulgaris

Vesicle A small, superficial fluid-filled blister, generally <0.5 cm in size.
seen in: herpes zoster, pompholyx

Bulla A larger fluid-filled blister, >0.5 cm in diameter (pl. bullae).
seen in: bullous impetigo, bullous pemphigoid

Cyst A thin fluid or semisolid filled sac that lies within the skin. Cysts are typically fluctuant on palpation.
seen in: epidermal inclusion cyst, cystic acne

Wheal A transient, often erythematous papule or plaque with well-circumscribed borders. Wheals are elevated due to edema and are often itchy.
seen in: urticaria

Acknowledgments

Thank you to my coworkers Elizabeth Enschede, Mandy Sacher, and Mariana Shimelfarb for your support and for calling me into exam rooms to look at skin conditions (that might be good for the book!).

Thank you to the BIMG-Williamsburg medical assistants for keeping me on schedule even when you knew there was a patient with an interesting skin condition waiting for me behind the next exam room door.

Thank you Mom and Dad for your ever-present love, support, and encouragement.

Thank you Dave for being my rock through it all.

—Danya Reich

To Matty, best friend 25 years and counting, who makes sure it never gets too real.

To Mom, best friend 40 years and counting, who makes sure it gets real enough.

To Dr. Bari Cunningham, who trained me to be a care-giver first and a doctor second.

And To Squeaks who brings a smile to my lips, *Every Single Day*.

—Bobby Buka

Thank you to Dr. Reich and Dr. Buka for including me on this project, which has been an invaluable learning experience.

Thanks to my parents and sister for all the love, laughter, and support.

Many thanks to Dolapo for making me dinner and keeping me sane.

Lastly, thanks to the outstanding faculty and students at Imperial College London's School of Medicine.

—Corinna Psomadakis

Contents

Part I
Head and Neck

Chapter 1
Acne

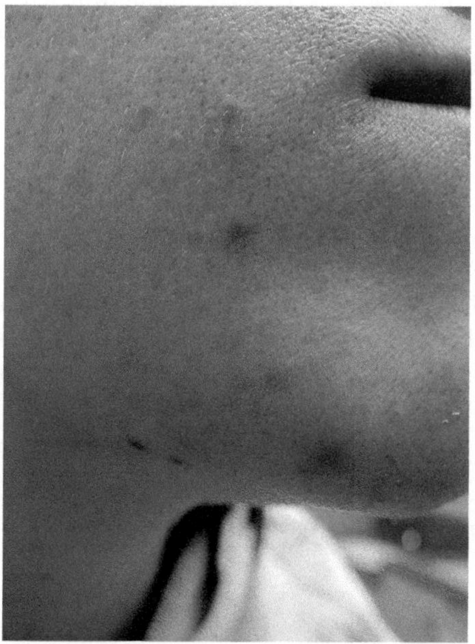

Fig. 1.1 Erythematous papules on the face, partially excoriated

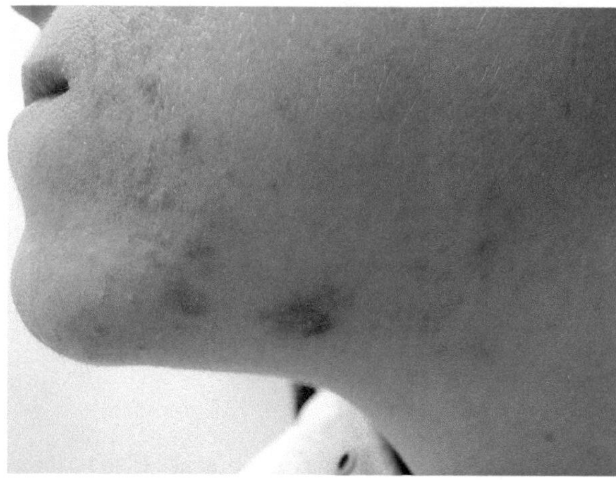

Fig. 1.2 Comedones periorally. Note also the larger acne cyst on left neck, an indication for systemic therapy

D. Reich et al., *Top 50 Dermatology Case Studies for Primary Care*,
DOI 10.1007/978-3-319-18627-6_1

Primary Care Visit Report

A 34-year-old female with no prior medical history presented with acne on her face. The patient was put on oral contraceptive (OCP) at the age of 16 for cystic acne and remained on OCP for the following 17 years, during which time her acne was well controlled. She discontinued OCP 1 year prior to visit because she wanted to get pregnant. Her acne flared about 8 months later. The acne was around her jawline, on her back, posterior neck, and behind her ears. She had not been using any acne medication as she found it dried her skin and made it flakey.

Vitals were normal. On exam, there was cystic acne on the patient's lower jaw and upper back.

She was treated with combination benzoyl peroxide/clindamycin gel (Benzaclin) 1–5 % twice daily. Retinoids were avoided due to the patient's desired pregnancy. The patient followed up 3 weeks later and her acne was improving on the Benzaclin; however, she noted her skin was drying and she had one additional pustular acne outbreak while on the medication. The patient was continued on Benzaclin only due to her desired pregnancy.

Discussion from Dermatology Clinic

Differential Dx

- Acne vulgaris
- Perioral dermatitis
- Folliculitis
- Rosacea

Favored Dx

Patient age and lesion distribution along the chin and jawline are suggestive of mild to moderate adult-onset, hormonal dominant acne.

Overview

Acne vulgaris is the medical term for common acne. It describes an extremely common condition affecting the pilosebaceous unit which consists of hair, hair follicle, arrector pili muscles, and sebaceous gland—a gland which secretes a lubricating oily matter called sebum into the hair follicle. Acne occurs when these hair follicles become clogged and represents a broad spectrum of lesions and severity. Its cause is multifactorial, with genetic predisposition, hormonal concentrations, change in quantity and quality of sebum secretion, colonization by the bacteria *Propionibacterium acnes*, and disrupted desquamation of keratinocytes all playing a role in its pathogenesis.

Acne is one of the most common dermatological complaints, with more than 80% of adolescents and adults developing acne at some point in their lives [1]. Teenage acne is more common in males than females; however, in age groups of 20 years and older, females are more often affected [2]. Recent data suggest that adult acne is becoming more common [2–4].

Presentation

The first presentation of acne usually coincides with the onset of puberty when androgens, especially testosterone and DHEA, stimulate sebaceous activity [5]; however, preadolescent acne is not uncommon. During adolescence, mixed comedones (whiteheads and blackheads) tend to initially appear in the centrofacial area (forehead, nose, chin), and later may spread to areas of high sebaceous gland activity, such as the remainder of the face, the upper arms, and the upper trunk.

A variety of lesions may present with acne and are classified as inflammatory or noninflammatory type. The precursor to all lesions is the microcomedone, which occurs when desquamated keratinocytes and sebum accumulate and clog pores (representing hair follicles). Microcomedones can unclog on their own, or evolve to become visible comedones. Comedones are noninflammatory lesions that are classified as open ("blackheads") when they are pigmented due to oxidation of cellular debris, or closed ("whiteheads"), which contain unoxidized material.

When comedones are left untreated, bacterial and hormonal factors, and poor exfoliation can lead to the proliferation of inflammatory lesions such as pustules, papules, cysts and nodules. Papules are inflamed comedones, pustules feature visible pus, cysts are large, inflamed pus-filled lesions, and nodules are large, firm bumps. Inflammation commonly occurs due to the colonization of follicles by *Propionibacterium acnes*, with the degree of inflammation variable depending on individuals' immuno-sensitivity to the pathogen. Additionally, inflammatory lesions occur when the follicle wall ruptures and the surrounding tissue becomes inflamed.

Lesions with severe inflammation carry the biggest risk of scarring, dyspigmentation, keloid formation, and development of true cysts.

Workup

Acne is diagnosed by clinical presentation. Blood tests to check for hormone levels (especially hyperandrogenism) are only indicated if patients demonstrate signs of an endocrine disorder (e.g., polycystic ovary syndrome most commonly, or

Cushing's syndrome), for example excessive body hair (hirsutism), or irregular/ infrequent menstrual periods. The recommended blood panel includes testosterone (free and total), LH, FSH, DHEA, and 17-hydroxyprogesterone. Abnormal test results warrant a referral to an endocrinologist.

Clinical assessment of acne should include severity grading. Although there is no standard scale to measure acne severity, some consensus has been achieved as to important aspects for consideration. When evaluating severity, physicians should consider the number and type of lesions, extent of distribution and involvement on facial and extrafacial sites, severity of inflammation, presence of pigmentary changes and scarring, and psychosocial effects on patient [5, 6]. These factors should help to classify an individual's acne as mild (i.e., minimal number of individual lesions), moderate (i.e., widespread whiteheads and blackheads with few cysts or nodules), or severe (i.e., scarring, nodules and/or cysts). It is important to ascertain from the patient whether the acne at the time of visit represents an average day, or whether they are experiencing a flare, as that may help dictate treatment.

Treatment

Acne medications account for 12.6% of the total cost of treating skin disorders globally [7]. Perhaps for that reason many different medications, including combination therapies, have been developed to treat acne. Left untreated, acne may spontaneously improve during late teenage years and early adulthood [2]; however, this carries a risk of scarring and is not always the case as acne can present for the first time, or persist, into adulthood. Treatment should focus on preventing the appearance of new lesions.

Acne can be treated with topical, systemic, and laser therapies. Topical treatments aim to decrease sebum production and reduce bacterial colonization, calm inflammation, and normalize the keratinization process [8]. Topicals generally fall into broader categories of antimicrobials (nonspecific activity against microbes), antibiotics (targeted activities against specific bacteria), and retinoids. Topical benzoyl peroxide (BPO) is a cornerstone of acne treatment that has antimicrobial, anti-inflammatory, and keratolytic effects. This can be used in combination with topical antibiotics or retinoids if monotherapy is inadequate; however, patients should be closely monitored for any irritation if both BPO and retinoids are used. Prescription azelaic acid gel or cream, and sodium sulfacetamide are further examples of antimicrobials that are useful in acne treatment, with the latter providing additional anti-inflammatory properties. All of the above topical treatments have demonstrated efficacy in treating mild acne [1, 8].

Topical retinoids are a class of medications that have been successful in treating comedonal acne. These include tretinoin, tazarotene, and adapalene. They have comparable efficacies; however, tazarotene demonstrates superiority in additionally reducing the number of inflammatory lesions and treating post-inflammatory hyperpigmentation [8]. Providers should note that tretinoin is rendered inactive in the presence of UV light, or oxidative products like benzoyl peroxide. When initiating retinoids, patients should be advised of potential irritation and initiate therapy slowly, by using the products every other day for the first week or 2. Although the systemic absorption of topical retinoids is minimal, they are strongly contraindicated in pregnancy. When retinoids alone are insufficient treatment, they can be used in conjunction with benzoyl peroxide (with BPO applied in the morning and retinoid at night in order to avoid retinoid inactivation by BPO), or topical antibiotics.

The primary topical antibiotic that is used in treating acne is clindamycin. Bacterial resistance has rendered the use of topical and oral erythromycin obsolete. Still, clindamycin should not be used as a monotherapy, and should be used in conjunction with benzoyl peroxide or retinoids in order to improve efficacy and minimize resistance.

Systemic therapies for acne include oral antibiotics, hormonal treatments, and isotretinoin. If topical treatments are not well tolerated, producing inadequate results, or if inflammatory lesions are numerous and severe, oral antibiotics can be prescribed. Doxycycline and minocycline are best tolerated and preferred over tetracycline due to decreased bacterial resistance [9]. A more recent approach with some demonstrated efficacy has been the use of subantimicrobial doses of doxycycline (20 mg twice daily for 6 months) with decreased bacterial resistance observed [9, 10].

Hormonal treatment for female acne includes oral contraceptives and spironolactone. Oral contraceptives that contain moderate to high levels of estrogen, e.g., Ortho Tri-Cyclen, Yasmin, and Estrostep, minimize sebaceous gland activity and can help control acne after 3–4 months of use [1, 9]. Spironolactone is an anti-androgen that is effective in 25–200 mg dosing [1, 7, 9]. Our practice generally prescribes doses of 50–100 mg daily, and 25 mg is sufficient for patients with milder cases of acne. Spironolactone is trialed in adult female patients with typical presentations of cystic acne along the jawline, as a treatment for the acne. If blood tests are performed and indicate abnormal hormone levels, they are referred to an endocrinologist for treatment of the hormone imbalance.

Oral isotretinoin is FDA-approved for severe, recalcitrant, nodular acne that has failed a more conservative treatment approach. It is the only known possible cure for acne, with cure rates up to 40 % [1, 9]. Isotretinoin is a known teratogen and thus patients in the USA need to be registered through the federally regulated iPledge program. Due to strict oversight of management, patients requiring isotretinoin therapy should be referred to a dermatologist for administration.

Laser and photodynamic therapy are increasingly popular alternatives to topical and oral acne treatment as they can help avoid some unwanted side effects. Fractional CO_2 lasers have been found to show up to 83 % improvement for some acne scars [11, 12], and pulsed dye lasers can improve inflammatory acne and reduce lesion counts [13].

In addition to the various treatment options reviewed above, any discussion of acne treatment warrants a mention of the historically controversial role of diet in acne. Randomized controlled studies on the topic are lacking, although recent research suggests foods with a high glycemic index, such as sugars and simple carbohydrates, and dairy (particularly skim milk) may play a role in its exacerbation [4, 14]. It should also be noted that smoking and stress can worsen acne as well [1, 3, 7].

Out of the treatment options discussed, the most appropriate course for the patient in this case was continuation of Benzaclin, as she was trying to become pregnant.

Follow-Up

Patients should be advised that most acne treatments require weeks to provide notable improvement, generally between 5 and 6 weeks to 3 months [7, 8]. Providers should follow up with patients after 4 weeks to assess improvement, as well as to discuss any unwanted side effects like dryness, or irritation. Treatment can be scaled back to every other day if there is excessive dryness or irritation. Alternatively medications like topical retinoids may be applied with moisturizer to help counter some of the side effects. If topical retinoids are well tolerated, dosages can be increased incrementally. If no improvement is noted on topical medications alone, patients can trial the addition of oral antibiotic therapy.

Questions for the Dermatologist

– *What is the first line of treatment for acne?*

First line therapy for acne would be an antimicrobial medication, most commonly an over-the-counter product that contains benzoyl peroxide. A first line prescription would be topical clindamycin. There are also prescription products that combine both benzoyl peroxide and clindamycin, which would make a good initial therapy.

– *Which acne treatments are safe during pregnancy?*

There are only two Category B medications available for acne treatment that are generally regarded as safe for use in pregnancy. Those are topical azelaic acid and clindamycin. There are mixed opinions about the use of benzoyl peroxide because animal studies have not been conducted; our practice doesn't recommend its use in pregnancy.

– *Which treatments are definitely not safe if a patient is trying to conceive?*

Our practice would not start a patient who is actively trying to get pregnant on oral isotretinoin therapy. For other oral medications, patients should stop immediately once they learn they are pregnant. We discontinue all oral medications upon conception rather than avoid these entirely.

– *Are there specific birth control pills that are better at treating acne?*

Estrogen-dominant oral contraceptives are preferred for treating acne.

– *What are the different kinds of acne and how are they best described?*

The main classification of acne is inflammatory versus noninflammatory. Inflammatory acne features red, juicy pimples (also known as pustules), or red nodules. This type of acne is best treated with antimicrobial medications. Noninflammatory acne features open and closed comedones, which are blackheads and whiteheads, respectively. These are best treated with the retinoid family of medications.

References

1. Nguyen TT. Acne treatment: easy ways to improve your care. J Fam Pract. 2013;62(2):82–9.
2. Collier CN, Harper JC, Cafardi JA, Cantrell WC, Wang W, Foster KW, Elewski BE. The prevalence of acne in adults 20 years and older. J Am Acad Dermatol. 2008;58(1):56–9.
3. Albuquerque RGR, Rocha MAD, Bagatin E, Tufik S, Andersen ML. Could adult female acne be associated with modern life? Arch Dermatol Res. 2014;306:683–8.
4. Mahmood SN, Bowe WP. Diet and acne update: carbohydrates emerge as the main culprit. J Drugs Dermatol. 2014;13(4):428–35.
5. Webster GF. Clinical presentation of acne. In: Zeichner J, editor. Acneiform eruptions in dermatology: a differential diagnosis. New York: Springer Science+Business Media; 2014.
6. Tan J, Wolfe B, Weiss J, Stein-Gold L, Bikowski J, Delrosso J, Webster GF, Lucky A, Thiboutot D, Wilkin J, Leyden J, Chren MM. Acne severity grading: determining essential clinical components and features using Delphi consensus. J Am Acad Dermatol. 2012;67:187–93.
7. Howard DM. Adult acne: overview and case study. Nurse Pract. 2014;39(8):12–5.
8. Kober MM, Bowe WP, Shalita AR. Topical therapies for acne. In: Zeichner J, editor. Acneiform eruptions in dermatology: a differential diagnosis. New York: Springer Science+Business Media; 2014.
9. Kardos Garshick M, Kimball A, Drake L. Systemic therapies for acne. In: Zeichner J, editor. Acneiform eruptions in dermatology: a differential diagnosis. New York: Springer Science+Business Media; 2014.
10. Skidmore R, Kovach R, Walker C, Thomas J, Bradshaw M, Leyden J, Powala C, Ashley R. Effects of subantimicrobial-dose of doxycycline in the treatment of moderate acne. Arch Dermatol. 2003;139(4):459–64.
11. Majid I, Imran S. Fractional CO_2 laser resurfacing as monotherapy in the treatment of atrophic facial acne scars. J Cutan Aesthet Surg. 2014;7(2):87–92.
12. Bhate K, Williams HC. What's new in acne? An analysis of systematic reviews published in 2011–2012. Clin Exp Dermatol. 2014;39(3):273–7.
13. Erceg A, de Jong EM, van de Kerkhof PC, Seyger MM. The efficacy of pulsed dye laser treatment for inflammatory skin diseases: a systematic review. J Am Acad Dermatol. 2013; 69(4):609–15.
14. Burris J, Rietkerk W, Woolf K. Acne: the role of medical nutrition therapy. Acad Nutr Diet. 2013;113(3):416–30.

Chapter 2
Actinic Keratosis

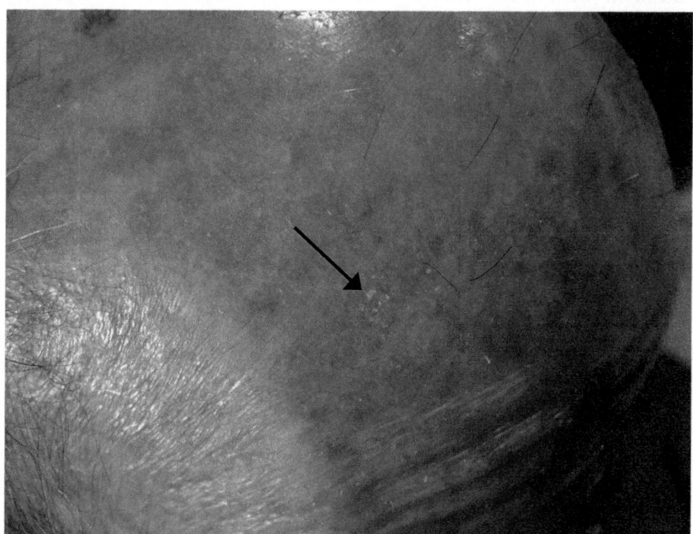

Fig. 2.1 Rough, scaly papule in the setting of poikiloderma (mottled atrophic, sun-damaged skin with areas of telangiectasia, hypopigmentation, and hyperpigmentation)

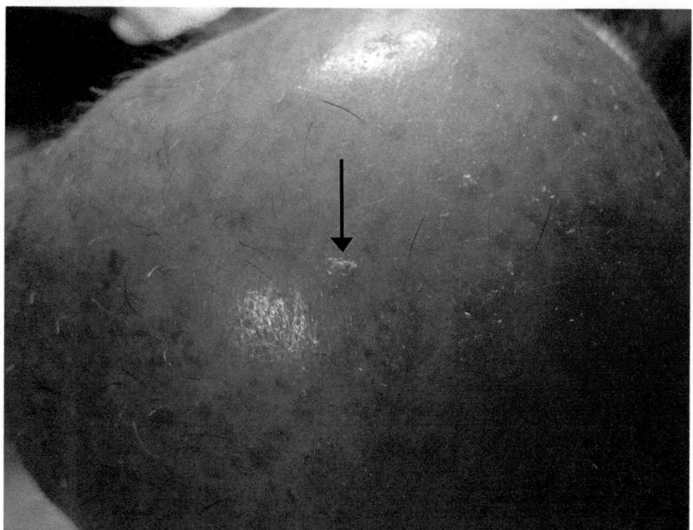

Fig. 2.2 Hyperkeratotic papule with scale on the vertex scalp

D. Reich et al., *Top 50 Dermatology Case Studies for Primary Care*,
DOI 10.1007/978-3-319-18627-6_2

Primary Care Visit Report

An 85-year-old male with past medical history of hypertension, atrial fibrillation, and coronary artery disease presented with a 5 mm area of thickened skin on his scalp. It had been present for "many years" and had not grown in size. It was neither itchy nor painful and did not bleed. He had not tried treating the lesion in any way and said "as long as it ignores me, I ignore it." The patient had been a lifeguard when he was in his late teens and twenties and also lived near the equator for 7 years and did not use sunscreen.

Vitals were normal. On examination, there was a 5 mm × 5 mm white scaly papular lesion on his anterolateral scalp.

This was diagnosed as actinic keratosis and the patient was treated with cryotherapy.

Discussion from Dermatology Clinic

Differential Dx

- Actinic keratosis
- Solar lentigo
- Squamous cell carcinoma
- Verruca vulgaris
- Bowen's disease

Favored Dx

The patient's age, history of sun exposure, and the location and appearance of the lesion are consistent with actinic keratosis.

Overview

Actinic keratoses (AK), also referred to as solar keratoses, are cutaneous neoplasms representing proliferation of abnormal keratinocytes. They are considered to be precursor lesions to in situ or invasive squamous cell carcinoma. While AK lesions do not progress to other types of skin cancers (basal cell or melanoma), they are strong predictors of these other types of skin cancers simply because patients with AK have sun damage and sun damage makes them more prone to any skin cancers [1]. The estimated risk of transformation of AKs to squamous cell carcinoma is 1 % per lesion per year, with an increased risk of up to 20% risk over the course of 10 years for individuals with multiple (>5) lesions [1, 2]. The estimated prevalence in the USA is 39.5 million [1]. They are the second most common dermatological complaint, with almost 100% of individuals above the age of 80 thought to be affected [1].

AKs primarily affect older men with fair-skin (Fitzpatrick phototype I and II) and a history of chronic exposure to UV radiation. Other risk factors are immunosuppression, history of prior AKs or skin cancer, and certain genetic conditions, such as xeroderma pigmentosum, Bloom syndrome, and Rothmund–Thompson syndrome [1]. Organ transplant recipients are at a higher risk of developing AKs [3]. UV exposure is the strongest causative factor in developing AKs, and it is thought to lead to mutations of the *p53* tumor suppressor gene [1, 4].

Presentation

Actinic keratoses typically present on sun-exposed areas of the skin, such as the face, neck, scalp, and upper extremities, particularly the dorsal hands. AKs affecting the lips are referred to as actinic cheilitis. AK lesions are rough, flat, and feature underlying erythema; however, the redness may be obscured by overlying adherent scale. AKs may be pruritic. Most lesions are under 6 mm in size, but left untreated they can extend to several centimeters. Lesions may progress to become hyperkeratotic. Individuals with AKs may have other characteristics of photodamage, including telangiectasias, sagging skin, lentigos, and dyspigmentation [1].

Workup

Actinic keratoses are diagnosed on clinical examination. Accurate diagnoses may be difficult due to the often subtle appearance, and they are more likely in specialist settings [1]. Suspected AKs may warrant a referral to dermatology.

Small lesions (<6 mm) do not require biopsy. Larger or thickened lesions should be biopsied to rule out deeper infiltration associated with greater malignant potential. Ulceration, pain, and bleeding are additional indications for biopsy.

Treatment

While most AKs do not progress to become squamous cell carcinoma (SCC), the majority of SCC lesions arise from preexisting AKs. It is not possible to predict which AK lesions will progress into SCC, thus all AKs should be treated to avoid the risk of malignant transformation.

Treatment of AKs does not affect the likelihood of new lesions presenting; however, it minimizes the risk of neoplastic transformation at the site of the treated lesion. AKs can be treated with cryosurgery, curettage with or without electrodesiccation, topical therapies, and procedures such as photochemotherapy, laser resurfacing, and deep chemical peels. Treatment should be selected based on number, thickness, and distribution of lesions, history of prior AKs or skin cancer, and patient preference [5].

Cryosurgery with liquid nitrogen is the most commonly utilized treatment modality, with reported clearance rates as high as 98 % after one to two sessions [5]. Efficacy is associated with longer freezing times; however, lesions treated for 20 s are associated with hypopigmentation upon healing [1, 5]. Recommended treatment is one freeze–thaw cycle of 10–15 s, achieving frost in a 1 mm ring surrounding the lesion. Long-term efficacy of cryotherapy is low and recurrence is high. Patients treated with cryosurgery may need to follow up with dermatology for further treatment and discussion of additional treatment options if their AK lesion does not fully heal, or if they have multiple lesions or recurrence.

No controlled studies have been done to evaluate clearance rates of curettage with or without electrodesiccation; however, it is an effective treatment method according to clinical experience. The procedure requires local anesthetic and is most appropriate for patients with few lesions, or with hyperkeratotic lesions [1].

Topical therapies for AKs include 5-fluorouracil (5-FU), imiquimod, and retinoids. 5-FU 0.5 % is applied to the entire affected area, meaning if there are multiple lesions, the cream should be placed throughout the area with lesions. This may be done once daily for up to 4 weeks or until erythema, erosion, crusting, and necrosis occur, at which time therapy should be discontinued. Hundred percent clearance of AKs was achieved in half of patients treated with 5-FU for 4 weeks [6]. Imiquimod is associated with up to 86 % full clearance rates when used three times daily over a course of up to 12 weeks [6, 7]. Imiquimod may also cause local irritation. Topical retinoids such as tretinoin and adapalene have demonstrated some efficacy in treating AKs, and are thought to prevent development of additional AKs [8, 9].

Patients with recurrent, abnormally thick, or numerous AKs should be referred to dermatology to discuss biopsy and treatment options. A specialist may be better suited to evaluate the need for procedural interventions including photochemotherapy, laser resurfacing, and deep chemical peels.

The abovementioned procedures should only be performed if the provider is confident in the clinical diagnosis of AK. If there is doubt about the diagnosis, a biopsy of the lesion in question or referral to a dermatologist are preferable. In addition, if the lesion is indurated, painful, ulcerated, or bleeding, or if the AKs fail to resolve after therapy or recur within 3 months of therapy, a biopsy should be done to rule out SCC.

Follow-Up

Patients treated with cryotherapy should be evaluated again after 2 weeks to monitor local healing. Recurrence of AKs is common, even if full clearance was achieved after initial treatment [5]. Patients with recurrent AKs should be referred to dermatology for discussion of the procedural interventions mentioned above.

UV radiation exposure is the strongest predictor of recurrence and development of malignancy, therefore preventing further lesions is tied to avoiding UV exposure. Patients should be advised to wear sunscreen daily, avoid sun exposure, and wear protective clothing, hats, and sunglasses. Vitamin D supplements may be taken if insufficiency is a concern [1].

Questions for the Dermatologist

– *How do you decide when to treat with creams vs. when to use cryotherapy?*

The decision relies on clinical judgment and is based on several factors. If I am doing "field therapy", treating numerous AKs in a single area, e.g., 20 lesions on the arm, it would be difficult to freeze all 20 of them. A cream that can be applied throughout the area would be a more reasonable approach to treatment. An individual lesion is easier to freeze because the area affected is minimal. Another factor is the patients' tolerance of down time. A blister from cryotherapy takes longer to heal. The location of the lesion may influence the decision as well. Some patients may not want longer healing times in highly visible areas like the face so in that case a cream would be a preferred choice. Finally, if the patient has tried creams already and the AKs do not respond, that would be an indication for in-office treatment with cryotherapy.

– *If the AKs regress, does the skin look normal after treatment with cryotherapy? Is there any scarring?*

There typically is no scarring with cryotherapy of AKs. It is possible for scarring to occur; however, it is very rare.

– *Do the creams cause scarring? Are there better cosmetic outcomes than with cryotherapy?*

The creams used to treat AKs do not cause scarring. There is no difference in cosmetic outcomes in the long term; however, there may be blistering initially with cryotherapy.

– *If you treat with creams or cryotherapy, are you foregoing biopsy? Are there any cases where biopsy is indicated? How would you decide whether to do a biopsy?*

AKs are typically very superficial and only involve the epidermis. If there is a hyperplastic AK, meaning it is abnormally thickened, there would be increased concern for developing squamous cell carcinoma, and a biopsy would be recommended. However, the average AK should be notably thin and would not require a biopsy.

– *Given AKs are caused by sun exposure, what do you recommend patients use for sun protection? Are there specific instructions for sun screening, such as how often to apply or what SPF to use?*

The recommendations are no different than those for the general population. We recommend daily use of sunscreen. SPF 30 is adequate as there is no incremental increase in sun protection with higher SPF. Physical sunblock, with zinc or titanium, is preferable to chemical sunscreen, which is inactivated by sunlight. Chemical sunscreens need to be reapplied regularly if someone is spending the day outdoors. Physical sublocks do not require regular reapplication except in cases when someone is active and sweating it off, or spending time in water and washing it off.

References

1. Duncan KO, Geisse JK, Leffell DJ. Chapter 113. Epithelial precancerous lesions. In: Goldsmith LA, Katz SI, Gilchrest BA, Paller AS, Leffell DJ, Wolff K, editors. Fitzpatrick's dermatology in general medicine. 8th ed. New York, NY: McGraw-Hill; 2012. Available from: http://accessmedicine.mhmedical.com.ezproxy.cul.columbia.edu/content.aspx?bookid=392&Sectionid=41138830. Accessed 27 Feb 2015.
2. Patel G, Armstrong AW, Eisen DB. Efficacy of photodynamic therapy vs. other interventions in randomized clinical trials for the treatment of actinic keratoses: a systematic review and meta-analysis. JAMA Dermatol. 2014;150(12):1281–8.
3. Togsverd-Bo K, Lei U, Erlendsson AM, Taudorf EH, Philipsen PA, Wulf HC, Skov L, Haedersdal M. Combination of ablative fractional laser and daylight-mediated photodynamic therapy for actinic keratosis in organ transplant recipients—a randomized controlled trial. Br J Dermatol. 2015;172(2):467–74.
4. Neto PD, Alchorne M, Michalany N, Abreu M, Borra R. Reduced P53 staining in actinic keratosis is associated with squamous cell carcinoma: a preliminary study. Indian J Dermatol. 2013;58(4):325.
5. Goldenberg G, Perl M. Actinic keratosis: update on field therapy. J Clin Aesthet Dermatol. 2014;7(10):28–31.
6. Jorizzo JL. Current and novel treatment options for actinic keratosis. J Cutan Med Surg. 2004;8 Suppl 3:13–21.
7. Krawtchenko N, Roewert-Huber J, Ulrich M, Mann I, Sterry W, Stockfleth E. A randomised study of topical 5% imiquimod vs. topical 5-fluorouracil vs. cryosurgery in immunocompetent patients with actinic keratoses: a comparison of clinical and histological outcomes including 1-year follow-up. Br J Dermatol. 2007;157 Suppl 2:34–40.
8. Ianhez M, Fleury Jr LF, Miot HA, Bagatin E. Retinoids for prevention and treatment of actinic keratosis. An Bras Dermatol. 2013;88(4):585–93.
9. Micali G, Lacarrubba F, Nasca MR, Ferraro S, Schwartz RA. Topical pharmacotherapy for skin cancer: Part II. Clinical applications. J Am Acad Dermatol. 2014;70(6):979.e1–12. quiz 9912.

Chapter 3
Impetigo

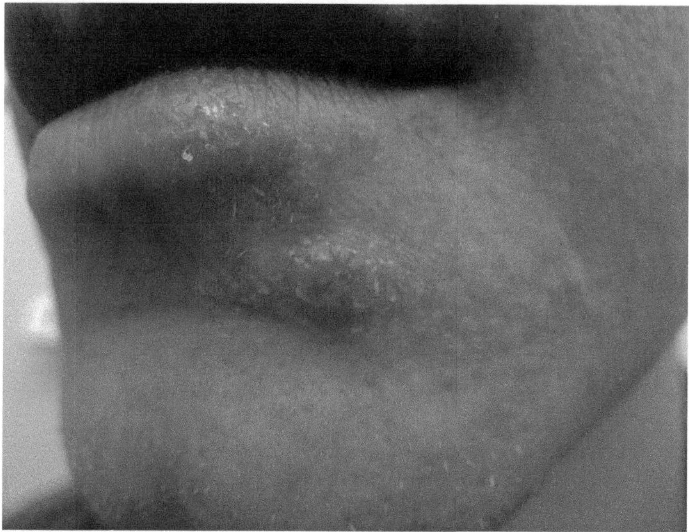

Fig. 3.1 Yellow crusted plaque at the left chin and lip, overlying pseudo-vesicular change

Primary Care Visit Report

A 30-year-old male with no past medical history presented with a "strange sore" on his face. It started 3 days prior to visit as a small non-itchy lesion, and progressively got larger. The day before the lesion appeared, the patient had been swimming in a river and bicycling. He put some over-the-counter hydrocortisone cream on it but it did not help.

Vitals were normal. On exam, there was a 4 mm × 4 mm papular lesion with some honey crusting on his left lateral lower lip; there was a 5 mm × 5 mm papular honey-crusted lesion with surrounding 1 cm × 5 mm erythematous papular rash on his left lateral chin area.

D. Reich et al., *Top 50 Dermatology Case Studies for Primary Care*,
DOI 10.1007/978-3-319-18627-6_3

The differential considered was impetigo versus herpes. The patient had no history of herpes nor did his wife. The honey-crusted appearance resembled impetigo so the patient was treated for impetigo with oral cephalexin 500 mg twice daily for 7 days and mupirocin ointment three times daily for 7 days.

Discussion from Dermatology Clinic

Differential Dx

- Impetigo
- Herpes simplex
- Tinea faciei
- Eczema

Favored Dx

Honey-colored crusted lesions are a telltale sign of impetigo.

Overview

Impetigo is a common and highly contagious superficial infection caused principally by *Staphylococcus aureus* and less frequently by β-hemolytic *Streptococci* bacteria. Impetigo is one of the most prevalent diseases globally [1], affecting mostly children and teenagers [2]. It is the most common bacterial infection seen in children and the third most common pediatric skin condition overall [3]. It is transmitted through direct contact, making it common in athletes [4]. Impetigo exhibits seasonal variations, with more occurrences in the summer, as well as in hot and humid climates [3, 5]. This variation could be due in part to the likelihood that more skin is exposed in warmer climates.

Impetigo can be classified as primary or secondary. Primary impetigo is direct bacterial invasion of previously normal skin. Secondary impetigo occurs at sites of minor skin trauma or on skin with compromised barrier function, and is more common in adults. This can occur due to an insult such as an insect bite or abrasion, or due to an underlying condition such as eczema, or cold sores caused by the herpes simplex virus.

Presentation

Two types of impetigo can be observed: nonbullous and bullous types. Nonbullous impetigo is more common, occurring in 70% of cases [3, 6], and mainly affects the perioral and perinasal skin. It initially appears as papules that progress to thin-walled vesicles surrounded by erythema. These become pustules that enlarge and then break down to form thick, adherent crust. This typically occurs over the course of about 1 week. Bullous impetigo is typically seen in young children, tends to affect the skin of the trunk, and involves vesicles which enlarge to become fluid-filled blisters that rupture within a few days of onset and leave a thin brown crust. Both types eventually develop a honey-colored crust covering the lesion, often surrounded by an erythematous halo. Impetigo tends to be a mild disease with few, if any, constitutional symptoms. Rarely, spread of the infection can lead to complications, including cellulitis, lymphangitis, septicemia, and scarlet fever.

Workup

Diagnosis can usually be made clinically; however, bacterial cultures are increasingly important as incidence of MRSA infections rises. Gram stains reveal gram-positive bacteria.

Treatment

Treatment options for impetigo include topical and oral antibiotics, and topical disinfectants. Some studies indicate that topical and oral antibiotics have a comparable efficacy in treating impetigo, while others demonstrate a slightly higher cure rate with topical mupirocin [2]. One advantage of topical antibiotics is that they have fewer side effects [2, 3, 7]. Mupirocin 2 % and retapamulin 1 % ointment are efficacious options, although mupirocin has demonstrated a higher cure rate [2].

When oral therapy is indicated (due to extensive involvement, severity or inadequate response to topical ointment), cephalexin and dicloxacillin are appropriate choices as MRSA is uncommon in impetigo. For penicillin or cephalosporin allergic patients, erythromycin or clarithromycin can be used. If MRSA is suspected, clindamycin, trimethoprim-sulfamexazole, or doxycyline are good choices.

Our practice recommends mupirocin 2 % cream or ointment twice daily for 1–2 weeks as a first-line therapy. In cases of recurrent impetigo where bacteria may be colonizing the axilla or anogenital region, patients can accompany topical therapy with disinfecting dilute bleach soaks. Bleach baths may be done once or twice weekly, dissolving ½ cup of bleach into a full bathtub as this can help reduce bacterial colonization rates. Bleach baths help to soften the superficial crusts on the lesions, exposing more of the infected lesion to subsequent treatment with topical antibiotics. The bleach water may be used on the face, with special caution to avoid getting any water in the eyes.

Follow-Up

Patients should be monitored for recurrent autoinfection. In that case, intranasal antibiotics may be warranted. Mupirocin nasal ointment applied twice daily for 5 days is recommended. In order to avoid further spreading, patients should be instructed to avoid scratching or touching the area, and avoid sharing towels. Topical antibiotics should be applied with cotton swabs, and patients should wash their hands frequently during treatment. Although impetigo is thought to be self-limiting, treatment is recommended in order to prevent its recurrence or spread. Following antibiotic treatment, most patients are clinically cured within 2 weeks.

Questions for the Dermatologist

– *Is it common for adults to get impetigo?*

Impetigo is common, and it does not only affect children; adults can get it too. Distinguishing between herpetic sores and impetigo is not always easy. Honey-colored crust is a clue suggestive of impetigo. Herpetic lesions appear initially as a cluster of vesicles superimposed on an erythematous base (which are often preceded by a prodromal clue like tingling) and later as round, well-circumscribed ulcers. Itching and pain can be associated with either herpes or impetigo. History of herpes would help with a definitive diagnosis, otherwise all other factors should be balanced before leading with one diagnosis.

– *Does impetigo require oral and topical treatment?*

The answer to this question depends on the severity of the infection. Severe impetigo may require oral antibiotic therapy. A non-complex case will most likely resolve with topical antibiotics alone. It is important to culture infected sites early so that if topical therapy fails, the bacterial strain has already been identified, and treatment can be followed with the appropriate oral antibiotics.

– *Did the patient's outdoor activities (swimming, biking) play any role in causing this?*

Wind and sunlight can incite herpetic outbreaks, which can lead to a secondary impetigo. As far as bacterial infection goes, unless there was local trauma there is no reason to suspect swimming, biking, and sweating alone would have caused the infection.

– *Some sources say to use mupirocin twice a day and some say three times a day. Is there danger in using mupirocin too often?*

Topical antibiotics can disrupt skin flora by killing good bacteria. Early studies do not show any added benefit to applying antibiotics for a third time daily which is why most sources recommend their use twice daily. The Infectious Diseases Society of America recommends using mupirocin twice daily.

References

1. Hay RJ, Johns NE, Williams HC, Bolliger IW, Dellavalle RP, Margolis DJ, Marks R, Naldi L, Weinstock MA, Wulf SK, Michaud C, J L Murray C, Naghavi M. The global burden of skin disease in 2010: an analysis of the prevalence and impact of skin conditions. J Invest Dermatol. 2014;134(6):1527–34.
2. Koning S, van der Sande R, Verhagen AP, van Suijlekom-Smit LWA, Morris AD, Butler CC, Berger M, van der Wouden JC. Interventions for impetigo. Cochrane Database Syst Rev. 2012;1, CD003261.
3. Cole C, Gazewood J. Diagnosis and treatment of impetigo. Am Fam Physician. 2007;75(6): 859–64.
4. Likness LP. Common dermatologic infections in athletes and return-to-play guidelines. J Am Osteopath Assoc. 2011;111(6):373–9.
5. Loffeld A, Davies P, Lewis A, Moss C. Seasonal occurrence of impetigo: a retrospective 8-year review. Clin Exp Dermatol. 2005;30(5):512–4.
6. George A, Rubin G. A systematic review and meta-analysis of treatments for impetigo. Br J Gen Pract. 2003;53(491):480–7.
7. Hartman-Adams H, Banvard C, Juckett G. Impetigo: diagnosis and treatment. Am Fam Physician. 2014;90(4):229–35.

Chapter 4
Alopecia Areata

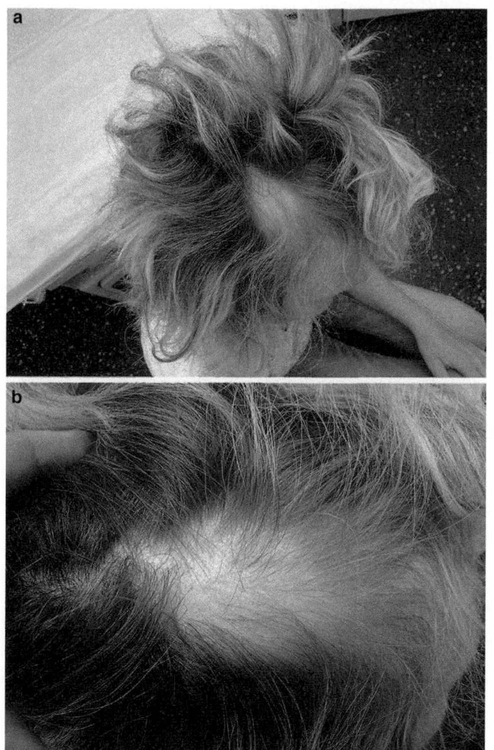

Fig. 4.1 (**a** and **b**) Smooth hairless patch with partial regrowth. Note well-demarcated edges

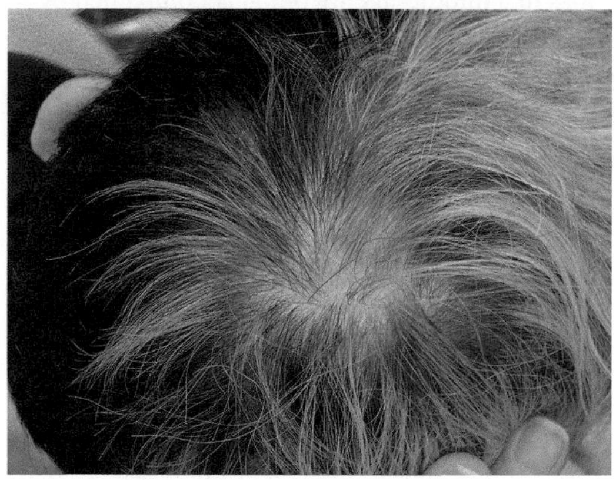

Fig. 4.2 Regrowth of terminal hair

D. Reich et al., *Top 50 Dermatology Case Studies for Primary Care*,
DOI 10.1007/978-3-319-18627-6_4

Primary Care Visit Report

A 45-year-old female with past history of scleroderma, autoimmune thyroiditis, and rheumatoid arthritis presented with two patches of hair loss on her scalp. The patient noticed an area with complete hair loss on the right side of her scalp which was small initially and gradually grew larger over the 10 days preceding her visit. She had also noticed a second bald patch forming in an adjacent area of the scalp. The patient reported a “prickly” feeling in the areas of hair loss.

Vitals were normal. On exam, there was a 5 cm × 3 cm area of alopecia in the right parietal scalp and a 3 cm × 1.5 cm area of alopecia in the superior occiput. The central area of alopecia patches had scant hair or hair follicles visible. Thinning hair was present at the periphery of the alopecia patches.

Given the patient’s history of multiple autoimmune diseases, she was referred to a dermatologist for biopsy and treatment of the alopecia.

Differential Dx

- Alopecia areata
- Telogen effluvium
- Tinea capitis
- Trichotillomania
- Traction alopecia

Favored Dx

Sudden onset hair loss in a middle-aged woman accompanied by additional autoimmune pathology is consistent with a diagnosis of alopecia areata.

Overview

Alopecia areata (AA) is an autoimmune disease marked by sudden onset, non-scarring hair loss. The condition results from damage to hair follicles in the anagen (growth) phase, driven by autoreactive CD8+ T-cells, that disrupts the normal hair cycle [1, 2]. Normal hair follicles go through periods of active hair growth (anagen), then follicular involution (catagen), and then rest (telogen). In AA, the peribulbar follicular inflammation causes the actively growing hair follicle to prematurely transition into catagen and telogen phases thus resulting in lack of hair growth/hair loss.

The etiology of AA is multifactorial, and involves genetic and environmental factors. The concordance rate in monozygotic twins is about 55 % [2]. There is family history of AA ranging in 10–42 % of cases, and that estimate is higher for early-onset AA [3]. AA is thought to be polygenic, and the involved gene loci may be located on chromosome 21, as there is an association with Down syndrome (trisomy 21) [3, 4]. The frequency of AA is equivalent across genders, and it can occur at any age, although it is more common in younger ages [3, 4]. The prevalence of the disease is about 0.2 %, and there is a 2 % lifetime risk of developing AA at some point [3–5]. AA is the most common cause of hair loss in childhood.

Alopecia areata is associated with a number of concomitant autoimmune diseases, including Hashimoto's thyroiditis, Grave's disease, Addison's, pernicious anemia, insulin-dependent diabetes mellitus, vitiligo, atopic diseases (including asthma, allergic rhinitis, and atopic dermatitis), and celiac disease [2, 3, 5]. The most common association is with Hashimoto's thyroiditis, although the minority of AA cases present with additional autoimmune disorders [3–5]. AA is also a common finding in vitamin-D deficient individuals [6, 7]. AA is organ-specific and limits its effects to the hair follicle, and sometimes the nails. Alopecia totalis is full loss of scalp hair, and it occurs in 5 % of individuals suffering from AA. Total body hair loss, or alopecia universalis, occurs in 1 % of AA patients at some point in the course of their disease [3]. Although the condition tends to be chronic, hair follicles are not permanently damaged, and hair regrowth is possible [2].

Presentation

Alopecia areata typically presents as asymptomatic, sudden-onset hair loss, most commonly on the scalp, beard, and eyebrows. The hair loss occurs in well-circumscribed round or oval patches. Sometimes patients describe stressful life events prior to onset [2]. A common characteristic of AA is the presence of "exclamation point" hairs, also called point noir hairs, which appear as black dots within the patch. The black dots represent hairs that were broken before exiting the follicle, and are subsequently pushed out.

In many cases AA presents with nail findings. Nail findings may precede, appear with, or follow AA onset. Typical nail findings are small pits or indentations, red spots on the lunulae, and/or vertical ridges. Nail abnormalities are associated with more widespread AA [4].

Workup

The presence of characteristic AA features of well-circumscribed bald patches, exclamation point hairs, and nail findings in the physical examination are usually sufficient to make a diagnosis. Positive family history would further support a diagnosis. There are no blood tests to confirm or rule out AA; however, if there is evidence to support a thyroid disorder (e.g., positive family history, exam findings), TSH and ANA tests would be relevant. A biopsy may be done if the diagnosis is unclear. Expected findings would be lymphocytic infiltrates surrounding the hair follicles, and a marked increase in catagen and telophase hair follicles [3].

Treatment

There is no cure for AA, and there is very little evidence-based guidance to help determine appropriate treatment [2, 3]. Treatment should be determined by disease extent, duration, and activity, as well as the potential distress it can cause to patients. In some cases, treatment may not be necessary, as 50 % of patients with limited disease lasting less than a year may experience spontaneous regrowth [8]. However, AA can have devastating psychological effects on patients, and they will likely prefer treatment. Part of the treatment discussion should include setting patient expectations, as treatment does not always work, and several studies define treatment success as >50 % hair regrowth [9]. There are numerous available treatment approaches, including topical, intralesional, and systemic corticosteroids, topical immunomodulators, biologics, minoxidil, anthralin, and photochemotherapy. First line treatments are topical and intralesional corticosteroids.

Super potent (class I) and potent (class II) corticosteroids have demonstrated success in treating mild AA [8, 9]. Multiple formulations (cream, lotion, ointment, foam, solution) are available, but one study indicated foam had superior therapeutic effects [8, 10]. Additionally, topical corticosteroids may be more effective when treatment occurs under occlusion [3, 11]. Clobetasol propionate 0.05 % (Class I) or betamethasone valerate 0.1 % foam (Class III) may be applied twice daily, or once nightly under occlusion of plastic wrap. In areas of the body that are difficult to wrap, for example the scalp, an adhesive like a bandaid or fabric tape may be used. This should occur on a discontinuous schedule to avoid extensive local skin atrophy, for example on 5 days per week for 4–6 months, depending on improvement. An alternative schedule is twice daily application for 2 weeks, followed by 2 weeks without treatment, for 4–6 months. One study found that Pacrolimus 1 % had equivalent efficacy as clobetasol 0.05 %, with fewer side effects [8]. Hair regrowth may be observed within anywhere from 6 to 24 weeks.

Intralesional corticosteroid injections are first-line therapy for mild to moderate AA, with less than 50 % involvement [3]. It would not be appropriate treatment for individuals with alopecia totalis. Injections are administered at a concentration of 5–10 mg/cc and may help achieve local regrowth within 4–8 weeks [3]. Injections are administered every 4–6 weeks; however, many patients experience reversible atrophy of adjacent subcutaneous fat, which presents as dents in the skin at the injection sites. Repeated injections on the same sites may lead to permanent skin atrophy [4]. If no improvement is noted after four treatments, alternative approaches should be investigated.

Patients who do not respond to topical or intralesional corticosteroids may be referred to dermatology. Extensive disease, and patients with alopecia totalis or alopecia universalis should also be referred to a specialist, where alternate therapies may be explored.

Follow-Up

The clinical course of AA is variable and unpredictable. Most of the treatment studies have evaluated short-term outcomes, and those who studied outcomes beyond 6 months indicated that treatment does not influence the long-term prognosis of disease [9]. For patients with limited, patchy disease, the prognosis is better, and hair often spontaneously regrows. Increased severity, alopecia totalis, and alopecia universalis are associated with poorer prognosis [3, 4]. Overall, 25 % of patients with AA experience a single event of hair loss [3]. For most patients; however, it is a chronic, relapsing condition.

Questions for the Dermatologist

– *When you do bloodwork to rule out autoimmune systemic disorders and you find nothing abnormal, do you then just assume the AA is idiopathic? Or should the patient continue to have their blood checked for some time period afterwards?*

If there are no abnormal findings in the blood work, you would assume the condition is idiopathic. If the TSH and ANA tests were negative and there are no interesting findings in a review of systems, there is no need to redo blood tests. If there are additional symptoms to support presence of an autoimmune disorder, it would be worthwhile to order tests again.

– *If the patient is found to have autoimmune thyroiditis, is it necessary for that to get treated/controlled before the hair will grow back?*

No, treatment of any concomitant autoimmune disorder would not affect AA. AA has a higher prevalence in autoimmune and thyroid conditions. However, presence of Hashimoto's thyroiditis, for example, is only indicative of a propensity for autoimmune disorders generally.

– *Do any of the treatments (e.g., intralesional steroid injections and topical steroids) work any better than doing nothing and seeing if the hair grows back on its own?*

Yes, treatments have better results than no intervention. Intralesional steroid injections and topical steroids have double-blinded, placebo-controlled studies indicating benefits over no treatment. They can grow hair back faster, or make hair loss slower.

– *When the hair grows back, does it grow back with normal thickness and color, or does it grow back thinner?*

The hair often grows back thinner, or as short, fine vellus hair to begin with. The hair may be white initially but it will eventually repigment and become thicker.

– *If alopecia areata recurs, is it usually in the same spot as the first time? If it does occur in the same spot, does that make it less likely the hair will grow back?*

AA can appear anywhere on the body, including the beard in men, regardless of where the first patch occurred. Even if it recurs in the same spot, responders to therapy in the first go-round are more likely to respond to subsequent treatment.

References

1. Xing L, Dai Z, Jabbari A, Cerise JE, Higgins CA, Gong W, de Jong A, Harel S, DeStefano GM, Rothman L, Singh P, Petukhova L, Mackay-Wiggan J, Christiano AM, Clynes R. Alopecia areata is driven by cytotoxic T lymphocytes and is reversed by JAK inhibition. Nat Med. 2014;20(9):1043–9.
2. Hordinsky MK. Overview of alopecia areata. J Investig Dermatol Symp Proc. 2013;16(1): S13–5.
3. Otberg N, Shapiro J. Chapter 88. Hair growth disorders. In: Goldsmith LA, Katz SI, Gilchrest BA, Paller AS, Leffell DJ, Wolff K, editors. Fitzpatrick's dermatology in general medicine. 8th ed. New York: McGraw-Hill; 2012. Available from: http://accessmedicine.mhmedical.com.ezproxy.cul.columbia.edu/content.aspx?bookid=392&Sectionid=41138795. Accessed 23 Mar 2015.
4. Freyschmidt-Paul P, McElwee K, Hoffmann R. Alopecia areata. In: Hertl M, editor. Autoimmune diseases of the skin: pathogenesis, diagnosis, management. 3rd ed. New York: Springer; 2011. p. 463–96.
5. Lyakhovitsky A, Shemer A, Amichai B. Increased prevalence of thyroid disorders in patients with new onset alopecia areata. Australas J Dermatol. 2014. doi:10.1111/ajd.12178.
6. Mahamid M, Abu-Elhija O, Samamra M, Mahamid A, Nseir W. Association between vitamin D levels and alopecia areata. Isr Med Assoc J. 2014;16(6):367–70.
7. Kim DH, Lee JW, Kim IS, Choi SY, Lim YY, Kim HM, Kim BJ, Kim MN. Successful treatment of alopecia areata with topical calcipotriol. Ann Dermatol. 2012;24(3):341–4.
8. Hordinsky M, Donati A. Alopecia areata: an evidence-based treatment update. Am J Clin Dermatol. 2014;15(3):231–46.
9. Delamere FM, Sladden MM, Dobbins HM, Leonardi-Bee J. Interventions for alopecia areata. Cochrane Database Syst Rev. 2008;2, CD004413.
10. Tosti A, Iorizzo M, Botta GL, Milani M. Efficacy and safety of a new clobetasol propionate 0.05% foam in alopecia areata: a randomized, double-blind placebo-controlled trial. J Eur Acad Dermatol Venereol. 2006;20(10):1243–7.
11. Tosti A, Piraccini BM, Pazzaglia M, Vincenzi C. Clobetasol propionate 0.05% under occlusion in the treatment of alopecia totalis/universalis. J Am Acad Dermatol. 2003;49(1):96–8.

Chapter 5
Perioral Dermatitis

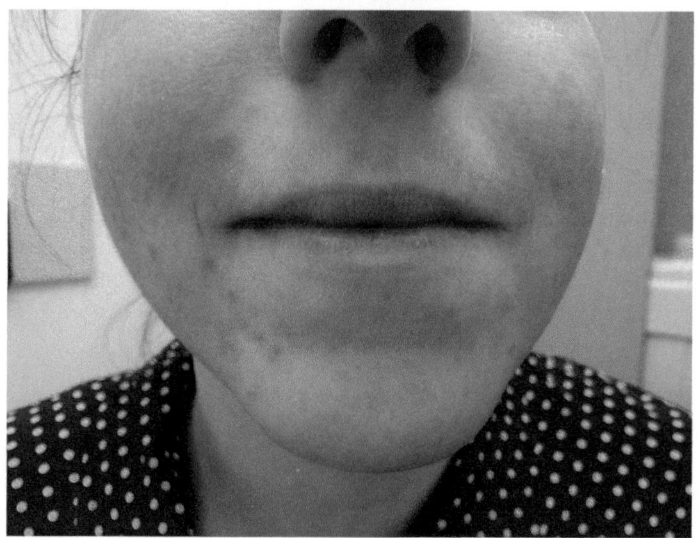

Fig. 5.1 Perioral papules with sparing of the vermillion border

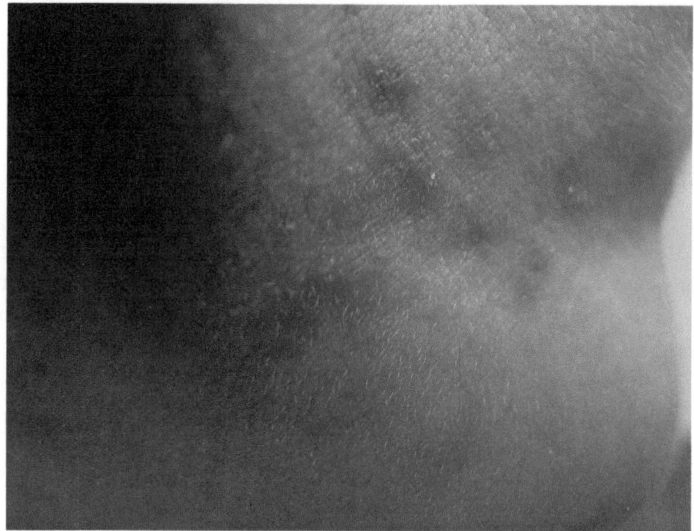

Fig. 5.2 Close-up perioral erythematous papules

D. Reich et al., *Top 50 Dermatology Case Studies for Primary Care*,
DOI 10.1007/978-3-319-18627-6_5

Primary Care Visit Report

A 29-year-old female with no past medical history presented with a rash on both sides of her mouth, chin, and nose. The rash had appeared intermittently over the past 5 months, but had been constant for the 2 weeks prior to this visit. She had not used any new facial products or soaps, nor made any changes to her diet. The rash was not itchy. She had not been able to figure out a pattern to the rash's emergence, nor any specific triggers.

Vitals were normal. On exam, there were scattered 3–4 mm erythematous papules lateral to both sides of her mouth, lateral to the left alar-facial groove, and on bilateral lateral chin.

This was treated as contact dermatitis with possible impetigo. The patient was instructed to use bacitracin ointment five times daily for 10 days. If no improvement was noted with bacitracin alone, the patient was instructed to add hydrocortisone lotion 1 % (Class VII) twice daily for 2 weeks.

Discussion from Dermatology Clinic

Differential Dx

- Perioral dermatitis
- Granulomatous periorificial dermatitis
- Rosacea
- Acne vulgaris
- Contact dermatitis

Favored Dx

Erythematous papular rash with perioral distribution suggests perioral dermatitis. The diagnosis given by primary care was contact dermatitis, and contact dermatitis is one of the causative factors associated with perioral dermatitis. However, no irritant or allergen was identified, and the rash distribution is limited to the perioral area, so dermatology reclassified the diagnosis as perioral dermatitis (with no impetigo).

Overview

Perioral dermatitis is an inflammatory papular eruption primarily affecting the skin surrounding the mouth. It sometimes also involves perinasal and periocular skin, in which case it may be referred to as periorificial dermatitis. There is a female predominance in adulthood, and it mainly affects women aged 15–25 years [1]. Perioral dermatitis presents in children under 13 years of age as well. There is no gender preference in children, and although earlier reviews suggested an African-American predominance, that is no longer thought to be the case [1, 2]. The granulomatous variant of perioral dermatitis (histology features granulomas and lymphocytic infiltrate), and periorificial involvement are more common in children [1–3].

The exact pathogenesis of perioral dermatitis is not known [1, 2, 4]. Topical steroid application is frequently implicated as a cause of perioral dermatitis, and patients may also experience flares when they attempt to discontinue steroid use [2]. The use of inhaled corticosteroids may be involved in pathogenesis in some cases [1, 3, 4]. Many other causes, such as *Demodex* mites, *Candida*, fusiform bacteria, and fluoridated toothpaste, have been implied; however, there is little evidence to substantiate them [1, 2, 4]. No association has been established between perioral dermatitis and hormones in young women [1].

Presentation

Perioral dermatitis presents with small, discrete, erythematous papules, pustules, and vesicles appearing on areas around the mouth, the nasolabial folds, and chin. The vermilion border is typically spared. In children it often involves other areas of the face, including the perinasal and periocular areas. There may be diffuse background erythema. The granulomatous variant may additionally feature yellow-brown papules and confluence of lesions [1]. The rash is often accompanied by pruritus, stinging, or burning sensations, which may be exacerbated by the application of moisturizers. Patient history may include recent topical steroid use on the face. Systemic involvement is very rarely associated [1, 3].

Workup

Diagnosis is made on clinical examination. A bacterial culture should be taken if there is suspicion of secondary infection. Patch testing does not reveal findings relevant to perioral dermatitis [1].

Treatment

While mild corticosteroids may improve symptoms in some patients, they are not recommended as treatment for perioral dermatitis as they are thought to be one of its causes. In cases where topical corticosteroid use is a causal factor, patients should slowly taper off treatment to avoid rebound flares [1, 2]. If any other causative agent has been identified, such as a topical irritant or cosmetic product, contact should be avoided. The cessation of products thought to precipitate perioral dermatitis is often referred to as "zero therapy" in the literature.

Perioral dermatitis is treated with a combination of oral antibiotics and topical metronidazole. Oral tetracycline, doxycycline, or minocycline is recommended over a course of 4–10 weeks depending on severity and response to treatment, with a 2–4 week taper at the end of therapy [1, 2]. Appropriate dosages are 50–100 mg twice daily for doxycycline and minocycline [4]. Oral tetracyclines (the class of antibiotics that include tetracycline, doxycycline, or minocycline) are contraindicated in children under 12 years of age. Oral erythromycin 250–500 mg twice daily is effective for children under 12 years, nursing mothers, and pregnant women [1, 2, 5]. The efficacy of oral antibiotics may be strengthened by adjunctive treatment with topical metronidazole 1 % twice daily. Topical metronidazole treatment alone may be adequate for mild cases of perioral dermatitis [1, 6]. Topical erythromycin and topical clindamycin are efficacious alternatives.

There have been some reports of efficacy of off-label treatment with topical calcineurin inhibitors [1, 2, 4, 7]. Pimecrolimus 1 % is especially effective in patients with suspected steroid-induced perioral dermatitis [7]. Another option for topical treatment is 20 % azelaic acid cream applied twice daily [1, 8].

Follow-Up

Topical corticosteroid use is the only identified precipitator of perioral dermatitis. Patients whose condition was triggered by corticosteroid use should avoid using them in the future. Perioral dermatitis is typically self-limiting and usually resolves within 2–3 months after treatment, or with cessation of corticosteroid use [1].

Questions for the Dermatologist

– *Is perioral dermatitis a variant of eczema?*

No, it is not. It is a largely idiopathic condition that causes a unique pattern of distribution around the mouth, nose, and sometimes eyes. There are a myriad of causes associated with perioral dermatitis, including fluoride in toothpaste and contact dermatitis. The one most frequently described is perioral dermatitis after steroid use.

– *Does dermatitis mean eczema, or is eczema a type of dermatitis?*

Dermatitis and eczema are synonymous terms, both describing inflamed skin. Unless there is another modifier word, like atopic, irritant, nummular, or xerotic, labeling a condition "dermatitis" or "eczema" alone does not provide a diagnosis. If I call something "eczematous dermatitis," it means I am not yet sure what it is. It describes a type of inflamed skin without putting it in a category.

– *Is perioral dermatitis bacterial in nature?*

No, it is not. A culture would not grow anything. Perioral dermatitis is an idiosyncratic immune reaction to any number of causes.

– *Why is perioral dermatitis treated with antibiotics if it is not thought to be bacterial?*

Cyclines are used to treat perioral dermatitis because of their anti-inflammatory effects. Cyclines have been shown to inhibit matrix metalloproteinases and cytokines, both of which are elevated in inflammation. The treatment dose for perioral dermatitis is lower than it would be for a bacterial infection.

– *What explains the rash coming and going?*

The patient was likely just getting reexposed to whatever her particular trigger is. Often times, you can look for causes of perioral dermatitis and not find any. Try to uncover any contact dermatitis, ask the patient to try non-fluoridated toothpaste, or look for the majority cause (steroid use) in the history. Sometimes patients are unknowingly using products with cortisone in them. Once the trigger is found, ask the patient to avoid it, and treat with oral antibiotics.

– *Is there something that triggers the rash that could explain why it persisted in the end?*

The rash is triggered by any number of things. Likely the patient was exposing herself to the trigger more regularly around the time of her visit than she had been while the perioral dermatitis was waning.

References

1. Lawley LP, Parker SS. Chapter 82. Perioral dermatitis. In: Goldsmith LA, Katz SI, Gilchrest BA, Paller AS, Leffell DJ, Wolff K, editors. Fitzpatrick's dermatology in general medicine. 8th ed. New York: McGraw-Hill; 2012. Available from: http://accessmedicine.mhmedical.com.ezproxy.cul.columbia.edu/content.aspx?bookid=392&Sectionid=41138787. Accessed 26 Feb 2015.
2. Tempark T, Shwayder TA. Perioral dermatitis: a review of the condition with special attention to treatment options. Am J Clin Dermatol. 2014;15(2):101–13.
3. Dessinioti C, Antoniou C, Katsambas A. Acneiform eruptions. Clin Dermatol. 2014;32(1):24–34.
4. Lipozenčić J, Hadžavdić SL. Perioral dermatitis. Clin Dermatol. 2014;32(1):125–30.
5. Nguyen V, Eichenfield LF. Periorificial dermatitis in children and adolescents. J Am Acad Dermatol. 2006;55(5):781–5.
6. Boeck K, Abeck D, Werfel S, Ring J. Perioral dermatitis in children—clinical presentation, pathogenesis-related factors and response to topical metronidazole. Dermatology. 1997;195(3):235–8.
7. Schwarz T, Kreiselmaier I, Bieber T, Thaci D, Simon JC, Meurer M, Werfel T, Zuberbier T, Luger TA, Wollenberg A, Bräutigam M. A randomized, double-blind, vehicle-controlled study of 1% pimecrolimus cream in adult patients with perioral dermatitis. J Am Acad Dermatol. 2008;59(1):34–40.
8. Jansen T. Azelaic acid as a new treatment for perioral dermatitis: results from an open study. Br J Dermatol. 2004;151(4):933–4.

Chapter 6
Seborrheic Dermatitis

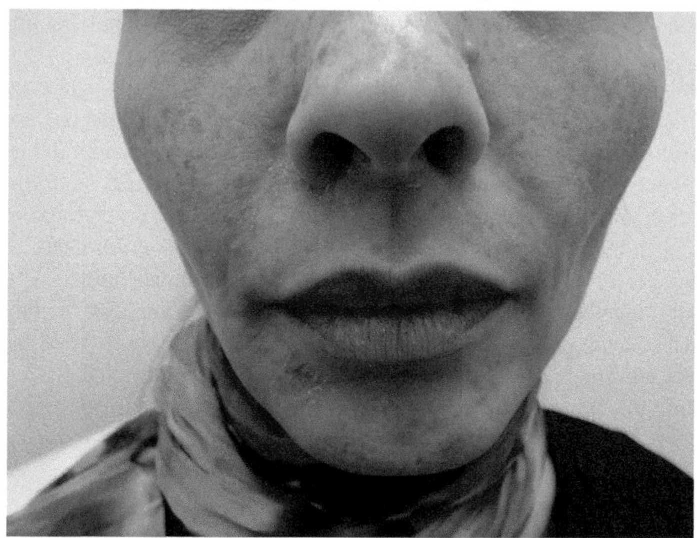

Fig. 6.1 Bilateral scaly erythematous, slightly greasy plaques typically found on the brow and nasolabial folds

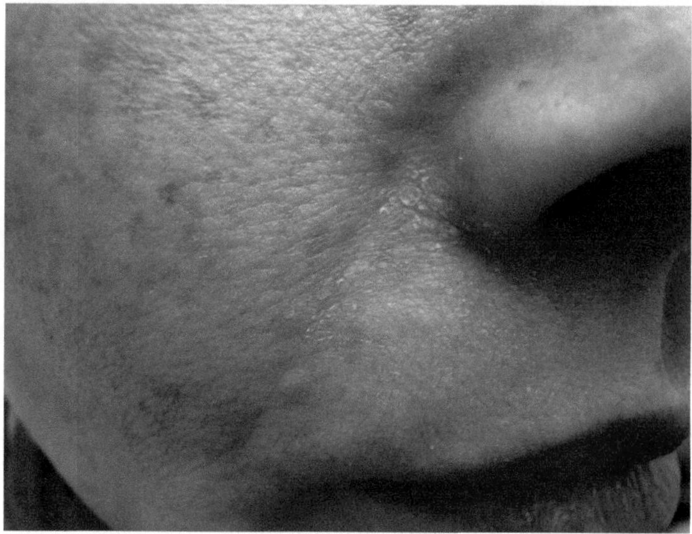

Fig. 6.2 Waxy plaque at the nasolabial fold

D. Reich et al., *Top 50 Dermatology Case Studies for Primary Care*,
DOI 10.1007/978-3-319-18627-6_6

Primary Care Visit Report

A 42-year-old female with past medical history of psoriasis presented with a rash on her face. She reported having similar outbreaks in the past, and they would resolve with application of tea tree oil. The present rash started about a week prior to visit, on the left nasal and cheek area. It was itchy, and she treated it by applying apple cider compresses, drinking coconut oil, and taking vitamins. The initial rash on the left side improved, but 3 days prior to visit a similar rash appeared on her right cheek, nasal area, and right chin, and progressively worsened since then. She tried one application of hydrocortisone valerate on the rash about 5 days prior to visit, and it did not help.

Vitals were normal. On exam, the right lateral alar crease had an erythematous scabbing rash, and the right nasolabial fold had a 1 cm × 3 cm erythematous papular rash. Her right lateral chin had a honey-crusted 1 cm × 1 cm erythematous papular rash, and her left alar crease featured a minimal erythematous papular rash.

This was treated as seborrheic dermatitis with overlaying impetigo, and the patient was prescribed hydrocortisone butyrate (Class V steroid) cream 0.1 % twice daily for 10 days for the seborrheic dermatitis and oral cephalexin 500 mg twice daily for 10 days plus mupirocin ointment 2 % three times daily for 10 days for the impetiginization.

Discussion from Dermatology Clinic

Differential Dx

- Seborrheic dermatitis
- Mild psoriasis
- Impetigo
- Dermatophyte fungal infection, e.g., tinea capitis, tinea faciei, tinea corporis
- Subacute lupus erythematosus
- Candidiasis

Favored Dx

Given the distribution and appearance of this rash, the favored diagnosis is seborrheic dermatitis, with one impetiginized area. However, seborrheic dermatitis and mild psoriasis are sometimes clinically indistinguishable when present on the face or scalp, and diagnosis is often times just a matter of how much scale is present, and how thick the plaques are. The term sebopsoriasis is sometimes used in those cases. Both facial seborrheic dermatitis and psoriasis can be successfully controlled with mild topical steroids, but may differ in their long-term management, as described below.

Overview

Seborrheic dermatitis is a common, chronic cutaneous condition involving areas of the body with active sebaceous glands, such as the scalp, face, chest, and back. Its pathogenesis is controversial [1], and it has been associated with presence of yeast of the genus *Malassezia*. Many factors contribute to its pathogenesis. *Malassezia* metabolites, such as oleic acid, compromise the permeability of the skin barrier, becoming more susceptible to irritants and triggering an inflammatory response [1]. Seborrheic dermatitis, also sometimes called seborrheic eczema, may be classified as a type of dermatitis, a fungal infection, or an inflammatory process similar to psoriasis.

Seborrheic dermatitis occurs in 1–3 % of immunocompetent adults [1]. It also occurs more commonly in immunocompromised populations, such as patients who are HIV positive or have AIDS (34–83 % incidence), those with chronic alcoholic pancreatitis, hepatitis C virus, cardiac transplants, or various cancers, and patients with neurological conditions, such as Parkinson's [1–3].

The onset of seborrheic dermatitis is commonly during infancy (when it is known as cradle cap), puberty, young adulthood, and past the age of 50. It is more prevalent in men than women [2, 3].

Presentation

Seborrheic dermatitis is characterized by red, flaking thin plaques. Presentation varies greatly in the degree of erythema, flaking, pruritus, and greasy appearance of lesions [2]. It tends to be exacerbated by cold, dry weather and may improve during summer months. Lesions may appear on the scalp, forehead, eyebrows, nasolabial folds, folds behind the external ears, ear canals, and suprasternal area. Presentation on the scalp is usually restricted to scaling and flaking. The retroauricular crease can have crusts and fissures.

Workup

The cause of seborrheic dermatitis is controversial, and many factors contribute to its development [2]. Accordingly lab workups may not necessarily be helpful. For example, a fungal culture may reveal the presence of Malassezia yeast; however, the yeast is present in most people regardless of whether they have seborrheic dermatitis. A bacterial culture would rule out impetigo.

Histologically, seborrheic dermatitis has a characteristic spongiosis, which is intercellular edema in the epidermis, that renders it distinct from psoriasis.

Treatment

Several different medications may be used to treat seborrheic dermatitis as there are many factors that contribute to its pathogenesis. Topical anti-inflammatory, such as corticosteroids and calcineurin inhibitors, antifungal, and keratolytic agents may be used. Topical azole antifungals are most effective in achieving long-term clearance, and topical steroids are most effective at reducing erythema, scaling and pruritus without unwanted side effects [4].

Combination therapy may provide the best approach to addressing multiple symptoms. Our practice prescribes ketoconazole 2 % cream and desonide 0.05 % cream (Class VI) twice daily for 2 weeks to treat seborrheic dermatitis on the face (applied in any order). Combination therapy alternating ketoconazole 2 % shampoo and clobetasol propionate 0.05 % shampoo each twice weekly for 4 weeks demonstrates higher efficacy than either shampoo alone in treating seborrheic dermatitis of the scalp [5].

Follow-Up

Seborrheic dermatitis tends to be a chronic and recurring condition. Treatment alleviates symptoms but does not provide a cure, thus long-term maintenance plans are necessary. Maintenance therapy has not been well researched; however, there are many options patients can try, including over-the-counter shampoos with pyrithione zinc, selenium sulfide, salicylic acid, tar, or antifungals (e.g., Neutrogena T/Sal or T/Gel, or Nizoral). These shampoos should be used between one and three times weekly, depending on initial severity and rate of recurrence. For facial seborrheic dermatitis, the most effective prophylaxis comes with intermittent application of mild topical corticosteroids 2–3 times weekly. Alternatively, ketoconazole 2 % cream may be applied to the affected areas once per week, or ketoconazole 2 % shampoo can be used as a facial wash once per week, which may be especially useful if there is eyebrow involvement. Men with moustaches and beards who experience seborrheic dermatitis may use ketoconazole 2 % shampoo daily on their facial hair until the rash resolves, and once weekly for maintenance. As discussed earlier, seborrheic dermatitis is often indistinguishable from mild psoriasis. If the diagnosis changes to psoriasis then the long-term management would be solely steroidal and not anti-fungal.

Questions for the Dermatologist

– *If this were seborrheic dermatitis alone (without impetigo), would it be appropriate to just treat with a topical steroid?*

Yes, topical steroids are a very successful treatment for seborrheic dermatitis. Mild topical steroids would be appropriate for use on the face.

– *Can seborrheic dermatitis resolve with topical steroid alone or does it need anti-fungal treatment as well?*

It can be controlled with topical steroids alone; however, it is likely to recur and usually requires long-term management.

– *What topical steroids can be used on the face and for how long?*

Topical steroids are classified from I to VII, with VII being the weakest. Usually class V to VII steroids are appropriately weak. Desonide 0.05 % is a good example. It may be used twice daily for up to 2 weeks to resolve acute inflammation, and can be used intermittently 2–3 times per week as long-term management.

– *What happens if topical steroids are used for too long, or too much, on the face?*

Lots of adverse effects can occur. Steroid-induced acne might be the first to appear. Thinning of skin, and telangiectasias (spider veins) would likely occur, followed by suppression of the hypothalamic–pituitary–adrenal (HPA) axis.

– *Does impetigo always require topical and oral antibiotic therapy?*

It would depend on severity. Severe cases of impetigo may require oral antibiotics, while mild cases would likely resolve with topicals. It is always important to culture suspected impetigo.

– *Do natural remedies like tea tree oil work? Are there alternative medicines that could help?*

There are data to suggest tea tree oil is an effective antimicrobial agent against yeast and bacteria. Our practice does not use it as a stand alone therapy. It can be considered as an adjunctive for those patients wanting a more holistic approach.

– *Is seb derm of the scalp the same as what is commonly referred to as dandruff?*

Yes, they describe the same condition. However, seborrheic dermatitis can also affect the penis, chest, or face and it is not usually called dandruff in those cases.

References

1. Dessinioti C, Katsambas A. Seborrheic dermatitis: etiology, risk factors, and treatments: facts and controversies. Clin Dermatol. 2013;31(4):343–51.
2. Gupta AK, Bluhm R. Seborrheic dermatitis. J Eur Acad Dermatol Venereol. 2004;18(1):13–26.
3. Wolff K, Johnson RA, Suurmond D. Chapter 2, Eczema/dermatitis. In: Fitzpatrick's color atlas & synopsis of clinical dermatology. 5th ed. New York: McGraw-Hill; 2005. p. 49–50.
4. Kastarinen H, Oksanen T, Okokon EO, Kiviniemi VV, Airola K, Jyrkkä J, Oravilahti T, Rannanheimo PK, Verbeek JH. Topical anti-inflammatory agents for seborrhoeic dermatitis of the face or scalp (Review). Cochrane Database Syst Rev. 2014;5, CD009446. doi:10.1002/14651858.CD009446.pub2.
5. Ortonne JP, Nikkels AF, Reich K, Ponce Olivera RM, Lee JH, Kerrouche N, Sidou F, Faergemann J. Efficacious and safe management of moderate to severe scalp seborrhoeic dermatitis using clobetasol propionate shampoo 0.05% combined with ketoconazole shampoo 2%: a randomized, controlled study. Br J Dermtol. 2011;65(1):171–6.

Part II
Upper Limbs

Chapter 7
Basal Cell Carcinoma

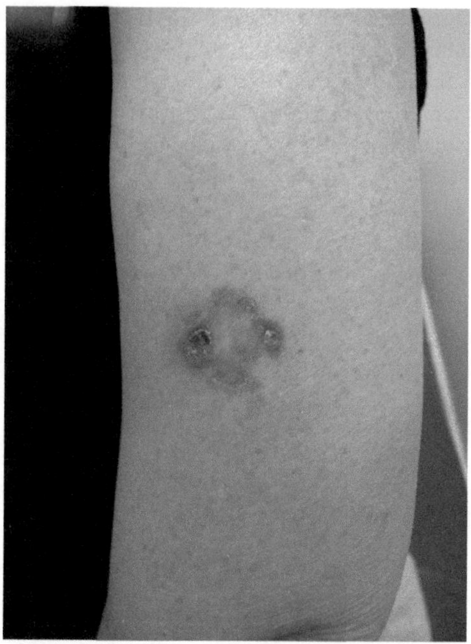

Fig. 7.1 From a distance, note the gross asymmetry of this lesion

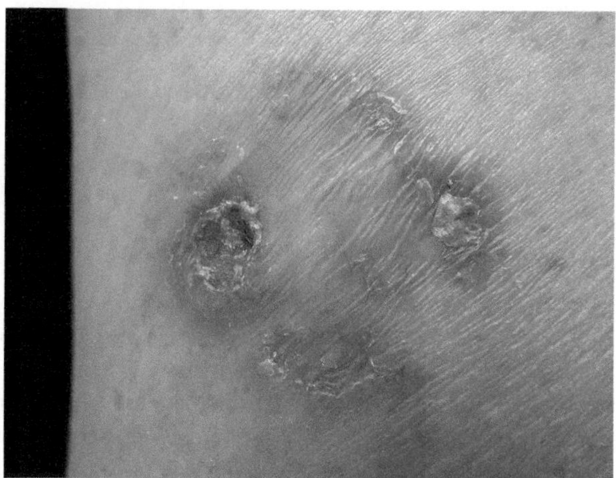

Fig. 7.2 Closer inspection reveals a scaly poorly-demarcated plaque with telangiectasias and an abraded surface

D. Reich et al., *Top 50 Dermatology Case Studies for Primary Care*,
DOI 10.1007/978-3-319-18627-6_7

Primary Care Visit Report

A 50-year-old female with no past medical history presented with a rash on her left upper arm that had been there, per the patient, "for at least 10 years." She said it changed in appearance sometimes but was always dry, scaly, and often itchy. The patient said she tried her best not to scratch it. She also reported that the lesion occasionally bled spontaneously. In the past, she had applied hydrogen peroxide and apple cider vinegar with no effect. She had also tried over-the-counter hydrocortisone cream and moisturizer, both of which made the scab and scale go away, revealing a red base.

Vitals were normal. On exam, on her left upper arm, there was a 2.5 cm × 2.5 cm erythematous, scaly plaque with irregular borders and peripheral scab.

The lesion was suspected to be psoriasis as the patient previously had a rash in her intergluteal cleft, which was diagnosed and treated as inverse psoriasis. However, she was referred to dermatology for further evaluation. At the dermatology clinic, the arm lesion was biopsied and found to be basal cell carcinoma. She subsequently underwent Mohs surgery to remove it.

Discussion from Dermatology Clinic

Differential Dx

- Basal cell carcinoma
- Amelanotic melanoma
- Bowen's disease
- Extramammary Paget's disease
- Squamous cell carcinoma
- Lichenoid keratosis

Favored Dx

In this case, biopsy was diagnostic of basal cell carcinoma (BCC). Psoriatic lesions would typically be more thickened. Long-standing pruritic, scaly lesions located in sun-exposed areas and accompanied by spontaneous bleeding, as well as the patient's fair skin and age, are aspects of the history and physical examination that would raise clinical suspicion of BCC in the absence of biopsy results. This patient's BCC appears to belong to the superficial subtype (discussed in more detail below), as the lesions are flat and scaly.

Overview

Skin cancers are the most commonly occurring type of cancer, with over one million diagnoses per year in the USA [1, 2]. BCC is a neoplasm of keratinocytes (an epidermal cell that produces keratin) of the lowest, or basal, layer of the epidermis, and accounts for 75–80 % of non-melanoma skin cancers [1, 2]. It affects men more commonly than women, and is considered a cancer of the elderly, although incidence is increasing overall particularly among younger women [1–4]. BCC predominantly affects fair-skinned people [2]. The actual incidence of BCC is difficult to estimate as non-melanoma skin cancers may not be included in cancer registry statistics [1, 5]. Additionally, in some countries only the first instance of BCC is reported, and recurrence as well as multiple lesions are common [3].

The pathogenesis of BCC is complex, and represents an interaction between genetic, phenotypic and environmental factors [5]. The main genetic abnormality in BCC is thought to be upregulation of the Hedgehog (HH) signaling pathway found on the *PTCH1* gene, which is responsible for normal tissue maintenance in adult life. UV radiation appears to induce mutations that inactivate *PTCH1*, *p53* and other tumor suppressor genes [2]. *PTCH1* mutations are present in 68–90 % of sporadic BCCs [2, 5].

Unlike squamous cell carcinoma which is related to cumulative sun exposure, BCC is believed to be associated with intermittent, intense sun exposure, and exposure early in life [1, 2, 4]. Although BCC most often presents on sun-exposed areas, UV exposure is not entirely predictive of lesion location, as BCC can also arise on areas of the body that are not typically sun-exposed [4]. The tendency to develop multiple lesions has a genetic link and may be suggestive of basal nevus syndrome [2]. Other risk factors for developing BCC include age, male sex, fair complexion, light-colored eyes, red hair, immunosuppressed status, and exposure to ionizing radiation [1, 2].

Presentation

Basal cell carcinomas typically present as dry, crusting, non-healing plaques that are pink to red in color. They can be pearly and translucent. They often feature small dilated blood vessels called telangiectasias and raised edges. Patients may complain of pruritus. Pain is associated with ulceration, depth of invasion, and the morpheaform variant of BCC—a variant with innocuous surface characteristics but deep, wide extension [6]. BCCs typically appear on sun-exposed areas of the head, neck, trunk, and extremities; however, they can occur anywhere. Patients may describe healing followed by recurrence of lesion, and bleeding spontaneously or after slight trauma. Larger lesions may feature partial necrosis. BCC tends to be destructive of local tissue and is usually not metastatic; however, long-standing, untreated BCC can invade subcutaneous layers, muscle, and bone.

There are five clinical subtypes of BCC, each presenting slightly differently. The most common subtype is nodular BCC, which typically occurs on the head and neck [2]. Pigmented BCC presents as a hyperpigmented, translucent nodule. Superficial BCCs are flat plaques that tend to occur on the trunk and resemble eczema. They are the second most common variant. Morpheaform BCC (also called infiltrating or sclerosing BCC) is a more aggressive variant that appears as a shiny, hypopigmented firm plaque most often located on the head and neck. This variant tends to be more painful [6]. Patients presenting with a scar without history of trauma should be evaluated for morpheaform BCC. Fibroepithelioma of Pinkus is a variant that looks similar to a skin tag, and usually presents on the lower back [2].

Workup

BCCs are diagnosed by shave or punch biopsy. Histopathology varies between subtypes and reveals basal cells with large nuclei, little cytoplasm, and stromal retraction.

Treatment

The goal of treatment is ensuring full removal of malignant tissue. Cryosurgery, topical chemotherapy such as imiquimod 5 %, electrodessication and curettage, surgical excision, and Mohs micrographic surgery are the main treatment modalities. Surgical treatment has the lowest failure rate and Mohs surgery specifically has the lowest recurrence rate [1, 2]. Treatment approach usually depends on the size, location, and depth of lesion.

Any lesions that generate suspicion of BCC should be biopsied, and if the lesion is small enough full removal should be attempted. Initial biopsy of the lesion may be performed in a primary care setting if the treating physician has experience performing biopsies. Patients can be referred to dermatology to discuss biopsy results that are confirmed BCC, or to perform the initial biopsy if needed. Any subsequent treatment should be undertaken by a dermatologist.

Follow-Up

Histologically confirmed complete excision of BCC is associated with <2 % local recurrence after 5 years [5]. Factors that are associated with recurrence, metastasis, and poor prognosis are lesions greater than 5 cm in size, location on ears or centrofacially, morpheaform subtype, poor delineation, incomplete excision, and histological features of infiltration, micronodular appearance, and perivascular or perineural involvement.

Patients with BCCs on the trunk are more likely to develop future lesions anywhere on the body, but especially on the trunk [7]. Other factors associated with poor prognosis are immunocompromised status, presence of multiple lesions, and involvement of lymph nodes, or metastasis [1, 2, 5]. Metastasis is very unlikely, occurring in fewer than 0.55 % of cases [2]. When it does occur, it usually affects sentinel nodes, or the lungs.

Patients with a history of BCC should be screened for new lesions twice yearly. Some precautions may be taken to help prevent new lesions, including wearing SPF daily, avoiding prolonged exposure to the sun or tanning beds, and wearing protective clothing.

Questions for the Dermatologist

– *What is the natural course of basal cell carcinoma if left untreated?*

The lesion persists and there is slow local tissue destruction.

– *The patient reported having the lesion for 10 years. Is it common for BCC to go undiagnosed for that long?*

It is fairly uncommon. Progression of lesions in this case are slower than average. Typically lesions are more painful and bleed spontaneously 6 months after they appear.

– *Does the process (i.e., inactivation of tumor suppressor genes) that gave rise to the BCC on her arm make it more likely for BCC to occur in other parts of her skin, like her leg?*

Patients with one BCC are more likely to develop others. Genetic changes to tumor suppressor genes are probably happening locally, and the lesions develop independently. However, they may be reflective of an environmental exposure such as UV radiation, which would affect multiple sites on the body. If those changes are happening in one area, they are more likely to happen in another.

– *If the patient gets more lesions in the future, would they be more likely to be BCC?*

Correct. A patient with primary BCC is at increased risk for developing subsequent BCC lesions.

– *Is there anything in the patient's history that is indicative of BCC, e.g. the lesions spontaneously bleeding?*

Irritation, bleeding, and the persistence of lesions would raise suspicion of BCC.

References

1. Rubin AI, Chen EH, Ratner D. Basal-cell carcinoma. N Engl J Med. 2005;353(21):2262–9.
2. Carucci JA, Leffell DJ, Pettersen JS. Chapter 115. Basal cell carcinoma. In: Goldsmith LA, Katz SI, Gilchrest BA, Paller AS, Leffell DJ, Wolff K, editors. Fitzpatrick's dermatology in general medicine. 8th ed. New York: McGraw-Hill; 2012. p. 1294–303.
3. de Vries E, Micallef R, Brewster DH, Gibbs JH, Flohil SC, Saksela O, Sankila R, Forrest AD, Trakatelli M, Coebergh JW, Proby CM, EPIDERM Group. Population-based estimates of the occurrence of multiple vs first primary basal cell carcinomas in 4 European regions. Arch Dermatol. 2012;148(3):347–54.
4. Xiang F, Lucas R, Hales S, Neale R. Incidence of nonmelanoma skin cancer in relation to ambient UV radiation in white populations, 1978–2012. JAMA Dermatol. 2014;150(10):1063–71.
5. Madan V, Lear JT, Szeimies RM. Non-melanoma skin cancer. Lancet. 2010;375(9715):673–85.
6. Yosipovitch G, Mills KC, Nattkemper LA, Feneran A, Tey HL, Lowenthal BM, Pearce DJ, Williford PM, Sangueza OP, D'Agostino Jr RB. Association of pain and itch with depth of invasion and inflammatory cell constitution in skin cancer: results of a large clinicopathologic study. JAMA Dermatol. 2014;150(11):1160–6.
7. Ramachandran S, Fryer AA, Smith A, Lear J, Bowers B, Jones PW, Strange RC. Cutaneous basal cell carcinomas: distinct host factors are associated with the development of tumors on the trunk and on the head and neck. Cancer. 2001;92(2):354–8.

Chapter 8
Digital Mucous Cyst

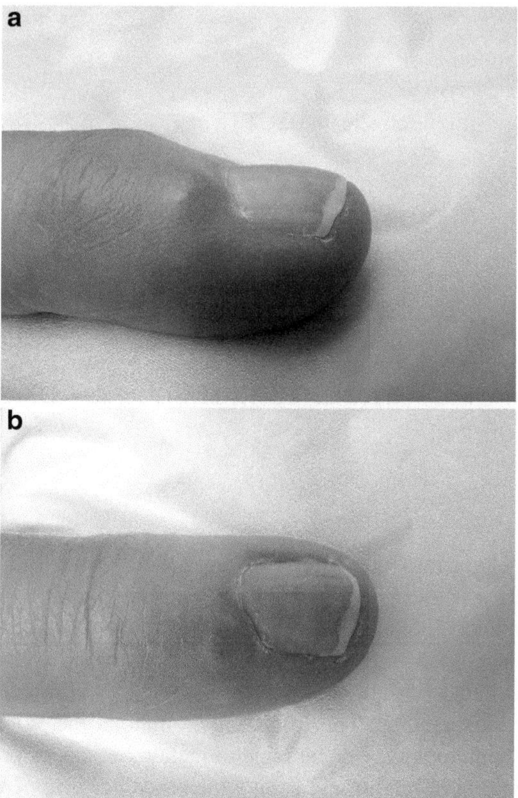

Fig. 8.1 (**a** and **b**) Proximal nail fold with firm, smooth subcutaneous nodule

Primary Care Visit Report

A 59-year-old female with no past medical history presented with a lesion on the pinky finger of her right hand. She first noticed the sore about 2–3 months prior. It was not painful, but it had started to distort her fingernail.

Vitals were normal. On exam, on the right hand fifth digit, just proximal to the nail bed, there was a 2 mm soft, non-tender, fluctuant mass with nail deformation.

This was treated as a digital mucous cyst, and the patient was referred to dermatology for surgical excision.

D. Reich et al., *Top 50 Dermatology Case Studies for Primary Care*,
DOI 10.1007/978-3-319-18627-6_8

Discussion from Dermatology Clinic

Differential Dx

- Digital mucous cyst (DMC)
- Periungual wart
- Acral fibrokeratoma
- Heberden's node
- Giant-cell tumor of tendon sheath (GCTTS)
- Gouty tophus

Favored Dx

Digital mucous cyst (DMC) is the favored diagnosis. The mass's presentation as non-tender and fluctuant, its persistence without change over 2 months, and its location on the proximal nail fold are all features consistent with DMC.

Overview

Digital mucous cysts, sometimes referred to as mucoid or myxoid cysts, are benign cysts of the fingers and toes. They lack epithelial lining, making them pseudocysts. They typically appear between the fourth and seventh decade, and are twice as likely to occur in women than men [1]. They are thought to arise from mucoid degeneration of connective tissue [2].

Two distinct forms have been described: myxomatous and ganglion type DMCs [1, 3–6]. The myxomatous type occurs due to metabolic changes in fibroblasts that lead to overproduction of hyaluronic acid, which then gets trapped, creates a cystic space and leads to a DMC. These are not connected directly to the adjacent joint. Ganglion type DMCs are associated with degenerative joint disease and occur more frequently in people with osteoarthritis. Ganglion type cysts are anchored directly to the affected joint (usually the distal interphalangeal joint) via a pedicle, and are filled with synovial fluid [3–5].

The two types are clinically indistinguishable, and a definitive diagnosis can only be made during surgery if a pedicle is observed, or by histopathology.

Presentation

Digital mucous cysts are translucent, round, dome-shaped lesions that appear on lateral or dorsal aspects of distal interphalangeal joints, or on the proximal nail folds of digits. They most frequently appear as solitary lesions; however, there have been a few reports of multiple DMCs [3]. They typically appear on fingers, although they also sometimes appear on toes [2]. DMCs tend to be under 1 cm in size. They are usually asymptomatic. They may sometimes discharge spontaneously, or cause reduced range of motion, pressure to the nail bed, nail deformities, and pain, especially as the cysts enlarge [1, 3].

Workup

Some of the differential diagnoses can be ruled out based on history. Acral fibrokeratomas are usually preceded by local trauma; tumors (GCTTS, histiocytoma) would exhibit rapid growth.

Digital mucous cysts tend to be compressible, can be transilluminated, and express clear or yellow viscous, jelly-like contents when incised. White structures appear on compression, consistent with increased collagen [2, 7]. If diagnosis is unclear, imaging studies (plain X-ray, MRI, CT, ultrasound) may be done to determine the nature of the growth.

If a biopsy is performed to rule out malignancy, histopathology of mucous cyst would reveal a cystic space with mucinous content, increased fibroblasts in the dermis, and no apparent lining of the cyst wall [3].

Treatment

DMCs are benign and may not require treatment. Asymptomatic cysts can be monitored. Some digital mucous cysts may spontaneously resolve. If patients are bothered by cosmetic appearance, they experience discomfort, or the DMC is causing nail deformity or functional impairment cysts may be treated. Treatment options include incision and drainage, intralesional steroids (e.g., triamcinolone acetonide 5–10 mg/ml), sclerotherapy (e.g., 1 % sodium tetradecyl sulfate), cryosurgery, electrodesiccation, CO_2 laser, and surgical excision. Of these the most effective is surgical excision, with cure rates up to 100 % [1, 4–6, 8, 9].

A conservative approach of incision and drainage followed by steroid injection is favored. This may be done in a primary care setting [6]. I&D usually requires several treatments as fluid tends to re-accumulate, and leads to cure rates of up to 72 % [5, 6]. Steroid injection alone is associated with high recurrence rates [6]. Cryosurgery has a 56–86 % cure rate [5]. It requires unroofing and draining the cyst, and freezing down to the cyst base. Frost should be maintained for about 10 s, which can be achieved by spraying continuously for about 4–5 s, then allowing it to thaw. This freeze-thaw cycle should be repeated 2–3 times per visit. Patients desiring treatment by sclerotherapy, electrodesiccation, CO_2 laser, or surgery should be referred to dermatology or hand surgery.

Follow-Up

The literature on DMCs suggests a possible risk of infection, although the link is controversial [5, 8, 9]. Patients should be instructed to report back to the office if they notice any tenderness, redness, or swelling consistent with inflammation.

If patients are dissatisfied with the treatment modality or progress, they may be referred to one of the above specialists for more aggressive therapy. Patients choosing conservative treatment should be made aware of the likelihood they may need to return for multiple treatments. In most cases, any nail abnormalities return to normal after the DMC has resolved, or when the nail grows out [8].

Questions for the Dermatologist

– *Is the I&D done on digital mucous cysts different than the I&D done for abscesses or paronychia? Could the I&D have been done in a primary care office?*

Digital mucous cysts are incised and drained in the same way, and this procedure can be performed in primary care. However, they have a higher recurrence rate when they are treated in this manner, which is one of reasons to excise them rather than I&D.

– *Will the nail bed become normal again after the cyst has been drained and removed?*

The nail itself will grow out normally as long as the nail matrix was not traumatized. There may be dystrophy if the DMC caused trauma to the nail matrix.

– *Can digital mucous cysts become infected? Do they ever require antibiotics?*

DMCs do not tend to become infected. Antibiotics would only be warranted if a secondary infection occurred after manipulation of the DMC.

– *If the cyst starts draining on its own, does it require further I&D, or is it considered to be resolving?*

If the cyst starts draining on its own, it may not require further treatment. Monitoring the area of recurrence would be an acceptable approach.

References

1. Park SE, Park EJ, Kim SS, KIM CW. Treatment of digital mucous cysts with intralesional sodium tetradecyl sulfate injection. Dermatol Surg. 2014;40(11):1249–54.
2. Salerni G, Alonso C. Images in clinical medicine. Digital mucous cyst. N Engl J Med. 2012;366(14):1335.
3. Hur J, Kim YS, Yeo KY, Kim JS, Yu HJ. A case of herpetiform appearance of digital mucous cysts. Ann Dermatol. 2010;22(2):194–5.

4. Hernández-Lugo AM, Domínguez-Cherit J, Vega-Memije ME. Digital mucous cyst: the ganglion type. Int J Dermatol. 1999;38(7):533–5.
5. de Berker D, Lawrence C. Ganglion of the distal interphalangeal joint (myxoid cyst): therapy by identification and repair of the leak of joint fluid. Arch Dermatol. 2001;137(5):607–10.
6. Zuber TJ. Office management of digital mucous cysts. Am Fam Physician. 2001;64(12): 1987–90.
7. Loder RT, Robinson JH, Jackson WT, Allen DJ. A surface ultrastructure study of ganglia and digital mucous cysts. J Hand Surg Am. 1988;13(5):758–62.
8. Johnson SM, Treon K, Thomas S, Cox QG. A reliable surgical treatment for digital mucous cysts. J Hand Surg Eur Vol. 2014;39(8):856–60.
9. Arenas-Prat J. Digital mucous cyst excision using a proximally based skin flap. J Plast Surg Hand Surg. 2014;11:1–2.

Chapter 9
Periungual Warts

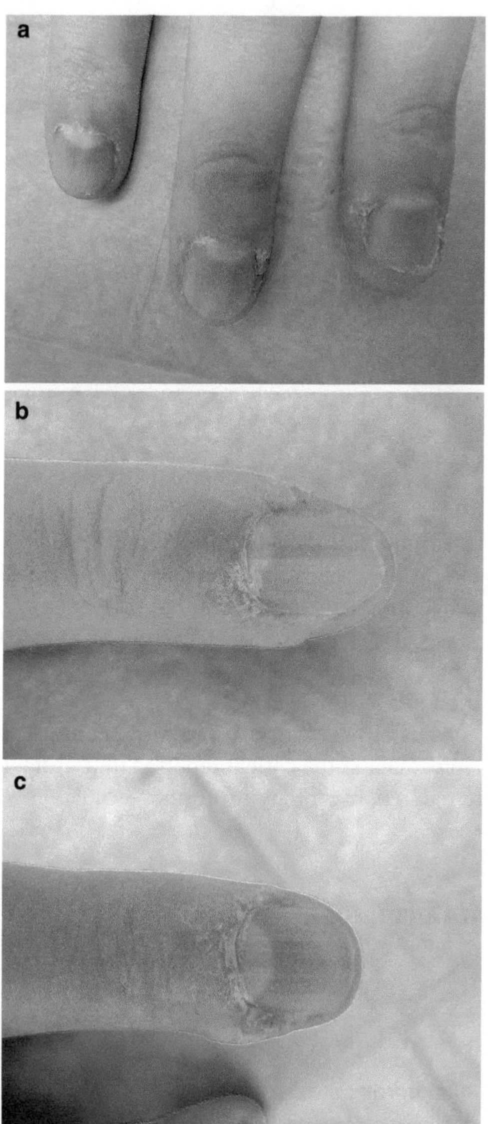

Fig. 9.1 (**a**–**c**) Hyperkeratotic, firm, verrucous papules periungal

D. Reich et al., *Top 50 Dermatology Case Studies for Primary Care*,
DOI 10.1007/978-3-319-18627-6_9

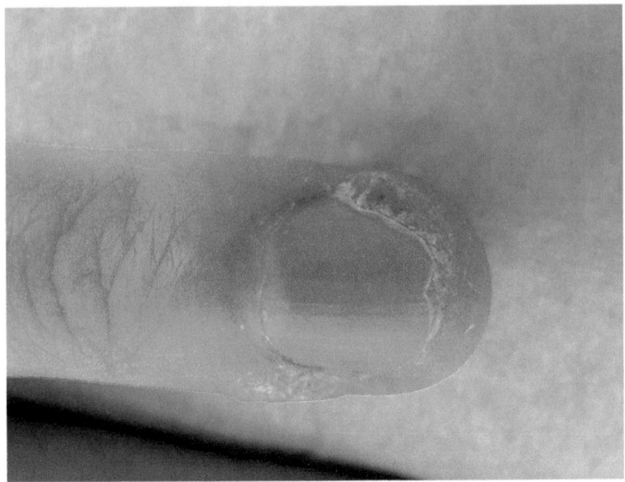

Fig. 9.2 Lesions that extend subungually can be particularly challenging to treat

Primary Care Visit Report

A 32-year-old male with no past medical history presented with redness, scaling, and induration around his fingernails for 1 year. He had previously been prescribed terbinafine cream, which improved the redness but the periungual rash persisted.

Vitals were normal. On exam, verrucous, well-demarcated, skin-colored to lightly pigmented papules and erythema were present on the periungual areas of all digits. Some induration and scaling was noted.

The differential considered was warts (or verrucae) alone versus verrucae accompanied by fungal involvement as the patient reported improvement with terbinafine. The patient was referred to dermatology for further evaluation.

Discussion from Dermatology Clinic

Differential Dx

- Periungual warts
- Acquired periungual fibrokeratoma
- Lichen planus
- Angiokeratoma
- Onychomatricoma
- Periungual callus
- Squamous cell carcinoma

Favored Dx

Some of the patient's lesions feature the dark, central puncta typical of common warts. The appearance and history is consistent with verrucous lesions.

Overview

Cutaneous warts are more prevalent in men than women. The median affected age in both genders is during the third decade, but prevalence peaks in school-age years. Palms and feet are the most commonly affected sites although they can occur anywhere on the body [1]. Warts may appear more frequently in immunosuppressed populations, such as organ transplant recipients, or those with HIV infections, and demonstrate more extensive involvement and recalcitrance in those cases.

Cutaneous warts are caused by human papillomavirus. Over 150 different strains have been identified, but HPV 1, 2, 4, 7, 27, 57, and 65 appear to be frequently linked with cutaneous warts [2, 3]. Rarely, types 16 and 18 can cause periungual warts and are considered high risk for transforming into squamous cell carcinoma.

Presentation

Periungual warts are warts that appear adjacent to nails of the hands and feet. Warts typically present as small, rough, cauliflower-like papules. Black puncta, tiny dots representing blood vessels, often appear at the center of the hyperkeratotic, dome-shaped lesions. These may also cause pinpoint bleeding if the growth is shaved down. Warts in children may resolve spontaneously over a period of several months to a year, while they may persist for several years in adults.

Workup

Clinical examination is usually sufficient for diagnosis. Biopsy should be performed in immunocompromised patients, or in recalcitrant, long-standing warts to rule out high risk strains of HPV, Bowen's disease, and squamous cell carcinoma [4].

Treatment

The approaches to wart treatment include topical, intralesional, and laser therapies. Surgical options include electrodesiccation, a tissue destruction technique using electrical current, and excision but are not first-line due to risk of scarring and the likelihood of recurrence [5]. The elected therapy should take into account patient age and immunity, tolerance for discomfort, lesion size and number, and desired speed to resolution.

Cryotherapy with liquid nitrogen is a very common and successful approach to therapy. It can be directly sprayed or applied with a cotton tipped applicator, depending on patient age, as younger children may have difficulty tolerating extensive spraying, and location of lesion. Clearance rates can be as high as 85 % and perhaps higher when warts are pared down to get rid of thickened, dead skin prior to freezing [6, 7]. Spray should be applied at a 90° angle, 1–2 cm away from the skin. Frost can be achieved by spraying continuously for about 4–5 s then allowing the skin to thaw for about 10 s. This freeze–thaw cycle should be repeated 2–3 times per visit. Treatment may require several sessions before the wart resolves. In our practice, we average three treatment sessions.

Topical 50 % salicylic acid has a lower clearance rate at approximately 24 % and thus does not appear to be more effective than cryotherapy [7, 8]. It may be used for patients desiring a more conservative treatment approach. Imiquimod 5 % cream is an immune response modifier than may be successful when used as a combination therapy with salicylic acid or other destruction methods (e.g., paring, cryotherapy), but unlikely to produce complete clinical clearance on its own [9].

Intralesional candida antigen causes upregulation of immune responses which are thought to then target warts. Candida injections have been found to achieve clearance in 74 % of patients, and are particularly useful in recalcitrant warts [3]. Candida injections can cause local erythema and pruritus. Intralesional bleomycin injections at a concentration of 1 mg/ml demonstrated complete resolution without recurrence after a year in one study [10]. Bleomycin works as a chemotherapeutic agent that interferes with the reproduction of viral cells. Injections should not be administered more than two times per site over the course of treatment in order to avoid risk of local necrosis and Raynaud's disease.

Patients may be referred to a dermatologist for treatment with pulsed dye laser (PDL). PDL targets the microvasculature that supplies verrucous growths. When the blood supply is eliminated, the warts become necrotic and eventually fall off. PDL treatment is advantageous because patients do not experience much pain and there is low risk of scarring; however, clearance rates are lower, at 34 %, after an average of 2–4 treatments [3, 5].

Follow-Up

The specifics of patient follow-up will depend on the course of treatment elected; however, all patients should return for reevaluation 2 weeks after initial therapy to monitor progress. Cryotherapy and PDL should be repeated every 2 weeks until warts have resolved. Candida and bleomycin injections may clear warts after one treatment, but warts should be monitored under a dermatoscope to confirm no residual puncta are visible. Some patients may opt to take conservative approaches like salicylic acid treatment, or occlusion under duct tape, in which case they may be instructed to return for treatment if the warts grow too bothersome.

Questions for the Dermatologist

– *Do warts often have a superimposed fungal infection?*

No. However, if the position of a wart is lifting the nail plate, that would predispose the area to a secondary fungal infection by improving the access of that pathogen.

– *Do warts spread? Could this patient somehow be auto-infecting himself?*

Yes, warts can spread. Viral particles can be transmitted by scratching and picking. It is common to see children who are biting or sucking warts to later develop them on their lips.

– *What are the contact precautions, if any, for someone with warts?*

It is not necessary to isolate patients with warts. They are transmittable by prolonged skin-to-skin contact. Family members should be advised to wear sandals in the shower if the patient has plantar warts, and they should not share bath scrub brushes.

– *Are there any special considerations when doing cryotherapy on someone with warts on every finger? Is there a clinical indication for treating one hand at a time?*

The considerations should be discussed with the patient. There is no medical reason for treating one hand at a time, but patients have varying tolerance. Some patients may want the warts gone as soon as possible. Others may not be able to tolerate extensive treatment, and would prefer to take their time treating potentially blistering lesions.

– *Are there any specific precautions when using cryotherapy around the nail area so as not to cause any permanent nail disfiguring? i.e., do you do cryotherapy for shorter amount of time or a lesser number of freeze–thaw cycles?*

Nail growth comes from the nail matrix underneath the proximal nail fold. Freezing periungual warts, unless very aggressively with a wide area of tissue damage, is unlikely to impact that anatomic nail unit. With cryotherapy treatment on any region of the body, cycles with 4–5 s of continuous spraying followed by about 10 s of thawing aim to minimize tissue damage, which in turn avoids destruction of any underlying structures.

References

1. Kyriakis K, Pagana G, Michalides C, Emmanuelides S, Palamaras I, Terzoudi S. Lifetime prevalence fluctuations of common and plane viral warts. J Eur Acad Dermatol Venereol. 2007;21(2):260–2.
2. De Koning MN, Quint KD, Bruggink SC, Gussekloo J, Bouwes Bavinck JN, Feltkamp MC, Quint WG, Eekhof JA. High prevalence of cutaneous warts in elementary school children and ubiquitous presence of wart-associated HPV on clinically normal skin. Br J Dermatol. 2015. doi:10.1111/bjd.13216. Accessed 24 Oct 2014.

3. Herschthal J, McLeod MP, Zaiac M. Management of ungual warts. Dermatol Ther. 2012; 25(6):545–50.
4. Riddel C, Rashid R, Thomas V. Ungual and periungual human papillomavirus-associated squamous cell carcinoma: a review. J Am Acad Dermatol. 2011;64(6):1147–53.
5. Tosti A, Piraccini BM. Warts of the nail unit: surgical and nonsurgical approaches. Dermatol Surg. 2001;27(3):235–9.
6. Zimmerman EE, Crawford P. Cutaneous cryosurgery. Am Fam Physician. 2012;86(12): 1118–24.
7. Ko J, Bigby M. Randomized controlled trial of cryotherapy with liquid nitrogen vs topical salicylic acid vs wait-and-see for cutaneous warts. Arch Dermatol. 2012;148(7):840–2.
8. Kwok CS, Gibbs S, Bennett C, Holland R, Abbott R. Topical treatments for cutaneous warts. Cochrane Database Syst Rev. 2012;9, CD001781.
9. Ahn CS, Huang WW. Imiquimod in the treatment of cutaneous warts: an evidence-based review. Am J Clin Dermatol. 2014;15(5):387–99.
10. Soni P, Khandelwal K, Aara N, Ghiya BC, Mehta RD, Bumb RA. Efficacy of intralesional bleomycin in palmo-plantar and periungual warts. J Cutan Aesthet Surg. 2011;4(3):188–91.

Chapter 10
Paronychia

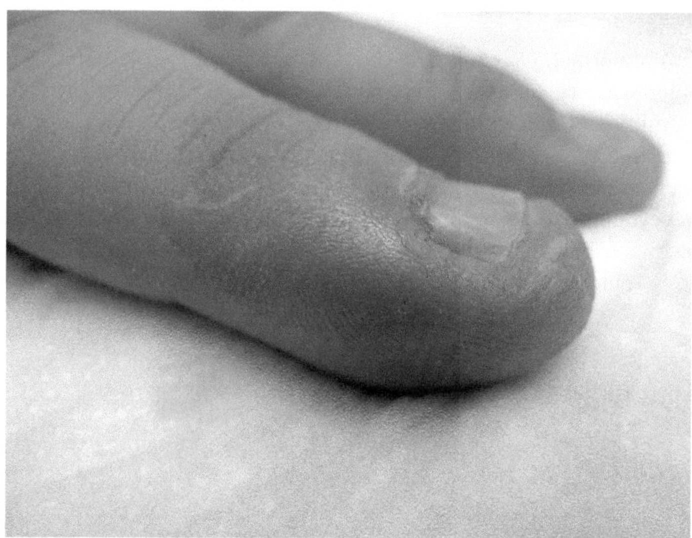

Fig. 10.1 Tender, boggy, erythematous tissue at right perionychium (Patient has applied iodine to account for yellow color)

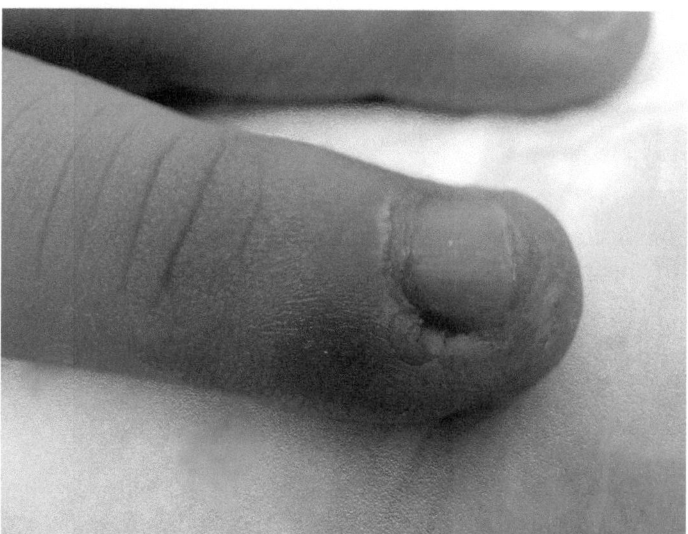

Fig. 10.2 Possible inoculation point noted at site of disrupted cuticle

D. Reich et al., *Top 50 Dermatology Case Studies for Primary Care*,
DOI 10.1007/978-3-319-18627-6_10

Primary Care Visit Report

A 32-year-old male with no past medical history presented with swelling of his right hand fourth finger, near his fingernail. It started the day prior to this visit, and he said he felt a lot of pressure in the fingertip. He tried icing it overnight with no improvement.

Vitals were normal. On exam, the skin lateral to the fingernail on his right hand fourth finger was erythematous, edematous, warm, and very tender to palpation. There was minimal fluctuance.

This was treated as paronychia. His finger was first soaked in warm water for 30 min, then an incision and drainage procedure was performed with a digital nerve block. However, no pus was expressed. The patient was sent home with instructions to soak his finger in warm water twice daily and to apply bacitracin to the area. He was asked to return to the office if the redness and swelling persisted or worsened.

Discussion from Dermatology Clinic

Differential Dx

- Bacterial paronychia
- Candidal paronychia
- Drug-induced paronychia
- Nail fold dermatitis
- Herpetic whitlow
- Ingrown nail

Favored Dx

Clinical examination and history are consistent with acute bacterial paronychia. It is apparent from physical examination that the patient is a nail biter, which is one of the predisposing factors for paronychia.

Overview

Paronychia is a common inflammation of the proximal nail fold and periungual soft tissues, which is classified as acute when it lasts fewer than 6 weeks, and chronic when it lasts greater than 6 weeks. The majority of cases are acute paronychia, which is most commonly associated with bacterial infection following mild local trauma, while chronic paronychia is associated with candidiasis. Predisposing factors for paronychia are exposure to chemical irritants, mechanical factors such as nail biting, picking, or finger sucking, and systemic conditions, such as diabetes and HIV [1, 2]. Less frequently, paronychia has been associated with use of certain medications, such as protease inhibitors, antiretrovirals, and chemotherapeutic agents.

The most common bacterial pathogen involved in acute paronychia is *Staphylococcus aureus*. *Streptococcus pyogenes*, *Pseudomonas aeruginosa*, and *Proteus* species are involved with less frequency [1–3]. Most cases of bacterial paronychia are caused by mixed flora, and paronychia that comes in contact with oral flora, as in nail biting and finger sucking, typically involves anaerobic bacteria [2, 4]. *Candida albicans* is often found in chronic paronychia. The pathogenesis of chronic paronychia is usually complex and multifactorial, and is currently thought to be an inflammatory process which may feature an overlying acute (i.e., bacterial) paronychia. Chronic paronychia is associated with excessive moisture, which may be the result of frequent immersion of the hands in water, as happens with occupational wet work. Paronychial herpes simplex virus lesions are referred to as herpetic whitlow.

Presentation

Acute paronychia presents as rapid-onset periungual erythema, swelling, and tenderness. Acute paronychia may develop within hours, and there may be ulceration and purulence. It usually presents on a solitary digit [2].

Chronic paronychia can lead to changes in the nails, such as thickening, ridging, and discoloration [1]. Chronic paronychia is not usually purulent, and it may be long-standing. More than one fingernail is often involved.

Workup

Physical examination and history are usually sufficient to make a diagnosis. A bacterial or fungal culture of contents expressed from the wound may be performed to confirm the offending pathogen; however, it is often not necessary.

Treatment

Treatment approach depends on whether the paronychia is acute or chronic, and the severity of inflammation. Acute bacterial paronychia may be treated with warm water compresses, and topical or oral antibiotics. Warm water compresses for 20 min up to three times a day may be sufficient treatment for mild cases of acute paronychia with minimal inflammation and no abscess. Their main role in treatment of severe cases is as adjunct therapy [1, 2]. Topical antibiotics such as mupirocin can be added to cases with more severe erythema, applied after each warm compress or soak. Oral antibiotics are appropriate for severe cases with severe inflammation [1]. For patients not exposed to oral flora (no nail biting and/or a paronychia of a toe), coverage of skin flora alone is appropriate—such as cephalexin 500 mg three or four times daily or dicloxacillin 250 mg four times daily. If oral flora exposure is present, amoxicillin/clavulanate 875/125 twice a day is appropriate. MRSA should be covered by the chosen antibiotic where there is a significant community MRSA presence [3, 4]. Clindamycin is a good option for MRSA coverage.

Alternately, although there is no evidence to the authors' knowledge of I&D having better or worse outcomes than oral antibiotics alone [2, 5], clinically it is common practice to perform an incision and drainage (I&D) on acute paronychia with an abscess. After appropriate local anesthesia (i.e., a digital block), a scalpel incision in the affected cuticle margin can relieve pressure and allow the patient some immediate symptomatic relief. Often incision and drainage can be sufficient to treat paronychia with abscess or oral antibiotics can be added after the I&D along with warm soaks which would help ensure the abscess would continue to drain. Oral antibiotics are typically prescribed for a 5 day course if an I&D is performed, or a 7–10 day course without I&D. Cases with nail irregularities can be referred to a dermatologist or hand surgeon.

Chronic paronychia, thought to be caused by prolonged exposure (often occupational) to water, features *Candida albicans* in up to 95% of cases [1]. The role of *C. albicans* in prolonging paronychia is unknown, and chronic paronychia is considered an inflammatory disorder. This variant may be treated with topical or oral (in severe cases) antifungals such as itraconazole and fluconazole; however, there is greater improvement when potent topical corticosteroids are used instead [6, 7]. A 2-week course of a potent topical steroid (Class I or II) is recommended for chronic paronychia. Additionally protective measures, such as wearing gloves, should be used in order to keep hands dry and away from irritants or allergens. If these treatments do not resolve the chronic paronychia, a course of antifungal therapy can then be added. Since chronic paronychia is now considered to be an eczematous process, it is equally important to address any underlying factors contributing to pathogenesis, including keeping hands dry in cases where excessive moisture is a causative factor, or treating systemic illness such as diabetes or HIV.

Follow-Up

Patients should be reevaluated after 1–2 weeks of treatment. Clinical improvement rather than cure may be the outcome for chronic paronychia. Avoiding environmental irritants, picking and biting habits, or other known triggers are essential in achieving a long-term cure. Recalcitrant cases should be referred to dermatology or hand surgery.

Questions for the Dermatologist

– *What conditions lead to paronychia? Is nail biting a factor?*

There are two forms of paronychia: acute and chronic. Nail biting can predispose someone to either form by exposing the nail fold to pathogens. Pathogens in the acute form are typically strep and staph, while in the chronic form it's *Candida*. The acute form presents acutely tender and swollen with purulence. The chronic form is characterized by a boggy, ragged cuticle. Wet work (e.g., restaurant food prep, new moms) can predispose people to the chronic form.

– *Is different treatment required for nail biters (i.e., different antibiotics)?*

The type of paronychia tends to determine the treatment. Acute paronychia would get treated with antibiotics, and chronic paronychia would get treated with topical steroids and/or antifungals. Nail biting could predispose someone to either form. However, acute paronychia in nail biters would warrant treatment with antibiotics that specifically cover oral flora.

– *When are oral antibiotics indicated?*

Oral antibiotics are indicated for acute paronychia, and in practice I almost always treat with oral antibiotics. Treatment purely with topical antibiotics is generally not successful because it is difficult for them to penetrate the nail fold. I use cephalosporins and penicillins to treat staph and strep paronychia. Some paronychias are caused by *pseudomonas*, most commonly following manicures. They can be identified by a blue-green hue to the purulence and lateral nail fold. Those cases can be treated with ciprofloxacin.

– *How do you know when to I&D? If it doesn't seem ready to I&D, what is the best treatment?*

The decision to I&D comes down to the extent of the abscess and edema. Acute paronychia is generally a tiny abscess. If it's very tender and very swollen, I will try to drain it. If it is only a little bit pink and tender, and it is not ready to I&D, I try oral antibiotics first. I also consider whether the patient can tolerate the potential pain of the procedure.

– *Are there common mistakes made when doing an I&D for paronychia?*

The strong part of the nail is proximal to the proximal nail fold. That is where the matrix is located, which would need to be avoided in such a procedure in order to avoid causing damage. Any procedure done on the side of the nail is well away from the matrix, so the risk of causing permanent dystrophy is low. I often need to try a couple of punctures before finding the pus pocket.

– *Can paronychia resolve with warm water soaks and topical antibiotics alone? Should anything be put in the water?*

Usually it cannot, but warm water soaks and hot compresses can be added as adjunctive therapy. It is helpful to massage the area after a 20-min soak or hot compress.

Massaging can get the abscess to open up on its own and drain. Treatment exclusively with hot compresses and warm water soaks is not recommended except in very mild cases, and should only be used if a patient is very resistant to using antibiotics. The next step if paronychia advances is dactylitis, where infection extends to the finger pad, and that is a much bigger problem. The compresses can be done with warm water, Burow's solution, or vinegar dissolved in a 1:1 ratio with warm water.

References

1. Shafritz AB, Coppage JM. Acute and chronic paronychia of the hand. J Am Acad Orthop Surg. 2014;22(3):165–74.
2. Rigopoulos D, Larios G, Gregoriou S, Alevizos A. Acute and chronic paronychia. Am Fam Physician. 2008;77(3):339–46.
3. Ritting AW, O'Malley MP, Rodner CM. Acute paronychia. J Hand Surg Am. 2012;37(5): 1068–70.
4. Tully AS, Trayes KP, Studdiford JS. Evaluation of nail abnormalities. Am Fam Physician. 2012;85(8):779–87.
5. Shaw J, Body R. Best evidence topic report. Incision and drainage preferable to oral antibiotics in acute paronychial infection? Emerg Med J. 2005;22(11):813–4.
6. Tosti A, Piraccini BM, Ghetti E, Colombo MD. Topical steroids versus systemic antifungals in the treatment of chronic paronychia: an open, randomized double-blind and double dummy study. J Am Acad Dermatol. 2002;47(1):73–6.
7. Hay RJ. The management of superficial candidiasis. J Am Acad Dermatol. 1999;40(6 Pt 2): S35–42.

Chapter 11
Interdigital Candidiasis

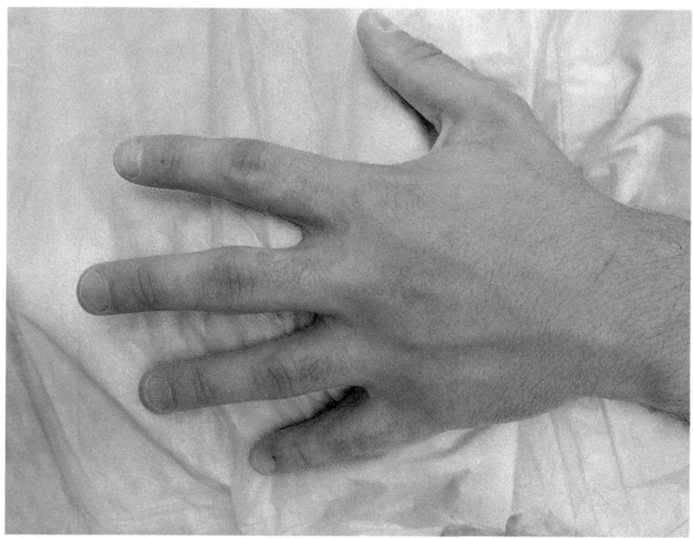

Fig. 11.1 Arcuate, erythematous scaly plaque between second and third digits

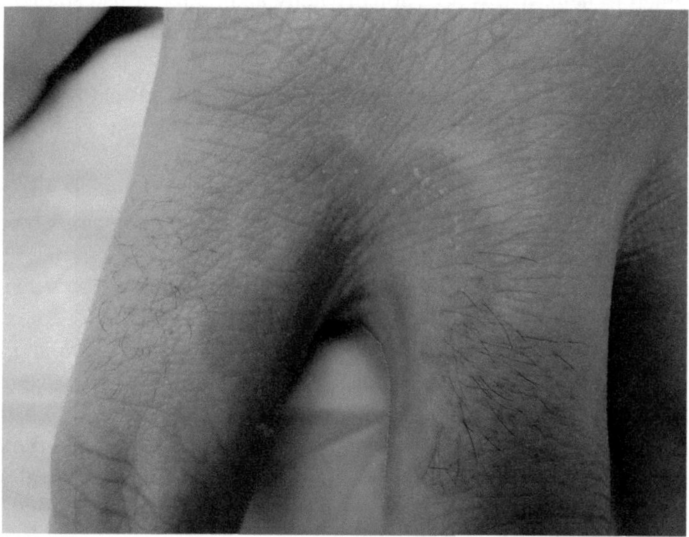

Fig. 11.2 Note the curvilinear edge of this expanding plaque

D. Reich et al., *Top 50 Dermatology Case Studies for Primary Care*,
DOI 10.1007/978-3-319-18627-6_11

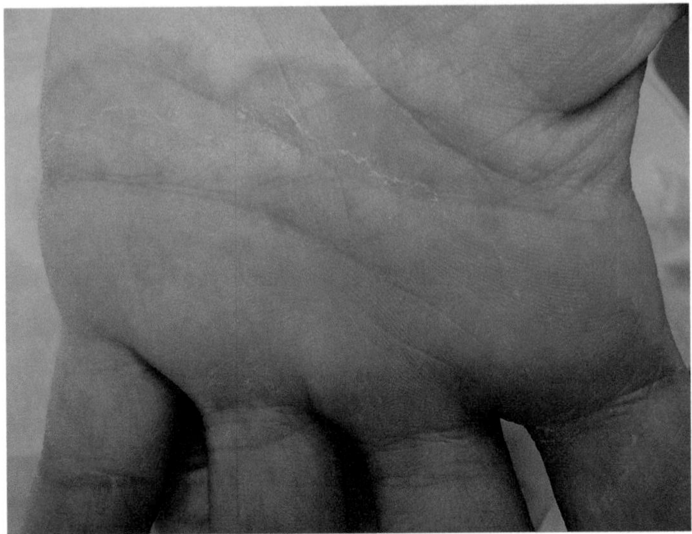

Fig. 11.3 Lesions extend to palmar aspect as well

Primary Care Visit Report

A 17-year-old male with no past medical history presented with a rash on his left hand that he had for a month prior to this visit. He had been applying Vaseline to it, which seemed to help. It was occasionally itchy and he felt it had started to affect the fingernail on his fourth finger. The rash was only on his hand and nowhere else on his body.

Vitals were normal. On exam, the distal portion of his left palm as well as the finger webbings of his left hand had an erythematous macular rash. The dorsal aspect of his left hand had a round erythematous, slightly scaly macular rash extending from the finger webbing between the second and third fingers to the proximal aspects of both fingers. This rash had a slightly darker erythematous border with slight central clearing.

This was treated as a fungal infection with econazole nitrate cream 1 % twice a day for 14 days.

The patient returned 4 months later for his annual physical exam and reported that the rash had improved with 14 days of antifungal cream. However, once he stopped using the cream, the rash recurred.

On exam at this return visit, the dorsum of his left hand had an erythematous scaly macular rash over the first, second, and third metacarpophalangeal joints, as well as in the finger webbings adjacent to those areas. The rash had an erythematous border with central clearing.

The patient was advised to restart the econazole nitrate cream 1 % twice daily but this time to use for a longer duration of 14–28 days.

Discussion from Dermatology Clinic

Differential Dx

- Interdigital candidiasis (AKA erosio interdigitalis blastomycetica)
- Tinea manuum
- Pompholyx
- Irritant dermatitis
- Allergic contact dermatitis
- Psoriasis

Favored Dx

Examination findings are consistent with interdigital candidiasis, a yeast infection of the finger webbings.

Overview

Interdigital candidiasis, also referred to as erosio interdigitalis blastomycetica (unrelated to *blastomyces dermatitidis*, the causal agent of a more severe, systemic fungal infection called blastomycosis), is a superficial fungal infection caused by any of the over 200 species in the *Candida* genus of yeasts, most frequently *C. albicans*. The interdigital variant, affecting the web spaces of fingers and toes, is the most common form of candidiasis [1].

Candida yeasts colonize an estimated 50 % of oropharyngeal passages of healthy individuals, and are commonly found as a component of normal skin and mucosal flora [2]. It is thought to be an opportunistic pathogen that causes infection on skin whose barrier function has been compromised. This can occur as a result of the maceration associated with chronic occupational exposure to moisture or sugar, as seen with bakers, bartenders, launderers, homemakers, or any person whose occupation involves repeatedly immersing the hands in water [3]. Wearing rings may also cause moisture retention that can lead to maceration [3]. Other predisposing factors are immunocompromised state, recent use of systemic antibiotics or corticosteroids, and warm, humid environment [1–3]. Diabetics are also predisposed to developing various yeast infections, including interdigital candidiasis [3].

Presentation

Interdigital candidiasis can affect the webbing of any of the fingers or, less frequently, the toes. It most frequently presents in the webbing between the third and fourth fingers of the hand. Interdigital candidiasis typically presents as an oval area of eroded (scaling) skin surrounded by an erythematous border. Scaling, erosion, and erythema can extend to the fingers and parts of the palm or dorsal hand. Maceration may also be seen, particularly when the condition is associated with prolonged exposure to water. The condition can be painful and pruritic.

Work-Up

Interdigital candidiasis is diagnosed based on typical examination findings, i.e. macerated erythematous patches appearing in interdigital areas. Skin scrapings and 10 % KOH test can confirm the diagnosis, by revealing hyphae, pseudohyphae, and spores associated with *Candida.*

Treatment

Treatment of interdigital candidiasis targets the offending yeast, potential gram-negative bacterial involvement, and correcting or eliminating aggravating factors, such as excessive moisture. Appropriate antifungal therapy for immunocompetent individuals is a topical azole antifungal cream, such as ketoconazole, applied twice daily for 2 weeks [2, 4]. Econazole is also a good choice as it includes some antibacterial coverage, and there is always a risk of opportunistic infection of macerated or fissured skin [5, 6].

Patients for whom excessive moisture is thought to be a causative factor may use an absorptive powder such as talc, or antifungal powders such as Desenex, Lotrimin, or Tinactin. Burow's aluminum acetate solution, commonly sold under the brand name Domeboro, is another option for addressing excessive moisture. A Domeboro packet is dissolved in cold water and then a cloth is soaked in the solution. It can be applied to the affected area for 15–20 min, up to three times a day. Any of the mentioned adjunctive treatments can be discontinued once the maceration has subsided. When an aggravating factor is identified, it is recommended the patient avoids or eliminates contact in order to minimize risk of recurrence.

Follow-Up

Interdigital candidiasis may be persistent and recurrent. Individuals will benefit from controlling any aggravating factors. Controlling diabetes, keeping hands dry, wearing gloves while immersing hands in water, and treating any immunocompromising conditions may help prevent recurrence when those factors are thought to play a causative role.

Questions for the Dermatologist

– *Is interdigital candidiasis different from other fungal infections?*

It is the same as any superficial candidiasis. It is a risk for food prep handlers and new moms. Macerated, wet interdigital spaces become an ideal environment for yeast colonization.

– *Since interdigital candidiasis can present in toe webbings as well, how can it be differentiated from tinea pedis?*

Erythema, maceration, and scaling of the feet are more likely to be caused by tinea pedis. It is not very common to see interdigital candidiasis on the feet. When it is seen, it usually affects multiple, or even all of the toe web spaces. Tinea pedis on the other hand is characteristically seen between the fourth and fifth toes. A further telltale sign of candidiasis would be a "satellite lesion", often a pustule, adjacent to the main affected area.

– *What can be learned from the fact that the patient's condition relapsed? Does it indicate longer treatment was needed? Or suggest a stronger potency medication should be used at the second visit?*

The patient was probably doing something that made him susceptible. If the topical did not work, the patient could have tried an oral antifungal. Topical antifungals do not come with varying potencies. After clearance, the patient could consider maintenance treatment with a topical azole once per week to keep candidal counts down.

– *Does response to a topical antifungal confirm a fungal diagnosis? Even though this patient relapsed, does his initial response to treatment suggest fungal etiology?*

Response to medication is a great clue. In cases where the diagnosis is unclear, trial and error with medications provides insight into the condition. Response to an antifungal points to a fungal infection.

– *What tests can be done to confirm diagnosis?*

A KOH test can be done, although it is not typically necessary. You would see "green balls" representing the yeast spores under the microscope.

– *Can interdigital candidiasis affect the fingernails?*

Although it seems intuitive the two conditions would track together, fingernail candidiasis is not typically seen. *Candida* is a rare causative agent of onychomycosis. I personally have never seen the two conditions present together in practice.

– *I treated the patient with econazole 1 % cream twice a day. You are recommending ketoconazole. How do you do decide which antifungal to use? Since they do not come in varying potencies, does one work better than the other for specific purposes or types of fungal infections or site of infection? For example, if econazole fails, is it worth trying a different cream in the azole family?*

Antifungals from the azole family have very similar effects. You could treat interdigital candidiasis with either. If there is no improvement with econazole after 2 weeks, it is unlikely you would get different results with ketoconazole, and it would be an indication to revisit the diagnosis.

References

1. Luo DQ, Yang W, Wu LC, Liu JH, Chen WN. Interdigital ulcer: an unusual presentation of Candida infection. Mycoses. 2011;54(6):e780–4.
2. Kundu RV, Garg A. Chapter 189. Yeast infections: candidiasis, Tinea (pityriasis) versicolor, and Malassezia (pityrosporum) folliculitis. In: Goldsmith LA, Katz SI, Gilchrest BA, Paller AS, Leffell DJ, Wolff K, editors. Fitzpatrick's dermatology in general medicine. 8th ed. New York: McGraw-Hill; 2012. p. 2298–307.
3. Adams SP. Dermacase. Erosio interdigitalis blastomycetica. Can Fam Physician. 2002;48:271, 277.
4. Hay RJ. The management of superficial candidiasis. J Am Acad Dermatol. 1999;40(6 Pt 2): S35–42.
5. Kates SG, Myung KB, McGinley KJ, Leyden JJ. The antibacterial efficacy of econazole nitrate in interdigital toe web infections. J Am Acad Dermatol. 1990;22(4):583–6.
6. Alsterholm M, Karami N, Faegemann J. Antimicrobial activity of topical skin pharmaceuticals—an in vitro study. Acta Derm Venereol. 2010;90(3):239–45.

Chapter 12
Blistering Dactylitis

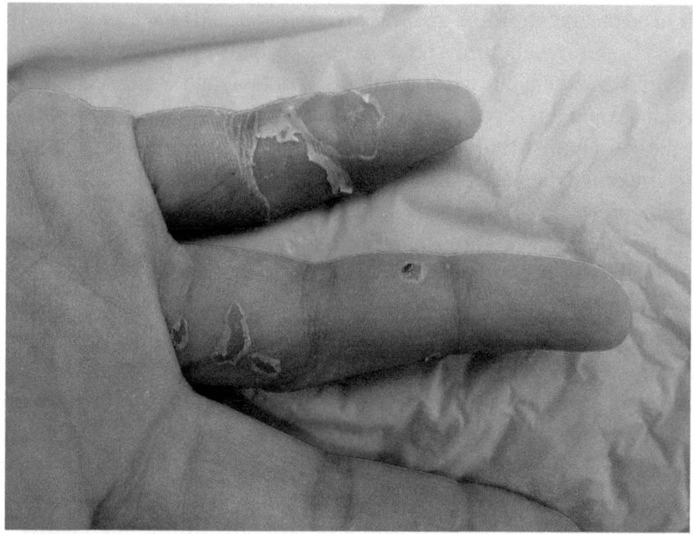

Fig. 12.1 Partial thickness shedding of digital skin with large collarets of scale

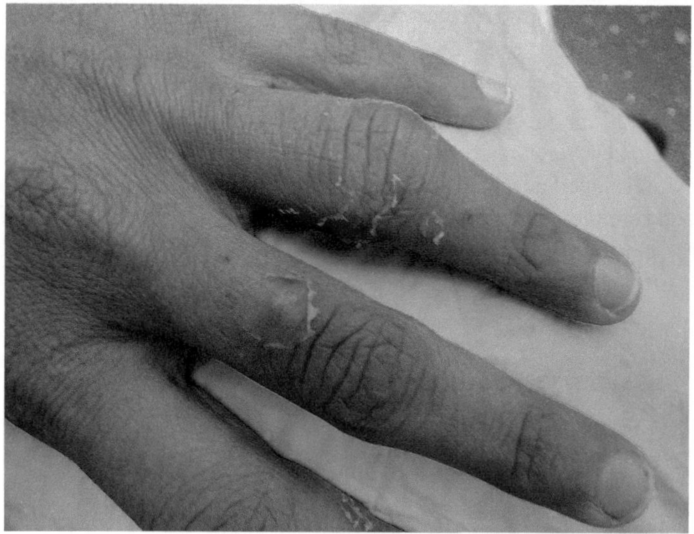

Fig. 12.2 Scale collarets are oftentimes an indication of an infectious process

D. Reich et al., *Top 50 Dermatology Case Studies for Primary Care*,
DOI 10.1007/978-3-319-18627-6_12

Primary Care Visit Report

A 37-year-old female with no past medical history presented with redness and peeling skin on bilateral hands and fingers after sustaining a dog bite 2 weeks prior. The patient was bitten on both hands when she jumped in to separate a dog fight. The patient initially went to an emergency room and was given tetanus and rabies vaccines. Three days later, her fingers were swelling so she went back to the ER and was admitted for 3 days of IV antibiotics (vancomycin and ampicillin/sulbactam) and was discharged on amoxicillin/clavulanate and doxycycline, which she was taking at the time of this visit.

While the pain and stiffness in her fingers had improved somewhat, the patient remained concerned because she noticed the night prior that certain areas had become "red and bumpy" and about 4 h later, the skin on her fingers began to peel. The patient had no fever or chills, and felt fine otherwise.

At the time of this visit, the patient was status post three rabies vaccinations on Day 0, Day 3 and Day 7 and was due for the fourth vaccine, though she found out from its owner that the dog who bit her was up to date on its rabies vaccinations.

Vitals were normal. On exam, on bilateral hands, there were multiple erythematous lesions with erythematous bases at the sites of the dog bites. There was peeling on the periphery of many of the lesions, and many were indurated and tender to palpation.

Specifically, the right hand pinky finger had erythema and tenderness to palpation spanning the full circumference of her finger (dorsal and ventral aspect) at the distal-interphalangeal joint and extending proximally with limited active range of motion (but full passive range of motion) at the distal-interphalangeal joint. At the periphery of the erythema, the skin was peeling. The left thumb had a 1.5 cm × 1.0 cm erythematous lesion with peeling skin at the periphery, with some induration and tenderness to palpation. The left fourth finger had a 3.0 cm × 1.5 cm erythematous, tender and indurated lesion with peeling at the periphery at the proximal-interphalangeal joint. She had limited active range of motion at this joint (normal passive range of motion). No warmth on any of the lesions. Peripheral pulses were normal.

Since the patient was already on antibiotics yet continued to have further worsening of pain and developed new areas of erythema and peeling, I was concerned about an abscess and referred her immediately to a hand surgeon for further evaluation. The hand surgeon examined her and was not concerned for an abscess but did recommend her for physical therapy.

Discussion from Dermatology Clinic

Differential Dx

- Blistering dactylitis
- Epidermolysis bullosa simplex, localized type
- Bullous impetigo

Favored Dx

The open lesions following dog bites most likely contracted a bacterial infection, resulting in blistering dactylitis.

Overview

Blistering dactylitis is a condition indicative of a superficial infection caused by β-hemolytic streptococcal bacteria, or by *Staphylococcus aureus*, both of which are commonly found in dog saliva.

Animal bites are common, with over one million animal bites occurring annually [1]. It is estimated that half of all Americans will experience a mammalian bite during their lifetime, and dog bites account for the majority of reported bites (80–90 %) although the infection rates are low (2–20 % of bites) [2]. Children are more likely to be bitten than adults, and are more likely to experience injuries to the neck and face versus adults who are more commonly bitten on the upper extremities. Bites on the hand are the most likely to develop infections [3].

Presentation

Patients in the acute blistering phase of blistering dactylitis present with superficial, tender blisters over the fat pads of the palmar aspects of the fingertips. Fingers may be erythematous and swollen, and blisters can ooze. The acute blistering phase may be very short-lived, and patients may not notice bullae, especially if they are small or burst soon after onset. Lesions tend to be asymptomatic; however, some patients may complain of pain and tenderness in the area, and they may be febrile.

Workup

Obtain a bacterial culture of the blister fluid. Cultures should rule out MRSA infections, which are unlikely but can occur after dog bites.

Treatment

Blisters can be incised and drained [4], and the wounds should be irrigated. Rabies and tetanus vaccines should be administered, if indicated. The patient should start a course of prophylactic antibiotics, the type of which should be determined by bacteriology [1]. Penicillin or ampicillin are effective against many components of dogs' oral flora and doxycycline provides a good alternative in children older than 8 years [1]. The combination of amoxicillin and clavulanic acid has demonstrated efficacy in treating dog bites as well [1]. If cultures reveal MRSA, an appropriate substitute antibiotic such as trimethoprim/ sulfamethoxazole or doxycycline should be initiated.

Follow-Up

Patients should follow up at the end of their antibiotic course to ensure the infection has cleared. Further treatment may not be necessary, unless patients complain their symptoms have not resolved.

Questions for the Dermatologist

– *What do I need to be concerned about when it comes to dog (or other animal) bites?*

The three factors contributing to potential infection are the biting animal's oral flora, the bite recipient's skin flora, and environmental organisms. Rabies would be high on the list of concerns. Dog bites themselves would not cause tetanus, but breaks in skin following the bite increase the risk of exposure to *C. tetani*. Dogs' saliva can contain *Pasteurella*, *Staphylococcus*, and *Streptococcus* species, and, rarely, potentially fatal *Capnocytophaga canimorsus* [5]. Bacterial culturing should be part of the general workup. This is particularly important in animal bites with open wounds because bacteria can easily enter the wound. If no culture is taken and the prescribed antibiotic is not working, it will be less obvious which antibiotic to prescribe.

– *Does the peeling skin signify normal healing? Or is it something to be concerned about?*

The toxins produced by bacteria cause exfoliative dermatitis. The most reassuring sign is that normal skin is repopulating underneath the peeling skin. That is a sign of recovery.

– *Two weeks after a dog bite is there anything else I should be worried about beyond the actual bite?*

Ensure any tetanus concerns have been addressed, and find out if the biting dog's rabies vaccinations are current. Otherwise, the patient should be managed supportively.

– *In this case, the peeling did not occur until 2 weeks after the dog bites and after she has already been on 2 weeks of antibiotics. Is this common? Does this signify a super-infection from the initial dog bite, or just a new phase of the initial infection?*

Blisters that are seen in infectious blistering conditions are very superficial and rupture quite easily. It is possible that following bacterial infection, the patient briefly formed superficial blisters that collapsed and later began to peel. The patient may not have experienced a specific bullous phase; however, at some point the blisters were probably unroofed, and as the skin dried out it began to fall off and peel. Rather than signifying a super-infection, the peeling skin is more likely part of the initial infection.

References

1. Brook I. Management of human and animal bite wound infection: an overview. Curr Infect Dis Rep. 2009;11(5):389–95.
2. Griego RD, Rosen T, Orengo IF, Wolf JE. Dog, cat, and human bites: a review. J Am Acad Dermatol. 1995;33(6):1019–29.
3. Oehler RL, Velez AP, Mizrachi M, Lamarche J, Gompf S. Bite-related and septic syndromes caused by cats and dogs. Lancet Infect Dis. 2009;9(7):439–47.
4. McCray MK, Esterly NB. Blistering distal dactylitis. J Am Acad Dermatol. 1981;5(5):592–4.
5. Thomas N, Brook I. Animal bite-associated infections. Expert Rev Anti Infect Ther. 2011;9(2):215–26.

Chapter 13
Pompholyx

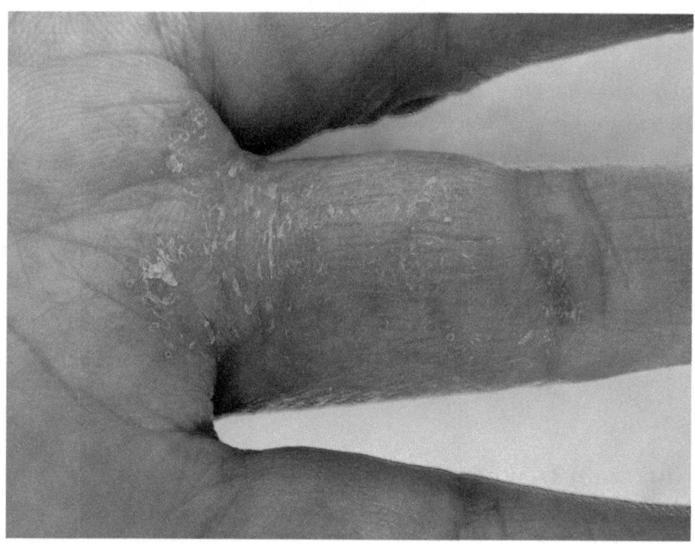

Fig. 13.1 Digits are preferentially affected with roughened plaques and prominent itch

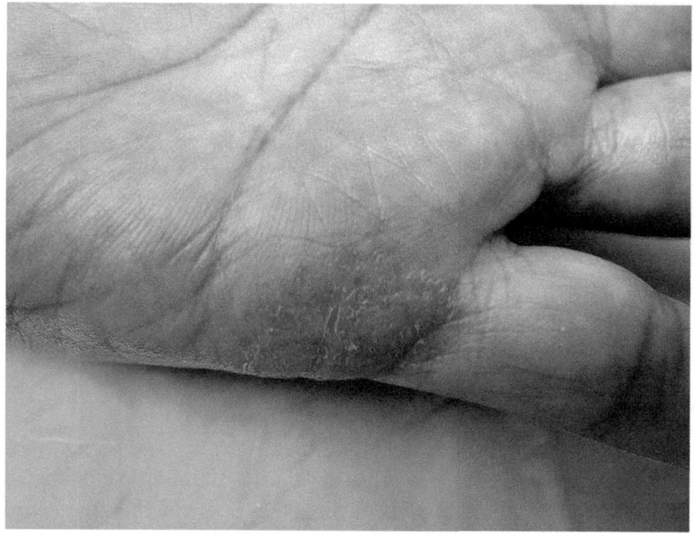

Fig. 13.2 Scale is found throughout this eczematous thin plaque

D. Reich et al., *Top 50 Dermatology Case Studies for Primary Care*,
DOI 10.1007/978-3-319-18627-6_13

Primary Care Visit Report

A 60-year-old female with past medical history of hypertension presented with a rash on her hand that she described as intermittently present since the birth of her son 36 years earlier. The rash was on the base of her right hand third finger, and on the lateral aspects of both of her hands. The patient had been using clobetasol on the rash for flares. She reported cycles of clearance for 2–3 weeks followed by recurrence.

Vitals were normal. On exam, on the palmar aspect of the patient's right hand, at the base of her third finger there was a 3 cm × 2 cm dry, scaly plaque and at the lateral base of her pinky finger there was a 2 cm × 2 cm dry, scaly plaque. On the patient's left hand, at the lateral base of the pinky finger on the palmar aspect, there was a 2 cm × 2 cm dry, scaly plaque.

This was treated as eczema. The patient had been using clobetasol proprionate (Class I steroid) fairly liberally for many years, but given the frequency with which she used it, she was prescribed desonide 0.05 % (Class VI steroid) cream twice daily for 14 days. A lower potency steroid was chosen to see if it would resolve the rash. The patient was also referred to dermatology.

Discussion from Dermatology Clinic

Differential Dx

- Pompholyx (AKA dyshidrotic eczema)
- Contact dermatitis
- Pustular psoriasis
- Scabies

Favored Dx

The desquamation noted on the patient's palms is consistent with the final stages of the vesicular eruption seen in pompholyx—eczema of the hands or feet.

Overview

Pompholyx is a type of chronic, vesicular dermatitis affecting the hands and sometimes the feet. It is also called dyshidrotic eczema, and it is characterized by small pruritic vesicles. Increased presence of eccrine sweat glands in the palms and soles of feet, as well as its link with hyperhidrosis, has led to the association of the vesicles in pompholyx with sweat glands [1]. These factors also make the condition more prevalent in warm weather.

The etiology of pompholyx is not known, although it has been linked with general eczema, contact allergies, hyperhidrosis, smoking, emotional stress, and immunological responses [2–4]. Immunocompromised populations, such as those with HIV infection, show a greater predisposition to pompholyx [1]. The condition can occur at any age but it shows peak prevalence between the ages of 30 and 40 years [2]. There is no gender preference.

Presentation

Pompholyx typically presents as a vesicular eruption on the palms, particularly the lateral aspects of fingers, and/or soles of feet. Palmar lesions alone occur in seven out of ten cases, palmoplantar lesions (on both hands and feet simultaneously) in two out of ten cases, and plantar lesions alone in one out of ten cases [2]. The tense, deep-seated, fluid-filled vesicles tend to be highly pruritic and may be accompanied by a burning sensation. Patients may report exacerbation of the burning sensation when they come in contact with water. The onset of small vesicles tends to be sudden. They may eventually coalesce and form a larger blister, and the lesions may spontaneously resolve. After the acute phase, patients experience desquamation on the affected skin. Recurrence is common.

Workup

Clinical diagnosis is usually sufficient. If there is a suspicion of contact dermatitis based on patient history, allergy patch testing may be done. Cases that are suspicious for bullous pemphigoid or epidermolysis bullosa, or where vesicles are hemorrhagic, should be referred to dermatology, where an immunofluorescence biopsy testing for the presence of antibodies may be performed. This biopsy requires a special transport medium (Michel's). Pompholyx of the feet should be evaluated for any dermatophytes as the compromised skin barrier becomes vulnerable to opportunistic infection. Dermatophytes may be detected by performing a KOH test on skin scrapings to look for hyphae.

Treatment

Treatment of pompholyx should be adapted to any suspected etiological factors. The targets of treatment are reducing inflammation, and suppressing pruritus. Oral antihistamines, such as hydroxyzine or diphenhydramine, may be prescribed to reduce itch. The standardized Dyshidrotic Eczema Area and Severity Index (DASI) has been developed to aid in management decisions. The DASI evaluates number of vesicles per square centimeter, erythema, pruritus, surface area affected, and desquamation [1]. High DASI scores may warrant combination therapy.

Topical strong corticosteroids (class I or II) are the mainstay of anti-inflammatory pompholyx treatment [5]. Fluocinonide ointment or clobetasol 0.05 % cream are examples of viable treatment options. Each should be used twice per day for up to 2 weeks, and patients should be warned of the long-term side effects of topical steroid use. The topical immunomodulator tacrolimus has demonstrated some success in treating pompholyx. Tacrolimus is a calcineurin inhibitor which, as a 0.1 % ointment used twice daily for 12 days, was found to be as effective as a corticosteroid, especially when combined with a prednisone taper [1, 5, 6]. If treatment with topical steroid or calcineurin inhibitor is unsuccessful, a 2-week oral prednisone taper can be prescribed at 0.5–1 mg/kg/day depending on severity [1, 5, 7].

Pompholyx has been associated with increased immune activity, and in some cases intravenous immunoglobulin (IVIg) has been used for treatment [8–10]. Thus systemic immunosuppressants, as well as treatment with psoralen and UVA light (PUVA) have demonstrated success in treating severe, recalcitrant pompholyx that is unresponsive to conventional treatment. Low dose methotrexate (12.5–25 mg) and cyclosporine (3–5 mg/kg/day) may be considered, although methotrexate may cause a wide range of side effects, and relapses are common with cyclosporine [1, 5, 11]. Light therapy has maximal immunosuppressive effects in the UV-A and UV-B range, and patients with chronic hand dermatitis who have used such therapy have shown improvement [1, 3, 5].

For patients whose symptoms are exacerbated by sweating, botulinum toxin A injections have helped resolve symptoms, likely due to their anhidrotic action [1, 5, 12]. The disadvantage of this approach is the requirement of injections in a sensitive area, and the potential cost.

Follow-Up

Pompholyx tends to be a chronic and recurrent condition for many patients. If initial topical treatment fails, patients may try oral prednisone therapy. After initial clearance, patients should be instructed to avoid any identified triggers as a preventative measure. For example, patients whose pompholyx is associated with a contact allergen may prevent future flares by avoiding the allergen. Those with hyperhidrosis can try using Burow's aluminum acetate solution between flares. Aluminum acetate is commonly sold under the brand name Domeboro, in packets that are dissolved in cold water. A cloth is soaked in the solution and applied to the affected area for 15–20 min, up to three times a day to control excessive sweating. Severe and recalcitrant cases may be referred to dermatology for further treatment.

Questions for the Dermatologist

– *Do you treat eczema and dyshidrotic eczema differently?*

Dyshidrotic eczema is a type of eczema that appears on the hands and feet. The treatment is the same as that for other types of eczema: strong emollient care with intermittent use of anti-inflammatory steroid creams to treat flare-ups. As with other eczema, if the baseline approach does not work, other means of immunotherapy should be trialed, e.g., light therapy or oral treatment.

– *How do you distinguish the two clinically?*

It is not necessary to distinguish between the two. Eczema of the hands and feet is the same as eczema elsewhere.

– *What should patients do between flares to control the condition?*

Increased work with water can cause flare-ups, and dyshidrotic eczema is often seen in barbacks and new mothers. Antiseptic waterless cleansers can also exacerbate the condition. Patients can avoid flares by frequently using emollients (e.g., Aquafor, Eucerin, Curel), thoroughly drying hands and moisturizing after cleansing. They should also be instructed to avoid washing affected areas too frequently, for too long, or with hot water.

– *In this case, the patient was switched from a class I steroid (clobetasol) to a class VI steroid (desonide). Is this unlikely to be a sufficiently potent class to treat pompholyx? Is it okay to keep someone on the higher potency steroid classes (I or II) for potentially chronic use with a recurrent condition like this?*

Desonide is probably not sufficiently potent to treat pompholyx. Furthermore, it confuses the treatment message. Using an approach where treatment is either on or off is more straightforward for patients. The treatment mode is either on, meaning the pompholyx is being controlled and we are aiming for rapid improvement with potent steroids, or treatment is off, meaning the patients are doing maintenance therapy with over-the-counter emollients and moisturizers that maintain the skin barrier's integrity. Treating with Desonide would partially improve the rash, but the patient would likely need to use the steroid more often. It is better to use class I potency steroids for active treatment, and when the rash gets better, discontinue the steroid and just do maintenance.

References

1. Wollina U. Pompholyx: a review of clinical features, differential diagnosis, and management. Am J Clin Dermatol. 2010;11(5):305–14.
2. Guillet MH, Wierzbicka E, Guillet S, Dagregorio G, Guillet G. A 3-year causative study of pompholyx in 120 patients. Arch Dermatol. 2007;143(12):1504–8.

3. Letić M. Use of sunglight to treat dyshidrotic eczema. JAMA Dermatol. 2013;149(5):634–5.
4. Lee KC, Ladizinski B. Dyshidrotic eczema following intravenous immunoglobullin treatment. CMAJ. 2013;185(11):E530.
5. Doshi DN, Cheng CE, Kimball AB. Chapter 16. Vesicular palmoplantar eczema. In: Goldsmith LA, Katz SI, Gilchrest BA, Paller AS, Leffell DJ, Wolff K, editors. Fitzpatrick's dermatology in general medicine. 8th ed. New York: McGraw-Hill; 2012. Available from: http://accessmedicine.mhmedical.com.ezproxy.cul.columbia.edu/content.aspx?bookid=392&Sectionid=41138711. Accessed 18 Nov 2014.
6. Sehgal VN, Srivastava G, Aggarwal AK, Sharma AD. Hand dermatitis/eczema: current management strategy. J Dermatol. 2010;37(7):593–610.
7. Usatine RP, Riojas M. Diagnosis and management of contact dermatitis. Am Fam Physician. 2010;82(3):249–55. Review.
8. Kotan D, Erdem T, Acar BA, Boluk A. Dyshidrotic eczema associated with the use of IVIg. BMJ Case Rep. 2013. doi:10.1136/bcr-2012-008001.
9. Vecchietti G, Kerl K, Prins C, Kaya G, Saurat JH, French LE. Severe eczematous skin reaction after high-dose intravenous immunoglobulin infusion: report of 4 cases and review of the literature. Arch Dermatol. 2006;142(2):213–7.
10. Miyamoto J, Böckle BC, Zillikens D, Schmidt E, Schmuth M. Eczematous reaction to intravenous immunoglobulin: an alternative cause of eczema. JAMA Dermatol. 2014;150(10):1120–2.
11. Egan CA, Rallis TM, Meadows KP, Krueger GG. Low-dose oral methotrexate treatment for recalcitrant palmoplantar pompholyx. J Am Acad Dermatol. 1999;40(4):612–4.
12. Wollina U, Karamfilov T. Adjuvant botulinum toxin A in dyshidrotic hand eczema: a controlled prospective pilot study with left-right comparison. J Eur Acad Dermatol Venereol. 2002;16(1):40–2.

Chapter 14
Arthropod Bites

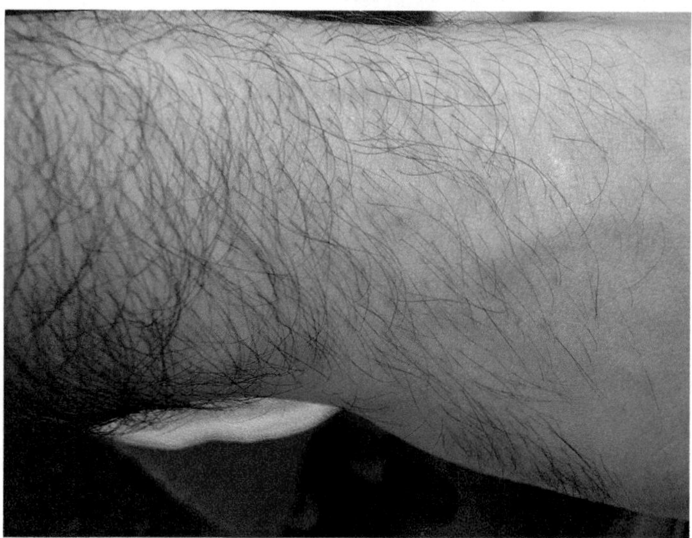

Fig. 14.1 Erythematous wheals with a raised, edematous central papule on the wrist

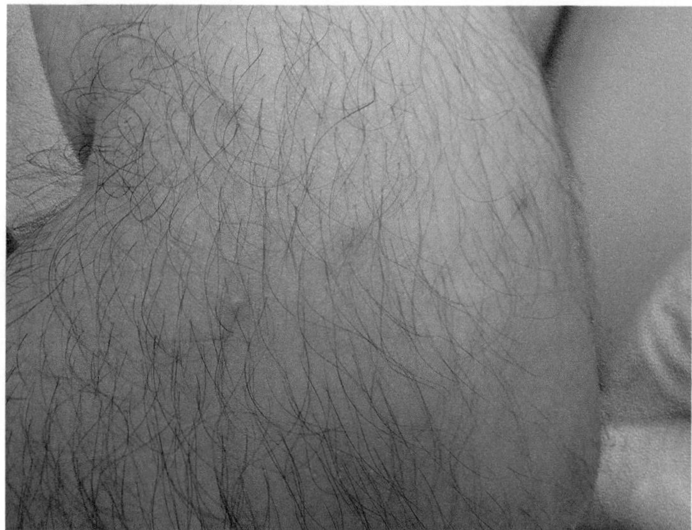

Fig. 14.2 Briskness of immune reaction will dictate the size of these lesions. It is, therefore, impossible to name the culprit based on the morphology of the lesion

D. Reich et al., *Top 50 Dermatology Case Studies for Primary Care*,
DOI 10.1007/978-3-319-18627-6_14

Primary Care Visit Report

A 26-year-old male with no past medical history presented with a rash on bilateral arms and wrists. The patient had woken up with the skin lesions 1 day prior. They were very itchy. They had gotten progressively worse since they appeared and seemed to become more symptomatic after he showered. The patient applied topical Benadryl cream which did not help.

Vitals were normal. On exam, there were multiple scattered erythematous papules with some excoriations on bilateral arms. There were no lesions in the web spaces of his fingers and no burrows. His right arm had an area of linear lesions, otherwise the lesions were diffusely scattered.

The lesions seemed to be bites; however, Primary Care was unsure of the source. The patient was treated for scabies with permethrin cream, and referred to dermatology in case the lesions did not clear up.

Discussion from Dermatology Clinic

Differential Dx

- Arthropod bites
- Scabies
- Urticaria
- Folliculitis

Favored Dx

On physical examination, the lesions appear to be arthropod bites. The phylum arthropods includes centipedes, millipedes, spiders, scorpions, and insects. The offending biter is difficult to identify without more details from the history, such as whether the individual has any pets (could suggest flea bites), if anyone else in the house has bites (scabies, fleas, or bed bugs), or whether he spent time outdoors with his arms exposed (mosquitoes, outdoor bugs). The distribution of the bites would not be typical of scabies, which tend to appear around the wrists and interdigital spaces. Furthermore, scabies lesions typically feature more extensive excoriation.

Overview

Arthropod bites are a significant cause of morbidity worldwide [1]. Arthropod bites and stings cause a range of symptoms in humans, ranging from mildly uncomfortable to life threatening. The majority of arthropod bites cause local reactions; however, some bites can cause toxic and anaphylactic reactions [2]. Many arthropods serve as vectors for diseases such as malaria, dengue, West Nile virus, Rocky Mountain spotted fever, Southern tick-associated rash illness (STARI), and Lyme disease.

The species of concern in the USA include the black widow and brown recluse spiders, the lone star, black-legged (*Ixodes scapularis*) and dog ticks, bed bugs, fleas, biting flies, and mosquitoes. Their significance is due to prevalence, severity of bite symptoms, or potential to transmit disease [1, 2]. Specifically, black widow spider bites cause severe muscle spasms and brown recluse spider bites can cause skin necrosis. Tick and mosquito bites are common, and the species are vectors for a number of diseases named above.

It is difficult to estimate the overall prevalence of bug bites, as many of them do not require any treatment. Systemic reactions from hymenoptera (insects such as bees, wasps, and hornets) stings have a lifetime prevalence ranging from 0.3 % in children to 7.5 % in adults [3, 4]. Fatalities associated with insect bites are very rare; however, some bites may require emergency management.

Presentation

Arthropod bites present in a variety of ways. Multiple bites will present as distinct pruritic lesions, often with a central punctum and surrounding erythema. Hymenoptera (e.g., wasps, bees) bites may be accompanied by pain, burning or stinging sensations, as well as local edema. Bed bug bites typically manifest in groups of three lesions (referred to as breakfast, lunch, and dinner lesions); however, such a pattern is not specific to bed bugs and cannot preclude other insects, as fleas are also known to cause a similar bite pattern (see Chap. 40 for more on bed bugs).

Scabies lesions usually involve papules with burrows containing a serpiginous line with a tiny black speck at the end, and present on the wrists, elbows, interdigital web spaces, and lower abdomen (see Chap. 41). Spider bites are more likely to present with extreme pain, although this again is not a symptom specific to spider bites. Any insect bite can cause vesicle formation. Although it is not necessarily the case, patients with bites from infesting, indoor bugs may report family members also experiencing bites. Bites from outdoor bugs are more likely to occur on parts of the body that are exposed to the environment, such as the neck and extremities.

Workup

Patient history is helpful in diagnosing bug bites, as they may recall a biting incident. Additionally, patients should be asked about outdoor activities, clothes worn and areas exposed during time outdoors, pets, and whether family members or roommates have also experienced bites.

If scabies are suspected, a scraping can be done and viewed under a microscope. Mineral oil is applied to a burrow or lesion, which is then scraped laterally with a number 15 blade. The scrapings are placed on a glass slide and viewed under a microscope. Microscopy may reveal eggs, mites, or fecal matter. Applying KOH to the slide may help visualize mite debris by dissolving keratin. Suspected cases of lice should include inspection of the hair shaft for any nits.

Treatment

Treatment of bites depends on the insulting arthropod and the accompanying symptoms. All bite wounds should be cleaned and remaining stingers, if any, should be removed using the edge of a bank card or butter knife to push them out. Tweezers are not recommended as squeezing the stinger may cause further venom release, although the amount of venom might be very small. Symptomatic relief should be provided either in the way of antihistamines to control itch, topical steroids to control inflammation, and ice packs or analgesics for pain [1, 2].

Bites such as the ones in this case are usually best treated with topical steroids. A medium potency steroid can be used on the limbs and trunk (excluding intertriginous areas), such as betamethasone valerate ointment 0.1% (Class III) applied to individual lesions twice daily for up to 2 weeks. Sedating antihistamines such as hydroxyzine may be taken by patients experiencing pruritus that interrupts their sleep.

Bites causing anaphylaxis should be treated with epinephrine or other vasoactive medications. Tick bites in geographical areas with high incidence of Lyme may be treated with a prophylactic 200 mg single dose of doxycycline if the tick species has been identified and was attached for more than 36 h [2]. Severe spider bites may require treatment with an antivenom. Secondary infection on bite sites should be treated with an appropriate antibiotic, as determined by a wound culture. Treatment for bed bug bites (which are also treated with topical steroids) and scabies are discussed in more detail in their respective chapters.

Follow-Up

Patient follow up is somewhat dependent on the offending insect. Although many mosquito-born diseases are concentrated in tropical and subtropical areas, they still occur in North America. Patients with recent travel history and mosquito bites should be aware of common symptoms of malaria and dengue. Uncomplicated bug bites should resolve within 1–2 weeks of treatment with corticosteroid, although post inflammatory hyperpigmentation may persist for several months.

Questions for the Dermatologist

– *Is there a way to tell which insect is doing the biting?*

No, unfortunately there is not. All bites are inflammatory reactions to saliva or an antigen present in the bite. There are some diagnostic clues. Flea bites tend to be smaller than bed bug bites, but this is not always true. History is most helpful in determining which bug is doing the biting. If bites are found following an outdoor activity like a picnic, they are probably outdoor bugs. Presence of blood on the sheets and new bites when the patient wakes up are suggestive of bed bugs. Bites in the dead of winter are more likely to be bed bugs. In that case patients should look for engorged bugs between 4 and 5 am, along the seams of their mattress.

– *How can insect bites be distinguished from other rashes?*

Rashes tend to spread out and extend to different parts of the body. Eczematous rashes may have indiscreet edges. They do not appear as discrete lesions the way bites do. Bites have clear demarcations and appear as individual lesions in groups.

– *Is there a way to tell whether the bites are caused by bed bugs? Scabies? Is there a lab test for any of the above?*

There is no lab test for different types of bug bites. Suspected scabies lesions can be scraped and viewed under a microscope to look for eggs and droppings. Scrapings are placed in mineral oil on a glass slide and viewed under a microscope on low power. Otherwise defer to history.

– *What is the best treatment for insect bites that are not scabies?*

The best treatment is topical steroids. Medium potency steroids can be used on the arms and legs twice daily for a short period of time, i.e., 2 weeks.

References

1. Schwartz RA, Steen CJ. Chapter 210. Arthropod bites and stings [Internet]. In: Goldsmith LA, Katz SI, Gilchrest BA, Paller AS, Leffell DJ, Wolff K, editors. Fitzpatrick's dermatology in general medicine. 8th ed. New York: McGraw-Hill; 2012. [cited 2015 Jan 21]. Available from: http://accessmedicine.mhmedical.com.ezproxy.cul.columbia.edu/content.aspx?bookid=392&Sectionid=41138941.
2. Juckett G. Arthropod bites. Am Fam Physician. 2013;88(12):841–7.
3. Baker TW, Forester JP, Johnson ML, Stolfi A, Stahl MC. The HIT study: Hymenoptera identification test—how accurate are people at identifying stinging insects? Ann Allergy Asthma Immunol. 2014;113(3):267–70.

4. Ruëff F, Przybilla B, Biló MB, Müller U, Scheipl F, Aberer W, Birnbaum J, Bodzenta-Lukaszyk A, Bonifazi F, Bucher C, Campi P, Darsow U, Egger C, Haeberli G, Hawranek T, Körner M, Kucharewicz I, Küchenhoff H, Lang R, Quercia O, Reider N, Severino M, Sticherling M, Sturm GJ, Wüthrich B. Predictors of severe systemic anaphylactic reactions in patients with Hymenoptera venom allergy: importance of baseline serum tryptase-a study of the European Academy of Allergology and Clinical Immunology Interest Group on Insect Venom Hypersensitivity. J Allergy Clin Immunol. 2009;124(5):1047–54.

Part III
Lower Limbs

Chapter 15
Tinea Pedis

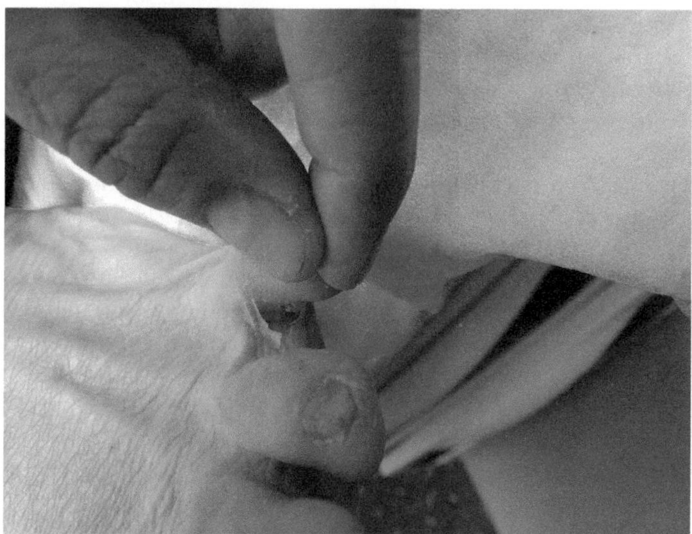

Fig. 15.1 Webspace maceration and itch are critical elements to making this diagnosis

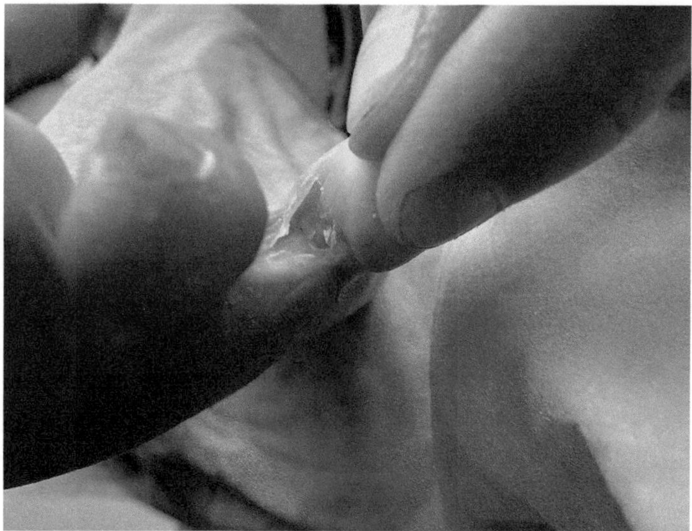

Fig. 15.2 Hyperkeratotic toenails present

D. Reich et al., *Top 50 Dermatology Case Studies for Primary Care*,
DOI 10.1007/978-3-319-18627-6_15

Primary Care Visit Report

A 37-year-old female with no past medical history presented with left foot pain which started acutely 2 days prior. At the visit, the pain was so severe she had trouble putting her shoe on. The pain was in the toe webbing between her left fourth and fifth toes. She had applied over-the-counter Lotrimin for athlete's foot but it did not help. She also had two thick yellow toenails on her left fourth and fifth toes, which had been like that for years.

Vitals were normal. On exam, there was a 5×5 mm yellow macular blister with some surrounding erythema in the toe webbing between the left 4th and 5th toes; there was trace edema and mild erythema on her 5th toe; there was some erythema on the dorsal aspect of the base of the 4th/5th toe webbing. The 4th and 5th toenails of the left foot were yellow, thickened, and ridged.

This was treated as an acute flare of tinea pedis, likely after longstanding onychomycosis. The patient was treated with 250 mg oral terbinafine for 2 weeks, as well as Burow's solution topically three times daily, and foot powder to prevent maceration and to keep the area dry. The patient was advised to follow up with podiatry if the blister worsened over the following few days while on treatment. With respect to the toenail fungal infection, the patient wanted to try natural remedies (i.e., tea tree oil) as opposed to staying on the terbinafine for 12 weeks.

Discussion from Dermatology Clinic

Differential Dx

- Tinea pedis
- Dyshidrotic eczema
- Pitted keratolysis
- Candidiasis
- Contact dermatitis
- Psoriasis

Favored Dx

Clinical examination, maceration between toe spaces, and presence of onychomycosis are suggestive of a fungal infection.

Overview

Tinea pedis, commonly known as athlete's foot, is a dermatophytic infection of the foot that causes scaling, flaking, itching, and maceration. It can sometimes lead to onychomycosis, or toenail fungus, which can be a source of reinfection in that the tinea pedis may be treated and cured, but the still existing onychomycosis can then lead to a recurrence of tinea pedis.

Tinea pedis is a condition that affects approximately 15 % of the global population [1]. Fungal infections generally affect men more than women. In the case of tinea pedis, the incidence is four times greater in men than women and increases with age [1]. Those who use communal pools, baths, and showers are more likely to develop an infection [2]. The dermatophytes that cause tinea pedis thrive in warm, humid environments, and are transmitted via direct contact, for example by retained skin in clothes, socks, or towels.

The typical disease process begins with dermatophytes adhering to epidermal keratins that are used as a nutrition source, followed by invasion and growth in the skin. Maceration, erythema, and hyperproliferation of the skin are among the symptoms that reflect the body's inflammatory response to infection.

Presentation

There are four distinct forms of tinea pedis: interdigital, hyperkeratotic "moccasin," bullous, and acute ulcerative type. More than one form can affect patients. The most common type is interdigital, which affects the webbing between toes and adjacent sole. Scaling and erythema on the lateral and medial aspects of the sole is referred to as moccasin-type because of its distribution. The bullous type is not common and it presents as vesicles on the soles of the feet. Most often tinea pedis will present with erythema, pruritus, scaling, and maceration in the plantar aspect of the foot.

Workup

Tinea pedis can be diagnosed on clinical examination. The diagnosis can be confirmed by detecting hyphae on epidermal scrapings in KOH preparation viewed under a microscope, or by taking a fungal culture of the macerated lesions. If patients have already used over-the-counter antifungal therapy, it is possible fungal culture results will be negative.

Treatment

Topical allylamines (i.e., terbinafine) and azoles are the most effective medications for treating tinea pedis. Allylamines are more efficacious than azoles, especially over longer periods of time (i.e., 4–6 weeks of therapy) [3]. Terbinafine 1 %, clotrimazole 1 %, or econazole 1 % twice daily are all acceptable options. Luliconazole 1 % daily for 1–2 weeks is a newer alternative that has demonstrated clearance of tinea pedis [4].

If oral therapy is indicated due to severity or recalcitrance, terbinafine is more effective than either griseofulvin or itraconazole [1]. A dose of 250 mg daily for 2 weeks has shown compelling mycological cure rates. In addition to medications, patients should be instructed to keep feet clean and dry. They should put their socks on before underwear in order to avoid spreading the infection to the groin.

Follow-Up

Patients should be reexamined after 2 weeks to assess clinical response. Continuation of topical therapy may be indicated if there is moderate progress. If infection is unresponsive, patients should consider initiating oral therapy. Those with full clearance should be advised to continue taking prophylactic measures such as wearing footwear in public pools and showers, thoroughly drying feet before putting on clean socks, applying antifungal powders like Lotrimin or Desenex to feet and shoes, and avoiding occlusive shoes.

Questions for the Dermatologist

– *Does onychomycosis often lead to tinea pedis or vice versa?*

Yes, it does. Left untreated, severe tinea pedis can migrate to the nail bed and lead to onychomycosis. The reverse can also happen with onychomycosis seeding tinea pedis.

– *With athlete's foot, is the mainstay of treatment to keep the area dry? Are oral medications and powders better than creams and lotions in terms of keeping the area dry (i.e., do creams/lotions add to the moistness of the area)?*

The mainstay of tinea pedis treatment is eradicating the dermatophyte. Prophylactic care during and after treatment requires keeping the feet dry and using powders. Antifungal creams or lotions (e.g., Lotrimin) may also be used as prophylactic therapy, and they would not contribute problematic moisture to the area. The specific formulation used should depend on patient preference. If there is excessive moisture, patients can try soaks with Burow's solution.

– *What is Burow's solution? And when/why is it used?*

Burow's aluminum acetate solution is a drying agent used for conditions with lots of suppuration (discharge, weeping, or pus). It can dry out suppuration in chicken pox, or pyoderma gangrenosum. If there's lots of moisture in a particular case of tinea pedis, you could use Burow's solution as an adjunctive treatment to help dry out the feet.

– *What foot powders are used? Prescription anti-fungal? Over-the-counter anti-fungal? Nystatin powder?*

I often recommend Zeasorb, an over-the-counter miconazole antifungal powder. Plain talcum powder is also a great drying agent.

– *When is topical treatment okay for tinea pedis, and when is oral treatment necessary?*

Our practice uses topical medications for tinea pedis. In the case of severe, recurring tinea pedis, or if onychomycosis is present, oral therapy is indicated. Oral terbinafine will work for both tinea pedis and onychomycosis, but they require different treatment durations. Onychomycosis requires about 3 months of terbinafine for toenails and 2 months for fingernails, while tinea pedis requires 2 weeks.

– *Does the severity of the patient's pain direct treatment differently?*

Yes. Severe pain makes a good case for use of oral therapy for faster clearance and minimizing risk of recurrence. Local wound care may also be required, as well as use of local anesthetic.

– *Given the severity of pain, and likely longstanding nature of infection, is there anything else to worry about with this patient?*

Most likely not. If the patient had a history of diabetes, the severity may indicate it is not being well managed. If the patient is otherwise healthy, she should be treated with a definitive therapy followed by prophylactic foot care.

– *With onychomycosis, is it worth trying topical medications first, or is it reasonable to go straight to terbinafine?*

Topical treatment for onychomycosis is effective after at least 1 year of use [3] 6% of the time. That's not a very compelling number for most patients. If patients have liver problems, or are uninterested in oral therapy, they can try topical antifungals, but clinical cure rates are fairly low.

– *If LFTs bump up while using terbinafine, how much of an increase is acceptable and how real is that risk?*

The answer to this question relies on the art of medicine as opposed to a hard and fast rule. A significant increase with no other explanation would be meaningful. Otherwise there would be no reason to discontinue oral therapy.

References

1. Bell-Syer SE, Khan SM, Torgerson TJ. Oral treatments for fungal infections of the skin of the foot. Cochrane Database Syst Rev. 2012;10:CD003584.
2. Schieke SM, Garg A. Chapter 188. Superficial Fungal Infection. In: Goldsmith LA, Katz SI, Gilchrest BA, Paller AS, Leffell DJ, Wolff K, editors. Fitzpatrick's dermatology in general medicine. 8th ed. New York, NY: McGraw-Hill; 2012. p. 2277–97.
3. Crawford F, Hollis S. Topical treatments for fungal infections of the skin and nails of the foot. Cochrane Database Syst Rev. 2007;3:CD001434.
4. Feng X, Xie J, Zhuang K, Ran Y. Efficacy and tolerability of luliconazole cream 1% for dermatophytoses: A Meta-analysis. J Dermatol. 2014;41(9):779–82.

Chapter 16
Pyoderma Gangrenosum

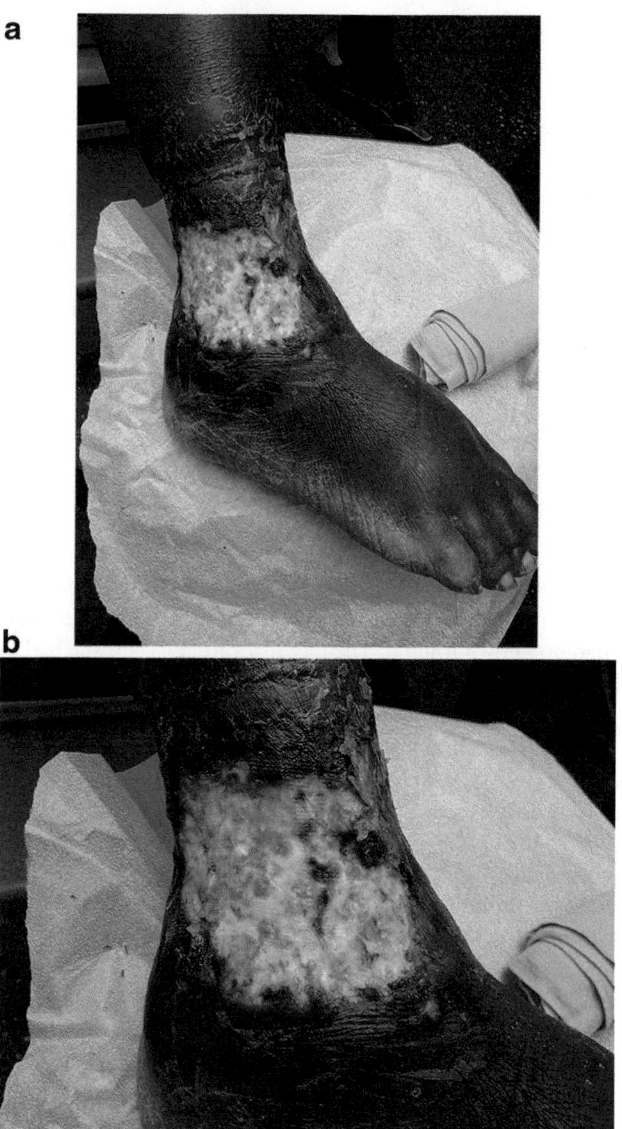

Fig. 16.1 (**a** and **b**) Painful ulceration with fresh granulation tissue and pinpoint bleeding

D. Reich et al., *Top 50 Dermatology Case Studies for Primary Care*,
DOI 10.1007/978-3-319-18627-6_16

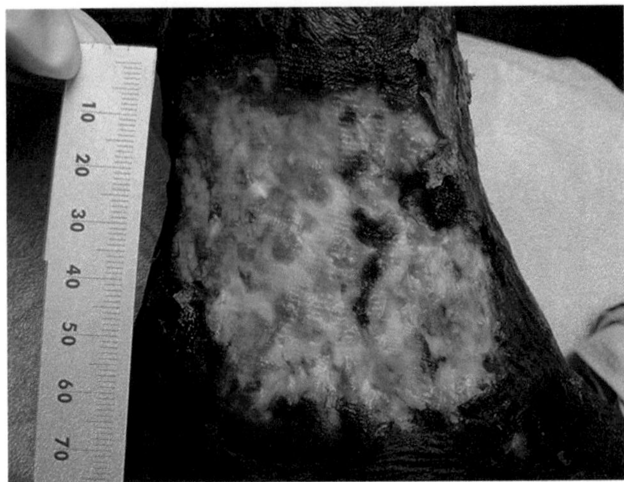

Fig. 16.2 Cribiform ulceration with "drop-off" or undermined edges

Primary Care Visit Report

A 69-year-old female with past medical history of hypertension and ulcerative colitis presented with right foot and ankle pain which she had been experiencing for about a week. She had no known trauma. The day prior to her visit, she had noticed some skin breakdown in the area. She had been applying over-the-counter antibiotic cream, Voltaren analgesic gel, and took some aspirin. About 8 months prior, the patient had started having crampy abdominal pain and blood in her stool. She was seeing a gastroenterologist for this.

Vitals were normal, except for elevated blood pressure of 150/80 mmHg. On exam, there was right ankle hyperemia, edema, and tenderness to palpation over the lateral malleolus with 1 cm of ulceration, and no lymphagitic streaking. Her complete blood count (CBC) revealed normal white blood cells, but significant anemia with a hemoglobin/hematocrit of 27.9/8.6.

This was initially treated as cellulitis with Bactrim DS BID for 10 days and topical Bactroban 2 % ointment TID.

Four days later, the patient returned with increased ankle pain and swelling, as well as a larger area of ulceration. At that point, her right foot and ankle had 2+ edema with a 2 cm pus-filled ulceration, which was exquisitely tender with surrounding erythema and warmth. The patient was sent to the Emergency Room for possible IV antibiotics given the lack of improvement on oral antibiotics.

She was admitted to the hospital and was treated with IV antibiotics for cellulitis without any improvement. The wound was surgically debrided and wound cultures showed no growth. She was then diagnosed with pyoderma gangrenosum and treated with oral prednisone and the wound started to improve.

These photos were taken 3 weeks after initially presenting at the Primary Care office.

Discussion from Dermatology Clinic

Differential Dx

- Pyoderma gangrenosum
- Cellulitis
- Antiphospholipid antibody syndrome
- Acute febrile neutrophilic dermatosis (Sweet syndrome)
- Arterial or venous insufficiency
- Verrucous carcinoma
- Cutaneous anthrax
- Blastomycosis

Favored Dx

A painful, deep ulcer with well-defined margins, with an associated history of ulcerative colitis is consistent with a diagnosis of pyoderma gangrenosum.

Overview

Pyoderma gangrenosum (PG) is an uncommon, chronic inflammatory skin condition characterized by neutrophilic infiltration of the skin and resulting in painful ulcers. The condition is immune-mediated; however, its exact cause is not known. While the name pyoderma suggests microbial etiology, PG is not infectious, though it is frequently misdiagnosed as such [1]. PG has recently been associated with mutations in the PSTPIP1, MTHFR, and JAK2 genes, and there are reports of familial cases without those mutations [2].

PG has a strong association with other autoimmune conditions, with underlying inflammatory bowel disease (IBD), seropositive and seronegative polyarthritis, and hematological disorders present in about 50 % of cases [2–4]. The likelihood is that the development of PG is multifactorial and represents a complex interplay between dysfunctional neutrophils, dysregulated inflammatory cytokines, and genetic predisposition [5, 7].

PG can affect people of any age but it most commonly affects those between the ages of 40 and 60, and it has a slight female predominance [3, 6, 7]. The incidence among the general population is estimated to be between three and ten patients per million per year [7].

Presentation

Pyoderma gangrenosum has several recognized variants, those being ulcerative, bullous, pustular, and vegetative. More than one variant can occur at the same time; however, one subtype tends to dominate the presentation. The variant that occurs most frequently, and the one discussed in this case, is the ulcerative subtype. Ulcerative, also sometimes called "common," PG tends to begin as an isolated papule or pustule that rapidly develops into a painful ulcer within 24–48 h. In 25–30 % of cases, the initial pustule develops at the site of previous trauma or injury such as venipuncture, laparoscopy, or a surgical site, a phenomenon referred to as pathergy [1, 3, 5, 6]. Up to 15 % of PGs occur at the site of abdominal stomas that have been placed for any reason (IBD or non-IBD etiology) [8].

PG presents as rapidly progressing, large, severely painful, weeping ulcer(s) with surrounding edema and erythema. The ulcer typically has a raised, serpiginous border with a dark purple "violaceous" edge. The base of the ulcer can be superficial or extend into subcutaneous fat and muscle, and typically features necrotic tissue within the base. PG can occur on any skin surface including the genitalia; however, it most commonly affects the lower limbs, reportedly in up to 80 % of cases [1].

Due to the association with systemic disease, individuals with PG may present with signs of being generally unwell. In addition to symptoms pertaining to PG itself, they may present with fever, fatigue, arthralgia, or myalgia.

Workup

Pyoderma gangrenosum is a diagnosis of exclusion that is generally made on a clinical basis. History plays a very important role in diagnosis, and careful attention should be paid to symptoms that accompany the systemic diseases frequently associated with PG. A non-healing ulcer that presents with gastrointestinal symptoms (diarrhea, abdominal pain, fatigue), hematological symptoms (fatigue, anemia, bruising), or arthritic symptoms (synovitis, arthralgia, myalgia) should raise suspicion for PG.

PG ulcers can be swabbed and sent for bacterial, fungal, and viral cultures. A biopsy is only needed to exclude alternate diagnoses as histopathologic findings are nonspecific for PG. The sample should be taken from the edge of the ulcer. There is no blood test to rule out PG; however, investigations for underlying systemic disease should be ordered when they are warranted by patient history, i.e., when accompanied by relevant systemic symptoms. Suspected pyoderma gangrenosum should be referred to a specialist.

Treatment

The treatment of PG is largely empirical as there are few controlled studies on this rare condition [7, 8]. The goals of treatment are to reduce inflammation, promote ulcer healing, and control any underlying disease. The approach to therapy involves topical and systemic medication, analgesia (e.g. acetaminophen or NSAIDs), and wound care. Potent topical corticosteroids alone may be adequate in very mild PG, and they are a useful adjunct therapy in more severe disease. Since this condition can result in large ulcerated and inflamed lesions, a higher potency topical steroid (Class I-II) is usually prescribed. One example is Clobetasol 0.05 % (Class I) which can be applied under occlusion of a non-adhesive dressing twice daily for up to 2 weeks.

For more severe PG, a high-dose systemic corticosteroid such as prednisone is the mainstay of treatment. The starting dose is 0.5–1.5 mg/kg/day, and that dose should be maintained until the ulcer begins to resolve. As the ulcer begins to heal, the dose can be tapered down. Alternatively, cyclosporine has demonstrated efficacy at 5 mg/kg/day either taken alone, or with a systemic corticosteroid [3, 8, 9]. Special caution should be taken when prescribing cyclosporine as it interacts with several medications, and patients will require monitoring.

Extensive or recalcitrant disease often responds to anti-tumor necrosis α medications. Infliximab and adalimumab are the two most commonly prescribed biologics. They have the added benefit of treating some of the potentially associated conditions, such as IBD or seropositive arthritis.

The ulcers of PG tend to be highly painful and great care should be taken when cleansing them. A mild rinse with saline provides adequate irrigation. Hydrocolloid dressings, or any non-stick dressing, can be applied to the ulcer to shield it from infection. The dressing use instructions should be carefully followed, and patients should be informed that severe PG ulcers often leave scars.

Follow-Up

Patients should be followed to ensure the ulcer(s) are healing. The ulcers of PG may take several months to fully resolve; however, individuals on systemic treatment tend to experience improvement within 24 h [9]. The course of the condition is difficult to predict. After one occurrence of PG, the condition may recur at any time. While control of any associated underlying disease helps to control PG, ulcers can reappear even in patients whose IBD is in remission. One way to prevent recurrence is to be careful to avoid any local injury, as PG is known to develop at sites of minor trauma. Treatment should be sought for any subsequent PG as soon as possible.

Questions for the Dermatologist

– *What is the association between ulcerative colitis and pyoderma gangrenosum?*

Any inflammatory bowel disease (IBD), including Crohn's and ulcerative colitis, carries a higher incidence of pyoderma gangrenosum.

– *Is PG diagnosed clinically or by biopsy?*

In some instances the presentation of PG can be obvious enough that it does not require biopsy. However, it is a fairly sophisticated diagnosis and, if in doubt, it should be confirmed by biopsy before initiating systemic therapy. This condition may be referred to dermatology for outpatient management.

– *What is the risk of recurrence?*

Once PG has occurred there is a higher likelihood it will return again. An ulcer can resolve after treatment; however, this is a challenging condition to treat and there is no definitive cure.

References

1. Binus AM, Qureshi AA, Li VW, Winterfield LS. Pyoderma gangrenosum: a retrospective review of patient characteristics, comorbidities and therapy in 103 patients. Br J Dermatol. 2011;165(6):1244–50.
2. DeFilippis EM, Feldman SR, Huang WW. The genetics of pyoderma gangrenosum and implications for treatment: a systematic review. Br J Dermatol. 2015;172(6):1487–97.
3. Powell FC, Hackett BC, Wallach D. Chapter 33. Pyoderma gangrenosum. In: Goldsmith LA, Katz SI, Gilchrest BA, Paller AS, Leffell DJ, Wolff K, editors. Fitzpatrick's dermatology in general medicine. 8th ed. New York: McGraw-Hill; 2012. p. 371–9.
4. Agarwal A, Andrews JM. Systematic review: IBD-associated pyoderma gangrenosum in the biologic era, the response to therapy. Aliment Pharmacol Ther. 2013;38(6):563–72.
5. Braswell SF, Kostopoulos TC, Ortega-Loayza AG. Pathophysiology of pyoderma gangrenosum (PG): an updated review. J Am Acad Dermatol. 2015;73(4):691–8.
6. Okhovat JP, Shinkai K. Pyoderma gangrenosum. JAMA Dermatol. 2014;150(9):1032.
7. Ruocco E, Sangiuliano S, Gravina AG, Miranda A, Nicoletti G. Pyoderma gangrenosum: an updated review. J Eur Acad Dermatol Venereol. 2009;23(9):1008–17.
8. Brooklyn T, Dunnill G, Probert C. Diagnosis and treatment of pyoderma gangrenosum. BMJ. 2006;333(7560):181–4.
9. Reichrath J, Bens G, Bonowitz A, Tilgen W. Treatment recommendations for pyoderma gangrenosum: an evidence-based review of the literature based on more than 350 patients. J Am Acad Dermatol. 2005;53(2):273–83.

Chapter 17
Cellulitis

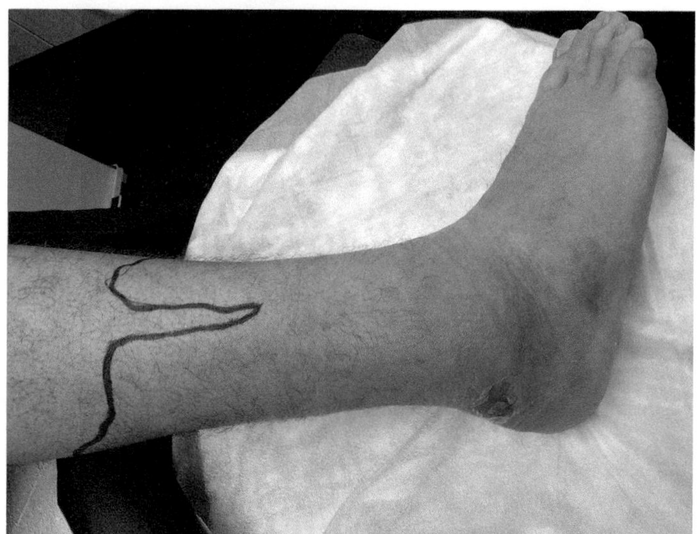

Fig. 17.1 Edges marked to gauge tracking of erythema and edema

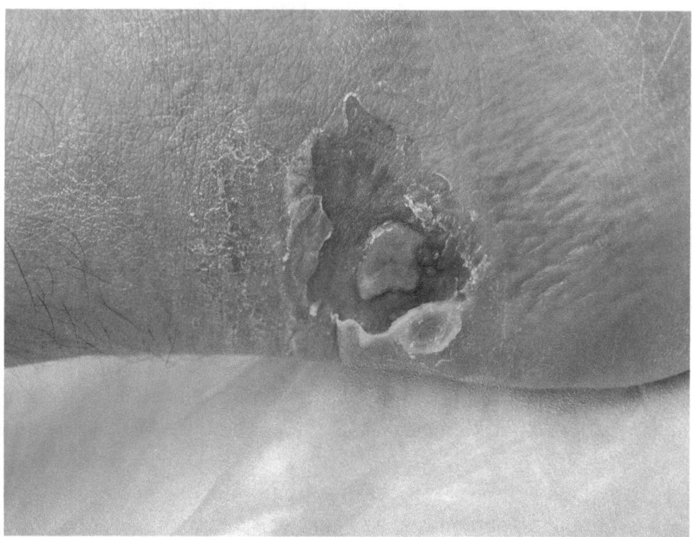

Fig. 17.2 Ulceration secondary to heavy third-spacing of fluid in tissue

D. Reich et al., *Top 50 Dermatology Case Studies for Primary Care*,
DOI 10.1007/978-3-319-18627-6_17

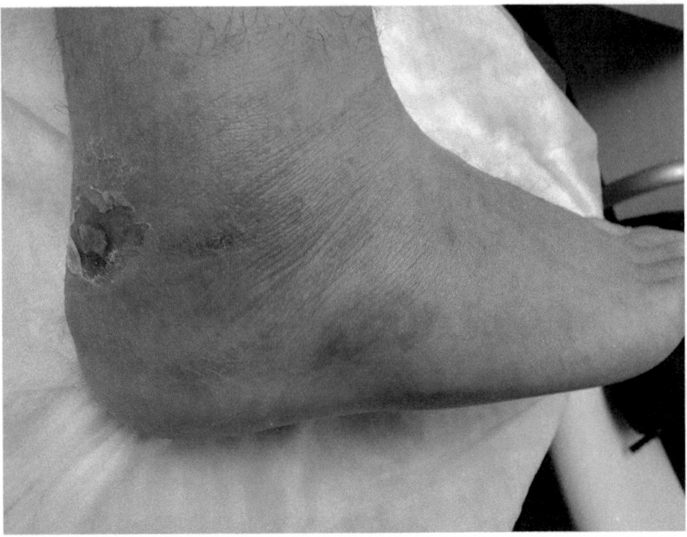

Fig. 17.3 Significant edema accompanies the erythematous rash

Primary Care Visit Report

A 24-year-old male with past medical history of staphylococcal and streptococcal skin infections and abscesses presented with an open lesion on his right posterior ankle accompanied by right leg erythema and edema. The patient reported that he had formed a blister in this same right heel 7 months prior. That blister healed, however the overlying skin did not fully return to normal. The patient said, "there was always a dark spot there after that."

Five days prior to this visit, his right foot and leg started swelling and becoming red, and the site of the prior blister opened up. The day prior to this visit, a "black spot" appeared adjacent to the open lesion, which then also "broke open," forming a large wound. He denied fever or chills, and felt otherwise well. The patient reported that the area had been much more painful 2–3 days prior to this visit, at which time he could not put on a shoe due to the pain and swelling. The pain had improved by the time of visit.

Vitals were normal. On exam, there was a 3.5 cm×2 cm weeping ulcer on the lateral Achilles area of his right heel, with surrounding blanchable erythema on his foot and ankle that extended to the mid lower leg. There was 1+ edema on the right lower leg.

This was treated as cellulitis progressing from an open abscess on the patient's posterior ankle. Since the patient had a history of staph and skin infections, he was treated for possible MRSA. The patient was prescribed oral sulfamethoxazole/trimethoprim 800–160 mg twice daily for 10 days, and topical bactroban 2 % three times daily to the open wound. The proximal border of the erythema was outlined with a permanent marker. The patient was advised to go to the Emergency Department if the erythema extended beyond the marked line or if any systemic symptoms developed as that could be an indication for intravenous antibiotic treatment.

Discussion from Dermatology Clinic

Differential Dx

- Cellulitis
- Abscess
- Erysipelas
- Impetigo
- Necrotizing fasciitis
- Stasis dermatitis

Favored Dx

Physical examination indicates cellulitis.

Overview

Cellulitis is a soft tissue bacterial infection caused mainly by gram-positive pathogens such as *Staphylococcus aureus,* MRSA, and β-hemolytic *Streptococci.* The infection occurs following breaks in the skin, commonly from surgical wounds, ulcers, or eczematous conditions.

Cellulitis is a common infection that complicates wounds, ulcers, and skin abrasions. It affects the dermis and subcutaneous tissue. The depth of involvement can be used to differentiate cellulitis from erysipelas, which is clinically very similar but affects superficial layers of the skin, and has well defined margins. The incidence of soft-tissue infections is high, accounting for as many as 10% of hospital admissions, and cellulitis is estimated to occur in 200 per 100,000 people but is variable depending on populations [1, 2]. Incidence of cellulitis is on the rise, mirroring the increase of MRSA infections.

Risk of developing cellulitis increases with age. It affects men and women equally [1]. Other risk factors for developing cellulitis of the lower limbs include history of cellulitis, lymphedema, venous insufficiency, tinea pedis, prior trauma, and chronic dermopathies [2, 3]. Cellulitis most frequently occurs in the legs, but can be seen in the face, trunk, and upper limbs. Breast cancer surgeries that involve lymph drainage can result in cellulitis of the upper limbs [4].

Presentation

Cellulitis presents as an erythematous, acutely tender, warm, and poorly demarcated inflammation of the skin. It most commonly affects the lower legs, and can be accompanied by edema, blisters, and necrosis in more severe cases [5–8]. The onset is fast and can occur within a matter of hours, and erythema can spread rapidly. Systemic symptoms like fever, chills, and malaise accompany cellulitis in 40 % of cases but are not necessary in making a diagnosis [2]. Many patients will present with history of trauma in the affected area.

Workup

Cellulitis is a clinical diagnosis. If the wound is purulent, cultures and sensitivities of the exudate should be collected to identify the responsible pathogen [7]. This can be particularly helpful for pediatric or immunocompromised patients, or in cases where an atypical pathogen is suspected [8]. Results may be complicated by natural colonizers or contaminants of the skin [5].

Treatment

Antibiotics are the cornerstone treatment for cellulitis. Antibiotics with anti-inflammatory effects, primarily macrolides and tetracyclines, may be helpful in treating accompanying symptoms. Antibiotic treatment should be active against β-hemolytic streptococci and *S. aureus*. Purulent cellulitis (i.e., with an associated abscess) should be treated with antibiotics that cover for MRSA such as clindamycin, trimethoprim-sulfamethoxazole, or doxycycline [7]. Non-purulent cellulitis (no purulent drainage and no associated abscess) can be treated with first generation cephalosporins since the offending pathogen is usually streptococcal or MSSA/staphylococcal [6]. Treatment course with oral antibiotics is 5–10 days. Severe cellulitis, or those cases accompanied by immunodeficiency, may require hospitalization and intravenous antibiotic treatment [4]. Pain relief medication is usually not required.

Marking the extent of erythema is useful for monitoring progress, and antibiotic coverage should be broadened if there is little improvement. Knowledge of MRSA in the community is helpful in choosing empiric treatment.

Follow-Up

Patients should return at the end of the treatment course to ensure resolution. Cellulitis involving the tibial area, obesity, chronic edema, smoking, and history of cancer are all risk factors for recurrence within 2 years [3, 6]. The rate of recurrence is higher in inpatients than outpatients [6]. In order to prevent recurrence, any underlying etiology should be treated as well. Elevating legs and wearing compression socks can help address poor venous circulation [9]. Cases of recurrent cellulitis suggest colonization of the nose, axilla, groin, or perianal area, which may be causing autoinfection. Culturing any of those areas and treating them with topical antibiotics if cultures are positive, e.g., with topical mupirocin twice times daily for 5 days, is recommended.

Questions for the Dermatologist

– *What were the 'black spots' that opened up and formed the lesions?*

Any black area in cellulitis would be necrosis. Otherwise it could perhaps be an area that has been bled into and appears very dark or maroon.

– *When an erythematous lesion is blanchable, what does that tell us about a diagnosis?*

It is not terribly informative. There is not much to be gained from pushing on lesions to see if they blanch. It is only helpful in trying to distinguish a vasculitis. If an area of vasculitis is pressed, which is referred to as diascopy, the area will not blanch because the blood is outside of the vessel. Any other erythematous lesion will blanch because there is still blood in the vessel.

– *Why do some people develop multiple abscesses? What else can be done to prevent abscesses from recurring?*

While *Staphylococcus epidermidis* is a normal skin colonizer, *Staphylococcus aureus* is not considered a normal component of skin flora and is treated as pathogenic. Streptococci are rarely seen on normal skin and can also cause skin infections. *S. aureus* and *Streptococcus* species can colonize the groin, axilla, and perianal area, and provide a source for future autoinfection. One of these areas may be cultured by rubbing the culture swab inside the nares or along the skin surface of the axilla, groin, or peri-anal area. If the cultures are positive, mupirocin should be applied to the inside of the nose, axilla, groin, and/or perianal area (depending on the areas cultured) two times daily for 5 days to help prevent recurrence. Bleach baths may be done once or twice weekly, where ½ cup of bleach is dissolved into a full bathtub, which can drop bacterial colonization rates. Whole-body washing with chlorhexidine can also be used, in combination with nasal mupirocin, to eradicate MRSA skin colonization.

– *Is there any recommendation for wound care of an open lesion other than treating with bactroban?*

A topical antimicrobial is sufficient, but wound wraps can help soothe pain and managing exudate from the wound. Xeroform and colloidal dressings are useful for open wounds.

References

1. McNamara DR, Tleyjeh IM, Berbari EF, Lahr BD, Martinez JW, Mirzoyev SA, Baddour LM. Incidence of lower-extremity cellulitis: a population-based study in Olmsted County, Minnesota. Mayo Clin Proc. 2007;82(7):817–21.
2. Dalal A, Eskin-Shwartz M, Mimouni D, Ray S, Days W, Hodak E, Leibovici L, Paul M. Interventions for the prevention of recurrent erysipelas and cellulitis (Protocol). Cochrane Database Syst Rev. 2012;4, CD009758.
3. McNamara DR, Tleyjeh IM, Berbari EF, Lahr BD, Martinez JW, Mirzoyev SA, Baddour LM. A predictive model of recurrent lower extremity cellulitis in a population-based cohort. Arch Intern Med. 2007;167(7):709–15.
4. Swartz MN. Cellulitis. N Engl J Med. 2004;350(9):904–12.
5. Lipworth AD, Saavedra AP, Weinberg AN, Johnson R. Chapter 178. Non-necrotizing infections of the dermis and subcutaneous fat: cellulitis and erysipelas. In: Goldsmith LA, Katz SI, Gilchrest BA, Paller AS, Leffell DJ, Wolff K, editors. Fitzpatrick's dermatology in general medicine. 8th ed. New York: McGraw-Hill; 2012.
6. Kilburn SA, Featherstone P, Higgins B, Brindle R. Interventions for cellulitis and erysipelas. Cochrane Database Syst Rev. 2010;6, CD004299.
7. Stevens DL, Bisno AL, Chambers HF, Dellinger EP, Goldstein EJ, Gorbach SL, Hirschmann JV, Kaplan SL, Montoya JG, Wade JC. Practice guidelines for the diagnosis and management of skin and soft tissue infections: 2014 update by the Infectious Diseases Society of America. Clin Infect Dis. 2014;59(2):e10–52.
8. Montalván Miró E, Sánchez NP. Cutaneous manifestations of infectious diseases. In: Sanchez NP, editor. Atlas of dermatology in internal medicine. New York: Springer; 2012.
9. Chlebicki MP, Oh CC. Recurrent cellulitis: risk factors, etiology, pathogenesis and treatment. Curr Infect Dis Rep. 2014;16(9):422.

Part IV
Nails

Chapter 18
Onychomycosis

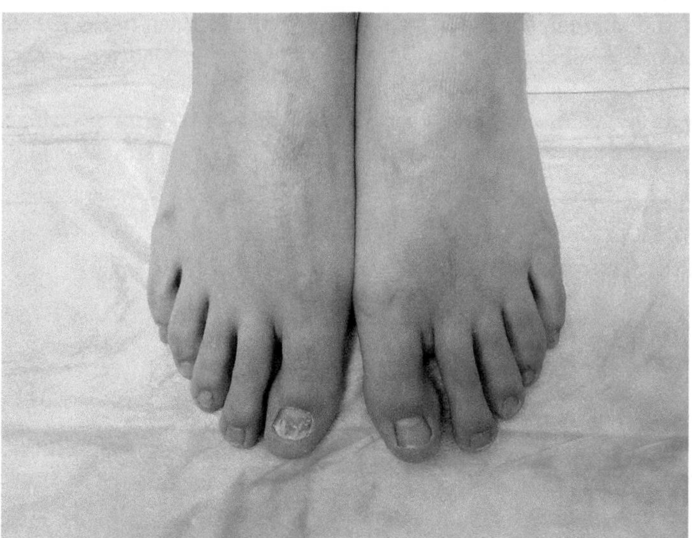

Fig. 18.1 Note not all toenails are typically affected

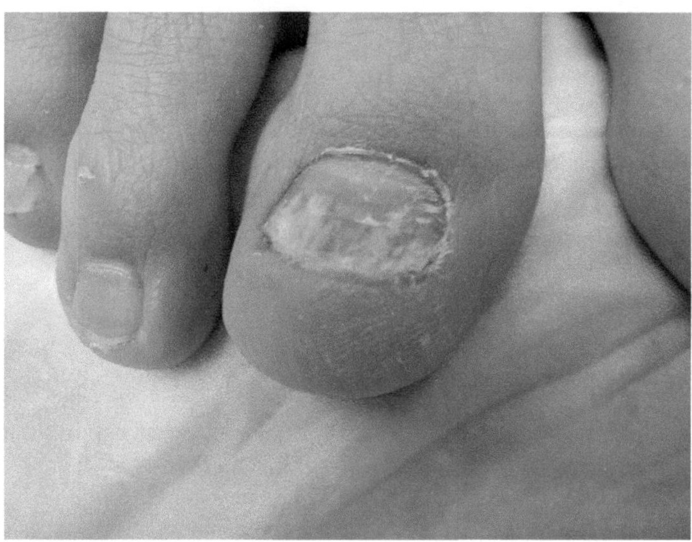

Fig. 18.2 Thickened nails with subungual debris, discoloration, and dystrophic nail plate

D. Reich et al., *Top 50 Dermatology Case Studies for Primary Care*,
DOI 10.1007/978-3-319-18627-6_18

Primary Care Visit Report

A 27-year-old female with no past medical history presented with a yellow, layered, scaly big toe toenail. Her toenail had been like that for almost 10 years; however, she had never treated it.

Vitals were normal. On exam, the right foot hallux toenail presented with thickening, scaling, peeling and yellow discoloration. The second toe of her left foot featured peeling of the distal skin of the toe.

This was treated as onychomycosis. A blood test for baseline liver function was ordered, and the patient was started on a 12-week course of oral terbinafine.

Discussion from Dermatology Clinic

Differential Dx

- Onychomycosis
- Psoriasis
- Lichen planus
- Trauma
- Onychogryphosis
- Subungual wart

Favored Dx

Physical examination is consistent with onychomycosis, distal subungual type. The peeling skin indicates underlying tinea pedis, which should also be treated.

Overview

Onychomycosis is a fungal infection of the nail by dermatophytes, yeasts, and non-dermatophyte molds. It is a common condition that affects 10–12 % of the population in the USA [1]. Incidence can be up to 25 % in some countries [2]. Prevalence increases with age, to affect up to 50 % of people above the age of 70, and it is increasing overall across all age groups [2–4]. Onychomycosis is often preceded by untreated tinea pedis which then spreads to the nail bed. Onychomycosis affects toenails more than fingernails, and tinea pedis accompanies onychomycosis in 30 % of cases [3]. Other risk factors are diabetes, immunocompromised state such as HIV, trauma, and poor peripheral circulation [3, 5].

The majority of onychomycosis cases are caused by the dermatophytes *Trichophyton rubrum*, *T. interdigitale*, and *T. mentagrophytes* [3–5]. The yeast *Candida albicans* is present in some fingernail onychomycosis, especially in cases of chronic paronychia. Immunocompromised status is a risk factor for developing candidal onychomycosis [6]. *Candida* is not thought to play a role in toenail onychomycosis. *Acremonium*, *Aspergillus*, *Fusarium*, and *Scopulariopsis* are nondermatophyte mold species that have been associated with fungal infection of the nail in rare instances.

Presentation

There are three clinically distinct subtypes of onychomycosis: distal subungual onychomycosis (DSO), proximal subungual onychomycosis (PSO), and white superficial onychomycosis (WSO). These have a clinically similar appearance, and are distinguished by the anatomical location of colonization. DSO affects the distal edge of the nail, PSO affects the proximal nail fold, and WSO results from direct invasion of the dorsal surface of the nail plate. DSO is the most common subtype overall, and PSO is more common in immunocompromised persons. PSO mostly involves *T. rubrum* and may be considered a sign of HIV [4].

Onychomycosis presents as thickened, opaque nail(s) with white, yellow, brown, or black discoloration. The nail(s) can feature shedding, onycholysis (separation of the nail from the nail bed), and subungual hyperkeratosis, marked by a chalk-like material that builds up under the nail [5]. All feature nail thickening, although WSO may not initially as the area beneath the surface of the nail may not yet be colonized [3]. WSO presents with superficial white spots on the nail plate. Fifty percent of cases of nail dystrophy have an underlying fungal etiology [3].

Workup

The diagnosis of onychomycosis should be confirmed by laboratory test prior to initiating oral treatment. Periodic-acid-Schiff (PAS) staining of a nail clipping is preferred as it is the most sensitive test for onychomycosis [7–9]. For this test, the affected nail is clipped just distal to its attachment to the nail bed, and the clipped nail along with its attached subungual debris are sent in 10 % formalin to the lab. A culture of the nail plate and subungual debris may be taken; however, it takes 3–6 weeks to obtain results [7]. If a culture is negative but the clinical suspicion is high, it should be repeated as culture results are associated with a high proportion of false negatives [8, 9].

A KOH test may be performed; however, it cannot identify the fungal species nor differentiate between dermatophyte, yeast, and mold infections. The subungual debris from the affected area is scraped onto a slide, KOH is added, and it is then viewed under the microscope. In cases of onychomycosis, KOH examination of subungual debris would reveal hyphae, pseudohyphae, or spores. KOH examinations and cultures are associated with more false negatives than PAS staining [6, 7]; however, KOH test has the advantage that it can be done rapidly in-office, at a low cost. A liver function test can be performed in advance of confirmed diagnosis in order to be able to potentially initiate oral antifungal treatment without having the patient return for this blood test.

Treatment

Management of onychomycosis should take into consideration the severity of infection, any associated tinea pedis, patient expectations vs. treatment efficacy, and potential for unwanted side effects. Tinea pedis should be treated to prevent recurrence of onychomycosis. In this case, the patient would benefit from the addition of a topical antifungal (such as ketoconazole 2 %). Treatment of tinea pedis is particularly prudent in diabetic patients who are at risk for developing cellulitis [3].

Topical therapy may be considered for patients with minimal nail involvement of the distal nail, in cases where onychomycosis spares the lunula and thus the nail matrix, or for whom systemic therapy is contraindicated. The cure rates for topical therapy are low [3–5]. Ciclopirox 8 % (Penlac) lacquer has been the topical agent of choice. It may achieve mycological cure (KOH and culture negative) in up to 36 % of cases, and clinical cure (clear nails) in 6–9 % of cases after daily application for 48 weeks [1, 3, 4, 10]. Regular debridement of the nails, by filing the surface and trimming the ends, prior to application may improve its efficacy [4, 10].

A newer treatment, the topical triazole antifungal Jublia (efinaconazole 10 % solution), was approved by the FDA in June 2014 for treatment of onychomycosis. Jublia has demonstrated a higher clinical cure rate of 17 %, and a mycological cure rate of 54 % after 48 weeks of daily application to nails with mild to moderate disease [11]. The cure rate of topical antifungals is much lower than systemic treatment; however, it eliminates the risk of toxicity and drug interactions.

Oral antifungals achieve mycological cure rates of up to 92 % after 12 weeks of treatment [1, 3, 10, 12]. Allylamines (e.g., terbinafine) and azoles are the classes of antifungals used to treat onychomycosis that has been confirmed by PAS staining. In most cases, where onychomycosis is caused by dermatophytes, terbinafine 250 mg daily for 12 or 16 weeks for toenails (6 weeks for fingernails) is more effective than itraconazole. For non-dermatophyte and yeast onychomycosis, itraconazole is recommended as it has a broader spectrum of coverage. Itraconazole is the drug of choice for fingernail onychomycosis, as fingernails are more likely to be infected by non-dermatophyte organisms, and cases known to be caused by *Candida*. Itraconazole may be given in pulsed (200 mg twice daily for 1 week every 4 weeks over a 12- or 16-week course) or continuous dose (200 mg daily for 3 months for adults) [1, 3, 13].

There is mixed evidence regarding improved efficacy of combination treatment with topical and oral antifungals [3, 10]. Recent investigations suggest there may be a role for Q-switched Nd:YAG 1064-nm laser treatment of onychomycosis [1, 7]. Patients who do not respond to conventional therapy may discuss this option with a dermatologist.

Follow-Up

Patients should be reevaluated after 1 month to assess improvement. It may take 3–12 months for nails to grow out and appear normal after mycological clearance is achieved. Severe infections affecting the nail matrix may cause scarring and permanent nail dystrophy [1]. After full clearance is achieved relapse rate is up to 30% [10]. This rate may be lowered slightly by using a 16-week treatment course. A liver function test should be performed at the end of treatment to ensure any possible elevation has been reversed.

Questions for the Dermatologist

- *When is it necessary to culture the nail? How is this done?*

Typically, clipping the nail and doing a PAS stain gives a good diagnostic yield. Nail cultures can be taken, although they delay diagnosis considerably. These are done by extracting subungual debris, using a curette.

- *Can you start treatment while awaiting the PAS or culture results?*

No, you should not initiate treatment without confirmed results. It is best practice to wait for the blood liver panel and confirmed onychomycosis report.

- *If the culture is negative but the clinical presentation is consistent with onychomycosis, is it appropriate to treat as such anyway?*

It is not appropriate to treat without diagnostic confirmation from PAS or culture. Adverse reactions are rare but they can be serious. Hepatotoxicity and drug interactions have been reported with oral antifungal use. If patients experience any effects on morbidity, for example liver inflammation, without diagnostic confirmation to support treatment, there could be medicolegal consequences for the prescribing physician.

- *What is the role of topical medications such as Penlac (ciclopirox lacquer) prior to initiating oral therapy?*

They do not serve much of a purpose. The cure rate of topical medications is very low. Their advantage is avoiding the rare systemic consequences of oral antifungals at the cost of efficacy.

– *Are there any herbal or home remedies that could help (e.g., tea tree or oregano oil)?*

Both of the listed examples are fungistatic, though not enough so to have an effect under the nail plate, where most hyphae reside. There has been some evidence that an over-the-counter mentholated ointment (Vicks VapoRub) can achieve partial cure and patient satisfaction, most likely by suffocating the offending aerobic fungi [3, 14].

– *If onychomycosis is improving but not fully resolved after 12 weeks of oral terbinafine, is it appropriate to treat for longer than 12 weeks?*

Most studies have been done for 12 weeks, with about an 80 % cure rate. At least one study was done that demonstrated further clearance after using terbinafine for 16 weeks (75.7 % vs. 80.8 %) [11]. Incremental improvement may be seen beyond 12 weeks; however, the patient would need to show significant improvement over those 3 months to warrant prescribing more. With little or no improvement after 3 months, the diagnosis would need to be questioned. Also, because the antimycotic medications bind to the keratin in the nail, improvement can continue for several more months even after the oral therapy has been stopped.

– *If you achieve mycological cure (negative culture or PAS after treatment) but not clinical cure (the nails are not clear after treatment), what happens next? Does the nail eventually grow out normally if the fungus is gone?*

Yes, in most cases, if mycological cure is achieved, the nail will grow out normally. This may take several months.

References

1. Lipner SR, Scher RK. Onychomycosis: current and investigational therapies. Cutis. 2014; 94(6):E21–4.
2. Hay RJ, Baran R. Why should we care if onychomycosis is truly onychomycosis? Br J Dermatol. 2015;172(2):316–7.
3. Schieke SM, Garg A. Chapter 188. Superficial fungal infection. In: Goldsmith LA, Katz SI, Gilchrest BA, Paller AS, Leffell DJ, Wolff K, editors. Fitzpatrick's dermatology in general medicine. 8th ed. New York: McGraw-Hill; 2012. p. 2277–97.
4. Rose AE. Therapeutic update: onychomycosis. J Drugs Dermatol. 2014;13(10):1173–5.
5. Ghannoum MA, Hajjeh RA, Scher R, Konnikov N, Gupta AK, Summerbell R, Sullivan S, Daniel R, Krusinski P, Fleckman P, Rich P, Odom R, Aly R, Pariser D, Zaiac M, Rebell G, Lesher J, Gerlach B, Ponce-De-Leon GF, Ghannoum A, Warner J, Isham N, Elewski B. A large-scale North American study of fungal isolates from nails: the frequency of onychomycosis, fungal distribution, and antifungal susceptibility patterns. J Am Acad Dermatol. 2000; 43(4):641–8.
6. Daniel III CR, Gupta AK, Daniel MP, Sullivan S. Candida infection of the nail: role of Candida as a primary or secondary pathogen. Int J Dermatol. 1998;37(12):904–7.
7. El-Tatawy RA, Abd El-Naby NM, El-Hawary EE, Talaat RA. A comparative clinical and mycological study of Nd-YAG laser versus topical terbinafine in the treatment of onychomycosis. J Dermatolog Treat. 2015;11:1–4.

8. Jung MY, Shim JH, Lee JH, Lee JH, Yang JM, Lee DY, Jang KT, Lee NY, Lee JH, Park JH, Park KK. Comparison of diagnostic methods for onychomycosis, and proposal of a diagnostic algorithm. Clin Exp Dermatol. 2015;40(5):479–84.
9. Weinberg JM, Koestenblatt EK, Tutrone WD, Tishler HR, Najarian L. Comparison of diagnostic methods in the evaluation of onychomycosis. J Am Acad Dermatol. 2003;49(2):193–7.
10. de Berker D. Clinical practice: fungal nail disease. N Engl J Med. 2009;360(20):2108–16.
11. Gupta AK, Simpson FC. Efinaconazole (Jublia) for the treatment of onychomycosis. Expert Rev Anti Infect Ther. 2014;12(7):743–52.
12. Gupta AK, Paquet M. Management of onychomycosis in Canada in 2014. J Cutan Med Surg. 2015;19(3):260–73.
13. Evans EG, Sigurgeirsson B. Double blind, randomised study of continuous terbinafine compared with intermittent itraconazole in treatment of toenail onychomycosis. The LION Study Group. BMJ. 1999;318(7190):1031–5.
14. Derby R, Rohal P, Jackson C, Beutler A, Olsen C. Novel treatment of onychomycosis using over-the-counter mentholated ointment: a clinical case series. J Am Board Fam Med. 2011; 24(1):69–74.

Chapter 19
Habit Tic Deformity

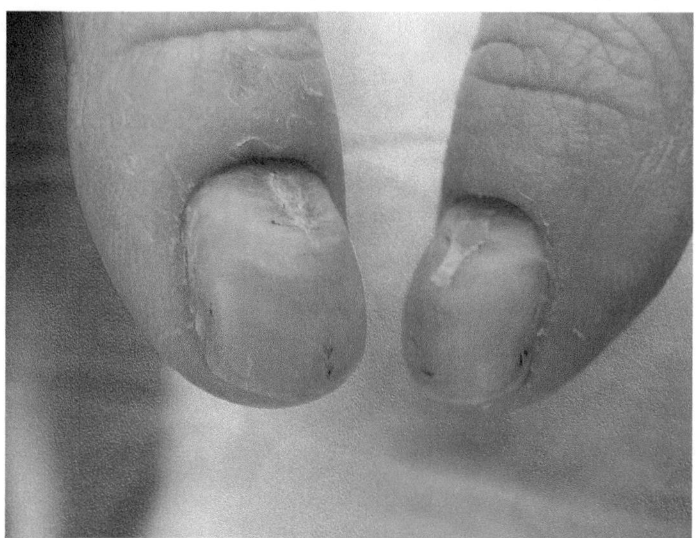

Fig. 19.1 Central canaliculi bilateral thumbs is pathopneumonic for this condition

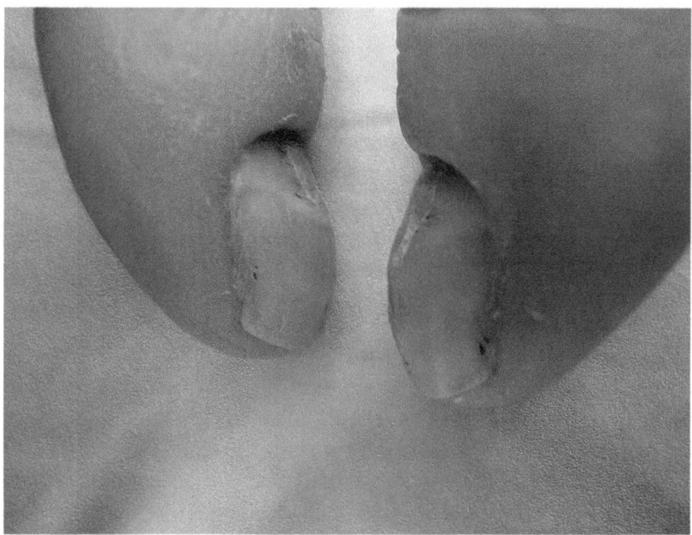

Fig. 19.2 Prominent clubbing results from local nail bed inflammation after repeated trauma

D. Reich et al., *Top 50 Dermatology Case Studies for Primary Care*,
DOI 10.1007/978-3-319-18627-6_19

Primary Care Visit Report

A 27-year-old female with past medical history of asthma, hypothyroidism, and depression presented with bilateral distortion of her thumbnails that started 2–3 years prior. She said that the base of her thumbnails started to "bubble," which then seemed to resolve on it's own until about 2 months prior. The thumbnail symptoms then began to recur, and were more severe again at the time of this visit, with parts of the thumbnails "tearing off."

Vitals were normal. On exam, the bases of her bilateral thumbnails featured deep grooves, some erosion, and dipping and spooning.

Fungal infection was considered, but the nails did not appear typical of onychomycosis. The patient was referred to dermatology, and photos were sent to a dermatologist who said it looked like there had been trauma to the nails. The patient had not mentioned anything about trauma when she presented, but when later asked whether she picked at her nails or cuticles, she described herself as a "voracious nail picker."

Discussion from Dermatology Clinic

Differential Dx

- Habit tic deformity
- Psoriasis
- Onychomycosis
- Median canalicular dystrophy

Favored Dx

Patient's picking habits indicate a habit tic deformity.

Overview

Habit tic deformity, also known as onychotillomania, is a traumatic injury of the nail caused by a nervous tic of pushing back, or picking the cuticle. It can also result from biting or picking the proximal nail fold. It is a common condition that presents mainly in adult patients. It is often an incidental finding rather than the primary purpose of an office visit [1]. The condition tends to affect the dominant thumb due to conscious or unconscious habitual picking by the ipsilateral index finger. It is thought to have an association with obsessive-compulsive disorder and anxiety [1–3].

Presentation

Habit tic deformity characteristically features a central nail depression, sometimes accompanied by multiple transverse parallel ridges. Thumbnails are most frequently affected, though any nail can be targeted by the tic [2]. In severe cases, the cuticles disappear, the proximal nail thickens and the lunulae, which are the crescent shaped white areas of the proximal fingernail, elongate. Patients may report the deformity has been present for several months or years.

Workup

Diagnosis is made on clinical examination and indication of picking or biting tic. If a causative injury is unclear, differentials should be investigated. To rule out psoriasis, elbows, knees, and family history should be investigated, and any nail pitting noted. Median nail dystrophy presents with a classic longitudinal split down the middle of the nail and does not feature cuticle changes. Paronychia would be accompanied by pain, swelling or redness. Lichen planus usually presents with nail splitting or atrophy. Onychomycosis would be ruled out with a nail biopsy.

Treatment

Habit-tic nail deformity has not received much attention in the literature. There is consensus that cessation of external trauma allows for normalization of the nail plate [1, 2]. As such, the target of treatment is the cessation of picking behavior. This can be achieved with physical barriers such as taping the nails to preventing picking. Patients may have objections to the cosmetic appearance of taped fingernails, resulting in low compliance [1].

The alternative approach to treatment would be targeting the underlying anxiety disorder. Serotonin reuptake inhibitors such as fluoxetine have been effective in treating habit-tic nail deformity [1–3]. Patients with underlying psychological concerns may be referred to a psychiatrist.

Follow-Up

Patients should be reevaluated after 3 or 4 weeks of therapy for improvement. If patients report changes in picking habits, normalization of the nail plate should be noted as it grows out. If deformity persists after behavioral modification, an alternative diagnosis should be considered.

Questions for the Dermatologist

- *How can the patient be helped to stop picking at her cuticles?*

Behavioral modification is one of the more challenging aspects of treatment that we come across in dermatology. Our role is to provide insight into a cause, but ultimately more assistance may be needed. Habit tic deformity is associated with obsessive-compulsive disorder, and psychiatrists are better suited to treat patients who would benefit from behavioral interventions or SSRI treatment.

- *Will the nails grow back normally if the picking stops?*

Yes, nails grow back normally once mechanical injury stops.

References

1. Ring DS. Inexpensive solution for habit-tic deformity. Arch Dermatol. 2010;146(11):1222–3.
2. Perrin AJ, Lam JM. Habit-tic deformity. CMAJ. 2014;186(5):371.
3. Vittorio CC, Phillips KA. Treatment of habit-tic deformity with fluoxetine. Arch Dermatol. 1997;133(10):1203–4.

Chapter 20
Subungual Hematoma

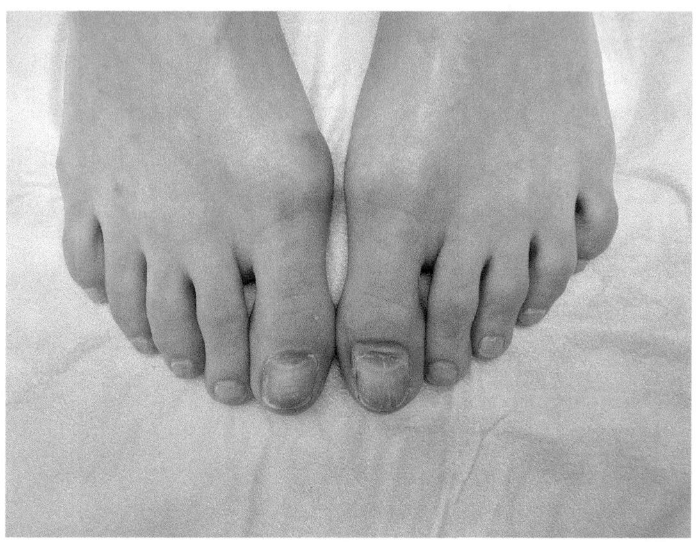

Fig. 20.1 Dusky maroon subungual color to the proximal nail bed bilaterally

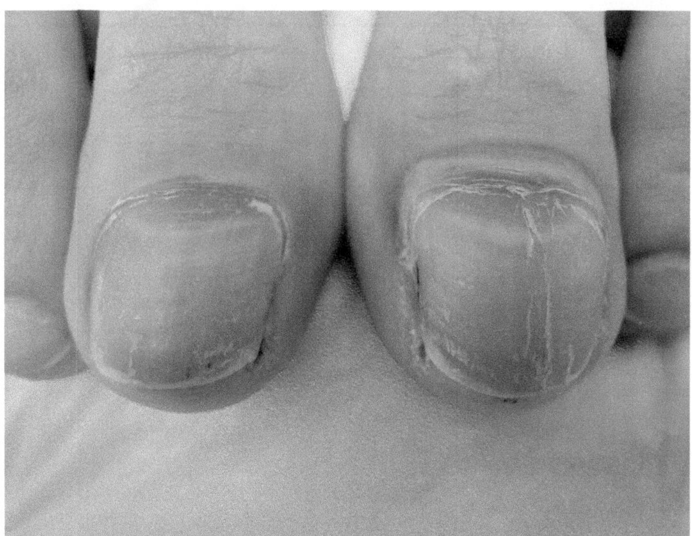

Fig. 20.2 Trephination of the hematoma is typically recommended for release of pressure and amelioration of pain if >50 % of the nail bed involved

D. Reich et al., *Top 50 Dermatology Case Studies for Primary Care*,
DOI 10.1007/978-3-319-18627-6_20

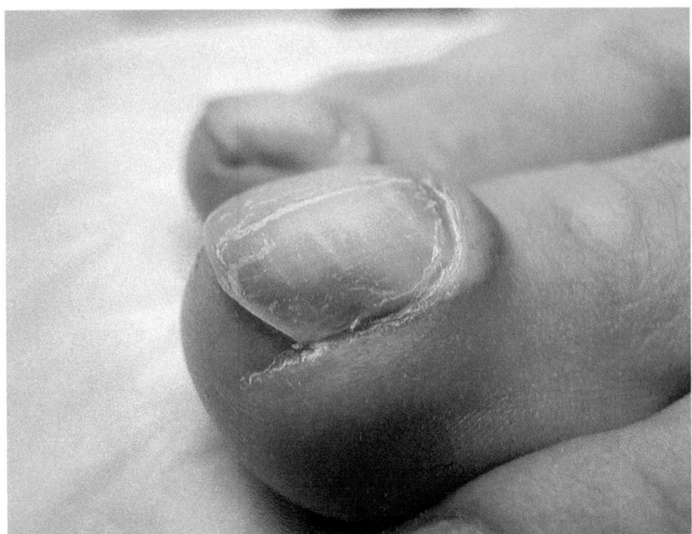

Fig. 20.3 Exsanguination extending to the lateral and proximal nail folds

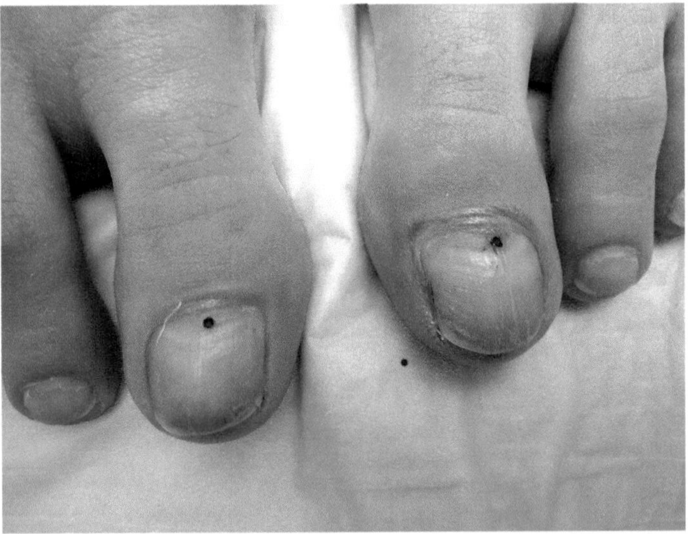

Fig. 20.4 Appearance just after trephination performed with heated paperclip

Primary Care Visit Report

A 33-year-old female with no past medical history presented with pain in both hallux toenails lasting 3 days. Three days prior, the patient had been walking in high heel shoes for 7–8 h. The morning after that, she noted that her bilateral hallux toenails were purple and red beneath the nails, and that the nails were elevated off the nail beds. There was no pain when she walked barefoot, but any pressure from socks or shoes irritated the area. The patient was a modern dancer who danced barefoot and was concerned because she "needed her toes." She was otherwise well.

Vitals were normal. On exam, bilateral hallux toenails with purple-hued nails were noted, with bilateral nails displaced superiorly, and bilateral cuticles appearing vesicular with clear fluid. Periungual and cuticle areas were non-tender. There was slight tenderness to palpation of bilateral nail beds with minimal pressure.

These were treated as subungual hematomas. The heated paperclip method was used to decompress the hematomas with a trephination procedure. The nail areas were cleaned with betadine, a paperclip was heated with a lighter until it was red hot, and then the heated end of the paperclip was placed onto each of the patient's hallux toenails in order to form small holes in them. As the heated paperclip was advanced, it melted the nail beneath it. When the paperclip was almost all the way through the nail, In order to avoid burning or puncturing the nail beds, an unheated 23-gauge needle was used to finish making the holes through the entire depth of the nails. With some light pressure applied to the nails, about 1 cc of serosanguinous fluid flowed from the hole in each toenail. The patient felt immediate relief. Bacitracin and gauze were applied to allow the fluid to continue to drain. The patient was also advised to soak her toes in warm water to allow for further drainage.

Differential Dx

- Subungual hematoma
- Melanoma
- Acral lentiginous melanoma
- Subungual nevus
- Onychomycosis

Favored Dx

The color and distribution of discoloration, patient history wearing tight-fitting shoes for an extended period of time, and successful alleviation of symptoms with trephination are consistent with subungual hematoma.

Overview

A subungual hematoma is a collection of blood and fluid under the fingernail or toenail, typically resulting from traumatic injury to the site. Subungual hematomas are a common problem in general dermatology [1]. They occur following crushing or traumatic injury to the nail. In toenails, they also occur in response to friction from tight-fitting shoes.

Subungual hematomas are usually straight forward to diagnose as there is a history of local trauma. Discoloration resembling that of a subungual hematoma but without the accompanying history of injury should be treated with particular care as melanoma is part of the differential. Subungual melanomas are often overlooked, and when they are finally identified they have progressed to later stages. They account for half of the melanomas in people with dark skin [2].

Presentation

Subungual hematomas present as dark blue, or reddish-blue discolorations beneath the nail plate, representing an accumulation of blood. This accumulation of blood is preceded by an acute injury, athletic activity, or friction from tight shoes. The nail plate may appear separated from the nail bed due to the subungual fluid. Patients may experience significant pain from pressure buildup under the nail.

Workup

Diagnosis of subungual hematoma is usually made on clinical examination. All 20 digits should be examined, and the size of discoloration noted. Patients should be asked about recent trauma, sports injuries, and when the discoloration appeared. An X-ray should be performed if there is a large area of discoloration with likely fracture. Dermoscopy of subungual hematoma should reveal red and blue globules distributed homogeneously in the nail plate [1, 3]. In contrast, if small (0.1 mm) granules of melanin are observed under dermoscopy, they may indicate instead the presence of a melanocytic (e.g., freckle, benign or dysplastic mole) lesion [1]. Dystrophy, destruction, and absence of the nail plate are signs of neoplasia [1]. If there is suspicion of melanoma, patients should be referred to dermatology to have a nail avulsion and biopsy.

Treatment

Sungungual hematomas can usually be managed with trephination when there is no nail bed laceration suspected [1, 4, 5]. This provides immediate relief from the discomfort associated with pressure buildup. Trephination can be performed with a hot paper clip, a sterilized needle (e.g., 18-gauge), a trephination device, electrocautery, or CO_2 laser [1, 2, 4–6]. The sharp trephinating tool should be twisted between the thumb and forefinger at a 45° angle until a small amount of blood is released. The hematoma can be drained by applying gauze and a small amount of pressure. Nail bed lacerations, or treatment with CO_2 laser, should be referred to dermatology as the nail plate may need to be removed [4].

Follow-Up

After drainage of the hematoma, patients should monitor any remaining nail pigmentation to ensure it grows out distally as the nail grows, as any underlying neoplasm would not migrate. If pigmentation remains, patients should be instructed to return for follow-up evaluation. Patients may take analgesics (unless they are contraindicated), soak the affected digit in warm water, and wrap gauze tightly so that it applies a light pressure if they experience further discomfort.

Questions for the Dermatologist

– *Do nails fall off after sustaining subungual hematomas? If so, do they grow back normally? How long does that process take?*

If there is greater than 50 % nail bed involvement, nails are likely to fall off on their own. It may take up to 3 months, but they do eventually grow back normally.

– *During nail regrowth is there anything particular to look out for, e.g., ingrown toenails?*

There is nothing in particular to worry about. If there were no problems with ingrown toenails previously, there is no reason to suspect the direction of growth will be compromised.

– *If there is damage to the nail bed, is there any additional treatment?*

Damage to the nail matrix is of greater concern. Damage to the nail matrix will likely result in dystrophic regrowth. It is relatively difficult to damage the nail matrix as it is located under the proximal nail fold; however, great care should be taken when trephinating the proximal nail as it is adjacent to the matrix.

– *Is it preferable to remove the entire nail following a hematoma, or is it better to drain it? Does the nail act as protection while it is attached, even if it will eventually fall off?*

It is not necessary to remove the entire nail. If there is greater than 50 % involvement of the nail bed, the nail should be trephinated and drained. This is because of pain associated with removing the entire nail rather than any protective function. If there is less than 50% involvement of the nail bed, it can be monitored and allowed to grow out naturally.

References

1. Braun RP, Baran R, Le Gal FA, Dalle S, Ronger S, Pandolfi R, Gaide O, French LE, Laugier P, Saurat JH, Marghoob AA, Thomas L. Diagnosis and management of nail pigmentations. J Am Acad Dermatol. 2007;56(5):835–47.
2. Tully AS, Trayes KP, Studdiford JS. Evaluation of nail abnormalities. Am Fam Physician. 2012;85(8):779–87.
3. Huang YH, Ohara K. Medical pearl: subungual hematoma: a simple and quick method for diagnosis. J Am Acad Dermatol. 2006;54(5):877–8.
4. Patel L. Management of simple nail bed lacerations and subungual hematomas in the emergency department. Pediatr Emerg Care. 2014;30(10):742–5.
5. Tzeng YS. Use of an 18-gauge needle to evacuate subungual hematomas. J Emerg Med. 2013;44(1):196–7.
6. Salter SA, Ciocon DH, Gowrishankar TR, Kimball AB. Controlled nail trephination for subungual hematoma. Am J Emerg Med. 2006;24(7):875–7.

Part V
Trunk

Chapter 21
Tinea Versicolor

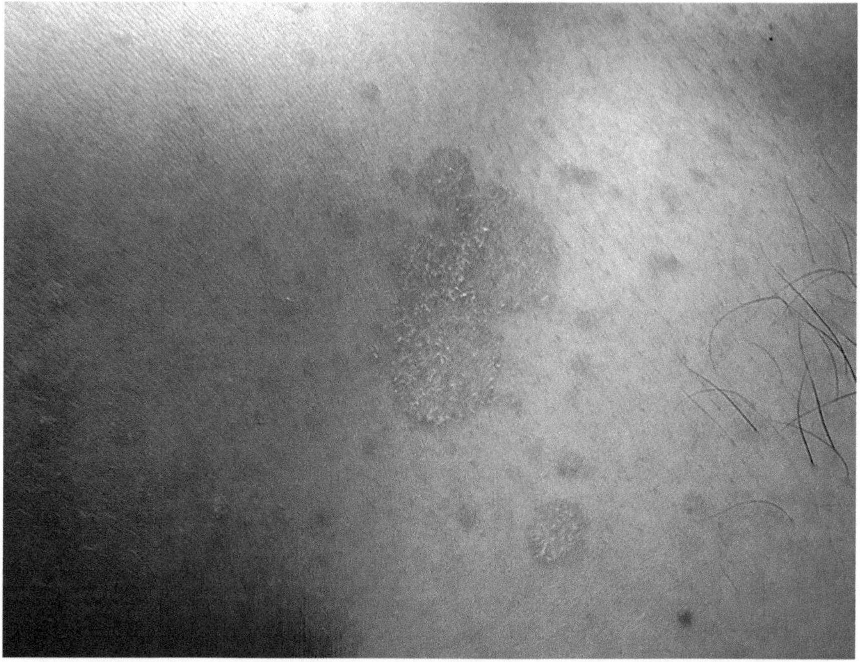

Fig. 21.1 Thin pink or brown plaques with fine scale may be coalescent or occasionally guttate (drop-shaped)

D. Reich et al., *Top 50 Dermatology Case Studies for Primary Care*,
DOI 10.1007/978-3-319-18627-6_21

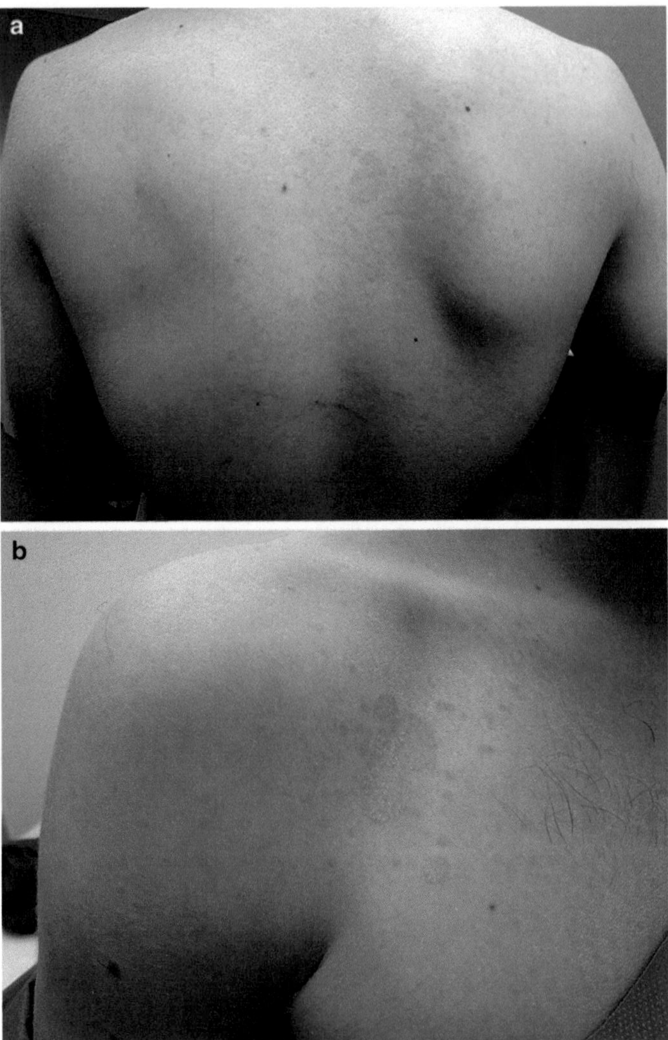

Fig. 21.2 (**a** and **b**) Chest and back are most commonly affected

Primary Care Visit Report

A 24-year-old male with no prior medical history presented with a rash on his chest, shoulders and back. The rash started in two spots on his left shoulder about 8 months prior. About 1 week prior to the visit, it spread to his chest. He did not report pruritus. He had not applied anything to the rash yet.

Vitals were normal. On exam, on the patient's chest, back, and flank, there were multiple scattered erythematous macular and papular lesions with irregular shapes and varied sizes. These lesions had well-delineated borders with mild central scale.

This was treated as tinea corporis based on the well-circumscribed lesions with central scale. The patient was prescribed 2 % ketoconazole cream once daily for 14 days.

Discussion from Dermatology Clinic

Differential Dx

- Tinea versicolor
- Tinea corporis
- Pityriasis rosea
- Confluent and reticulated papillomatosis
- Early stages of mycosis fungoides, a type of T-cell lymphoma

Favored Dx

Considering the patient's age, persistence of the rash, location of macules, and minimal pruritus, the favored diagnosis, as reclassified by dermatology, is tinea versicolor. Tinea versicolor is distinct from tinea corporis, and differs from all other tinea diseases (e.g., tinea pedis, tinea capitis) in that it is not a dermatophyte infection. However, they are treated in similar manners, with topical and oral antifungals, so in this case the 2 % ketoconazole would have been the appropriate treatment anyhow.

Overview

Tinea versicolor, also called pityriasis versicolor, is a benign superficial fungal infection characterized by scaly, hyperpigmented or hypopigmented lesions commonly found on the back, chest, and neck. Tinea versicolor is caused by an overgrowth of the lipophilic *Malassezia* yeast, which is a component of the natural skin flora.

Tinea versicolor is a common condition, most prevalent in tropical and sub-tropical climates, although seen in temperate climates as well. It can be recurrent, and may be seen waning in winter months and returning during the summertime.

Tinea versicolor is more commonly seen in males [1] and tends to occur during young adulthood [2]. It is not contagious, rather the yeast overgrows when favorable conditions are met. Exogenous factors contributing to its development include high heat and high humidity. Internal factors that favor this fungal overgrowth are greasy skin, excessive sweating, hereditary factors, corticosteroid treatment, and immunodeficiency [3]. To that end, people who exercise frequently or work physical jobs may be at higher risk of developing tinea versicolor.

Presentation

Tinea versicolor is typically found on the trunk, neck, and upper arms. Although it may not always be the case, tinea versicolor presents mainly as a hypopigmented rash on darker skin [1], and a hyperpigmented brown or red rash on lighter Caucasian skin. The lesions generally feature a fine scale and begin as round or oval macules or papules (if scaly), and may grow and coalesce to form larger patches or plaques. Some patients may present complaining of mild pruritus, but for most the condition is asymptomatic [2].

Workup

In most cases, tinea versicolor can be visually diagnosed according to the location and shape of the lesions [4]. If further confirmation is needed, sites may be examined under a Wood's lamp, which causes yellowish green fluorescence in about a third of cases. Gently scraping an active lesion using a scalpel or edge of a glass slide should generate a fine scale.

KOH test would reveal hyphae and spores. The scale scrapings should be placed on a glass slide and a small drop of 10 % KOH added before viewing under a microscope. Fungal cultures would not be beneficial as normal skin would also indicate presence of the yeast.

Treatment

Tinea versicolor may be treated with topical or systemic antifungals. Given the potential hepatotoxicity, drug interactions, and unwanted side effects such as GI problems and nausea, oral antifungals should be reserved for severe cases where the rash is resistant to topical therapy, recurrent, or covers a large surface area of the body.

The most effective topical treatments for eradicating tinea versicolor are imidazole creams. These would include ketoconazole, bifonazole, miconazole, and econazole [5]. They may be applied once or twice daily for 1–4 weeks, and data suggest higher concentrations of active ingredients and longer courses of therapy are most effective [5]. The author's practice typically uses topical 2 % ketoconazole twice daily for 2 weeks. Imidazole creams may be used in conjunction with a zinc pyrithione (e.g., Selsun Blue), selenium sulfide or sulfur salicylic acid shampoo [5], which can be used as a body wash daily for 1–4 weeks. It should be applied to the affected area for 5–10 min, then washed off.

In severe cases, systemic antifungals can be used. There are no established dosing guidelines to treat tinea versicolor orally; however, a single 400 mg dose of fluconazole [3], or alternatively two treatments of a 300 mg dose of fluconazole spaced 1 week apart effectively treat the condition [6]. The authors use 150 mg once daily for 5 days.

Follow-Up

After successful treatment, hypopigmetation or hyperpigmentation may persist for months; however, inactive macules will lack scale [5]. Tinea versicolor may require long-term prevention therapy as there is a likelihood of recurrence. The rash can recur in as many as 60 % of cases during the first year and 80 % during the second year [5]. Prophylactic therapies have not been well studied [7]; however, use of itraconazole 200 mg taken twice in 1 day, once monthly for 6 months, demonstrated efficacy [8] in preventing relapses. Patients may also use ketoconazole 2 % shampoo as a body wash on affected sites once weekly.

Questions for the Dermatologist

– *Is there a difference between tinea versicolor and tinea corporis?*

Yes, there is. Tinea versicolor is caused by an overgrowth of yeast that normally lives on the skin, while tinea corporis is a dermatophyte infection. Tinea versicolor is characterized by white, brown, or pink macules with fine scale. The macules tend to coalesce and cover large surfaces on the back and chest. The lesions of tinea corporis are solitary, often annular lesions, they have more distinct borders and they feature central clearing. Central clearing refers to a patch of normal skin surrounded by an abnormal border. Central clearing is characteristic of fungal infections but not tinea versicolor. The two conditions respond to similar treatments of topical antifungals; however, tinea versicolor tends to be recurrent and requires preventative therapy.

– *What could I miss if I misdiagnose?*

Confluent and reticulated papillomatosis (CARP) could be easily missed. CARP can look and feel very similar to tinea versicolor. It is typically a little bit darker and less scaly. It would lack the seasonal variation that is seen with tinea versicolor. CARP tends to be more hyperkeratotic and, in most cases, would not respond to antifungal treatment. CARP usually responds to oral antibiotics and topical retinoids.

– *How can I instruct patients to eradicate it, and do I need to?*

Tinea versicolor is harmless; however, patients may be bothered by its appearance or by associated pruritus. Many patients have recurrent tinea versicolor in warmer months, so it is not possible to eradicate completely. After the active infection is cleared (no longer generates scale), antifungal cream can be used prophylactically twice per month on the previous site of infection to keep it from returning. They can also use ketoconazole shampoo as a body wash once per week. Initial treatment with oral antifungals instead of topicals has a better duration of clearance.

– *How do I know when to treat with oral vs. topical medications?*

Tinea versicolor can be treated with topical medications alone. Patients who are treated with both oral and topical antifungals achieve longer-lasting clearance. Potential side effects of oral antifungals such as GI problems, nausea, or rarely hepatotoxicity, should be discussed with the patients.

– *Is terbinafine effective against TV? Or terbinafine can only be used for the TC and other true tinea/dermatophyte infections?*

Terbinafine is not effective against yeast infections, and tinea versicolor is an overgrowth of *Malassezia* yeast. Terbinafine is active against dermatophytes, and it is used to treat dermatophyte infections such as tinea corporis.

– *What is your go-to topical antifungal? Oral?*

Our practice uses medications in the -azole family for both. We prescribe topical 2 % ketoconazole twice daily for 2 weeks. Azoles are the oral medications of choice as they are less expensive and readily available.

– *Should I tell patients to continue treatment for a few days after the rash resolves? How long after they start the cream will they see resolution? How long should they use the cream before I say they are failing treatment?*

Patients should use the topical antifungal for another 2 days after there is no visible scaling. There is no harm in extending the treatment course. They should see a decrease in scale within a week of initiating treatment. If there is significant scale after 2 weeks, consider an alternate diagnosis, or initiating oral antifungals. After scales disappear, it could be months before pigmentation returns to normal.

References

1. Kallini JR, Riaz F, Khachemoune A. Tinea versicolor in dark-skinned individuals. Int J Dermatol. 2014;53(2):137–41.
2. Gupta AK, Ryder JE, Nicol K, Cooper EA. Superficial fungal infections: an update on pityriasis versicolor, seborrheic dermatitis, tinea capitis, and onychomycosis. Clin Dermatol. 2003; 21(5):417–25.
3. Faergemann J. Management of seborrheic dermatitis and pityriasis versicolor. Am J Clin Dermatol. 2000;1(2):75–80.
4. Kane KS, Ryder JB, Johnson RA, Baden HP, Stratigos A. Chapter 21. Cutaneous fungal infections. In: Color atlas & synopsis of pediatric dermatology. New York: McGraw-Hill; 2002. p. 528.
5. Hu SW, Bigby M. Pityriasis versicolor: a systematic review of interventions. Arch Dermatol. 2010;146(10):1132–40.
6. Yazdanpanah MJ, Azizi H, Suizi B. Comparison between fluconazole and ketoconazole effectivity in the treatment of pityriasis versicolor. Mycoses. 2007;50(4):311–3.
7. Gaitanis G, Magiatis P, Hantschke M, Bassukas ID, Velegraki A. The Malassezia genus in skin and systemic diseases. Clin Microbiol Rev. 2012;25(1):113–9.
8. Faergemann J, Gupta AK, Al Mofadi A, Abanami A, Abu Shareaah A, Marynissen G. Efficacy of itraconazole in the prophylactic treatment of pityriasis (tinea) versicolor. Arch Dermatol. 2002;138(1):69–73.

Chapter 22
Breast Cancer

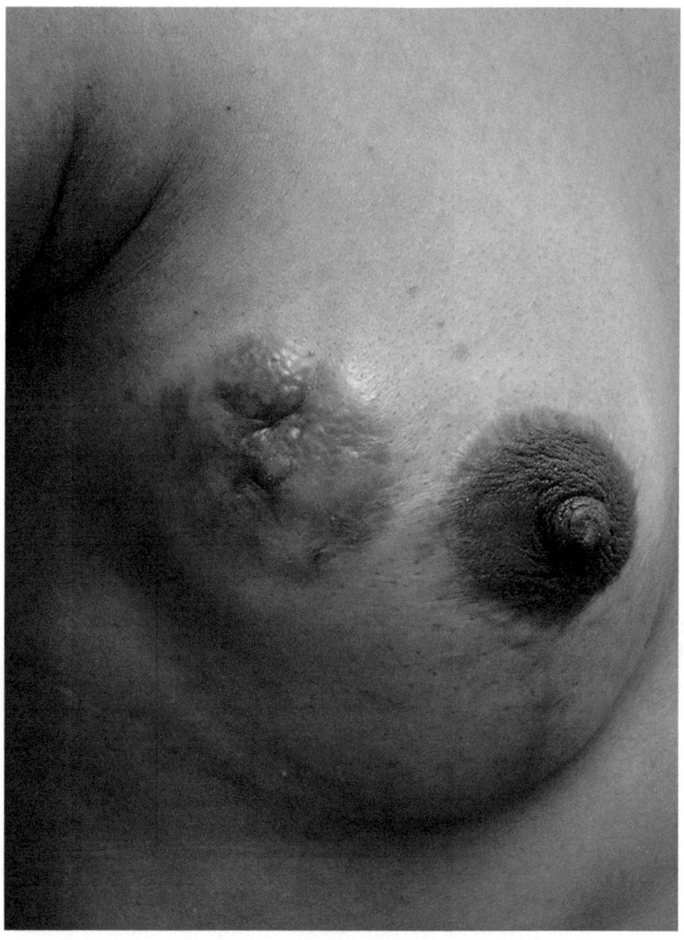

Fig. 22.1 Indurated, fixed, non-tender mamillated plaque at right outer breast

D. Reich et al., *Top 50 Dermatology Case Studies for Primary Care*,
DOI 10.1007/978-3-319-18627-6_22

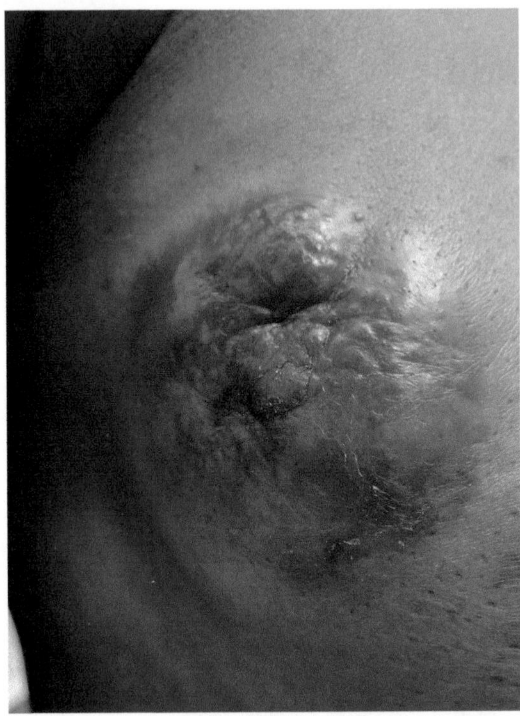

Fig. 22.2 Rapid growth over months is a concerning feature of any lesion

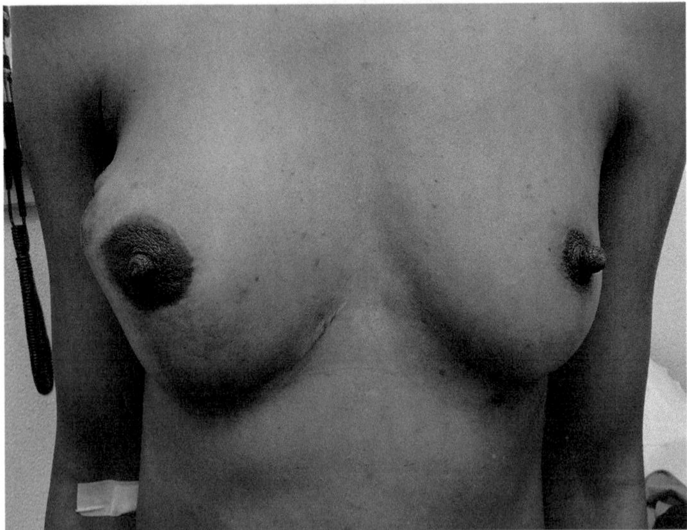

Fig. 22.3 Tissue retraction prominent at right breast

Primary Care Visit Report

A 37-year-old female with past medical history of Vitamin D deficiency presented for an annual physical exam. She was concerned about a lump in her right breast that she had first noticed about 2 months prior. She noted that the skin overlying the lump had become discolored over the past 2 months, it was sometimes tender, and the lump had been growing in size. She had no family history of breast cancer. At age 16, she had a benign breast lump in the same breast. The lump was removed at that time and an implant was placed in her right breast. The implant was then removed 2 years later, at age 18. Her last mammogram 2 years prior was normal.

Vitals were normal. On exam, around 10:00 of her lateral right breast, there was a 7 cm × 7 cm indurated area, with a central 5 cm × 3 cm area of discoloration. The lesion was purple-colored and erythematous, with central puckering.

The breast mass and associated skin changes were highly suggestive of breast cancer. The patient was referred to a breast surgeon the following day for biopsy. The mass was found to be cancerous, and the patient eventually underwent chemotherapy, a right modified radical mastectomy, and radiation therapy.

Discussion from Dermatology Clinic

Differential Dx

- Intraductal papillary carcinoma
- Metastatic carcinoma
- Paget's disease

Favored Dx

The changes in size and texture of the breast point to an internal malignancy, and the skin changes seen most likely represent local invasion of the skin by breast cancer.

Overview

Skin changes are associated with a number of internal malignancies, which can manifest in a variety of ways. These include local invasion of the skin by an adjacent cancer, metastasis to the skin from a distal cancer, and changes that are suggestive of various familial cancer syndromes. The skin changes seen in this case represent local invasion by an underlying breast cancer.

Breast cancer is the second most diagnosed cancer in women, with approximately 182,000 new cases per year [1, 2]. The incidence of breast cancer increases with age; however, breast cancer in younger women is associated with poorer outcomes. This is especially true of young black women, who experience early-onset and more aggressive cancers [1]. Other risk factors for breast cancer include prior history of breast cancer, family history, early menarche, age over 30 years at first childbirth, obesity, ionizing radiation exposure, and high socioeconomic status [2].

Skin changes may be visible in up to 2/3 of breast cancers in women [3, 4]. It has been suggested that the type of underlying breast cancer may be associated with specific skin changes [5]. Hormone receptor-positive breast cancer may be more frequently associated with ulceration and mass formation. Erythematous skin lesions, skin thickening, and infiltration of surrounding soft tissue may occur more frequently in triple negative (not positive for estrogen, progesterone, or HER2 receptors) and HER2-positive breast cancers [5]. Skin changes such as skin thickening, puckering, erythema, discharge, and distortion may also be caused by benign breast tumors [6].

Cutaneous metastases from distal cancers occur in approximately 5 % of all cancers, and they are the first sign of malignancy in 7.8 % of cases [7]. Cancers that are most likely to metastasize to a site on the skin distant from the primary tumor are: breast, colon, and melanoma in women, and lung, colon, and melanoma in men.

Presentation

Common changes of the nipple that are associated with breast cancer include dimpling, puckering, inversion, and discharge. Sometimes the changes are elicited on manipulation of the breast. Cutaneous changes associated with the adjacent breast tissue are puckering, flaking, pruritus, erythema, ulceration, vascularized cysts, telangiectasias, discoloration, textural changes such as dimpling (referred to as "peau d'orange," meaning skin of an orange), swelling, and changes in size. Cutaneous invasion by breast cancer may often present with pain.

A variant of metastatic breast cancer is the erysipelas-like eruption that occurs due to intralymphatic spread of the primary carcinoma. It is known as carcinoma erysipeloides [7]. Carcinoma en cuirasse (a rare form of cutaneous metastasis) presents with sclerosis and leathery texture changes. It may also involve nodules and ulceration. It can be present for many years prior to systemic involvement [7]. Inflammatory breast cancer, which accounts for 1–5 % of breast cancers, presents with edema, erythema, rapid increase of breast size, tenderness, color changes, and nipple inversion [8].

Workup

Both breasts should be examined in the upright and supine position for lumps, symmetry, and skin changes. Patients with unilateral skin changes consistent with local invasion of the skin should be referred to a breast cancer specialist, or surgeon for definitive diagnosis by biopsy.

Treatment

The appropriate treatment regimen for breast cancer will be determined by a breast surgeon as well as by an oncologist depending on the type of breast cancer found [9].

Follow-Up

The breast surgeon and oncology team determine follow-up screening for breast cancer patients. They will require more frequent examinations and mammograms to detect any potential recurrences.

Questions for the Dermatologist

– *What skin changes would raise suspicion for breast cancer?*

The one I see in practice most often is retraction, where the underlying tumor pulls the overlying skin. This gives the breast a warped contour. Induration, a thickened epidermal plaque, is also a common change.

References

1. Ademuyiwa FO, Gao F, Hao L, Morgensztern D, Aft RL, Ma CX, Ellis MJ. US breast cancer mortality trends in young women according to race. Cancer. 2014. doi:10.1002/cncr.29178.
2. Apantaku LM. Breast cancer diagnosis and screening. Am Fam Physician. 2000;62(3):596–602.
3. Devitt JE. How breast cancer presents. Can Med Assoc J. 1983;129(1):43–7.
4. Mahoney LJ, Bird BL, Cooke GM, Ball DG. Early diagnosis of breast cancer: experience in a consultant breast clinic. Can Med Assoc J. 1977;116(10):1129–31.
5. Kong JH, Park YH, Kim JA, Kim JH, Yun J, Sun JM, Won YW, Lee S, Kim ST, Cho EY, Ahn JS, Im YH. Patterns of skin and soft tissue metastases from breast cancer according to subtypes: relationship between EGFR overexpression and skin manifestations. Oncology. 2011;81(1):55–62.
6. Miltenburg DM, Speights Jr VO. Benign breast disease. Obstet Gynecol Clin North Am. 2008;35(2):285–300.
7. DeWitt CA, Buescher LS, Stone SP. Chapter 153. Cutaneous manifestations of internal malignant disease: cutaneous paraneoplastic syndromes. In: Goldsmith LA, Katz SI, Gilchrest BA, Paller AS, Leffell DJ, Wolff K, editors. Fitzpatrick's dermatology in general medicine. 8th ed. New York: McGraw-Hill; 2012. Available from: http://accessmedicine.mhmedical.com.ezproxy.cul.columbia.edu/content.aspx?bookid=392&Sectionid=41138876. Accessed 25 Feb 2015.
8. National Cancer Institute. Inflammatory Breast Cancer [Internet]. 2015 [cited 26 February 2015]. Available from: http://www.cancer.gov/cancertopics/factsheet/Sites-Types/IBC
9. Cady B, Steele Jr GD, Morrow M, Gardner B, Smith BL, Lee NC, Lawson HW, Winchester DP. Evaluation of common breast problems: guidance for primary care providers. CA Cancer J Clin. 1998;48(1):49–63.

Chapter 23
Juxtaclavicular Beaded Lines

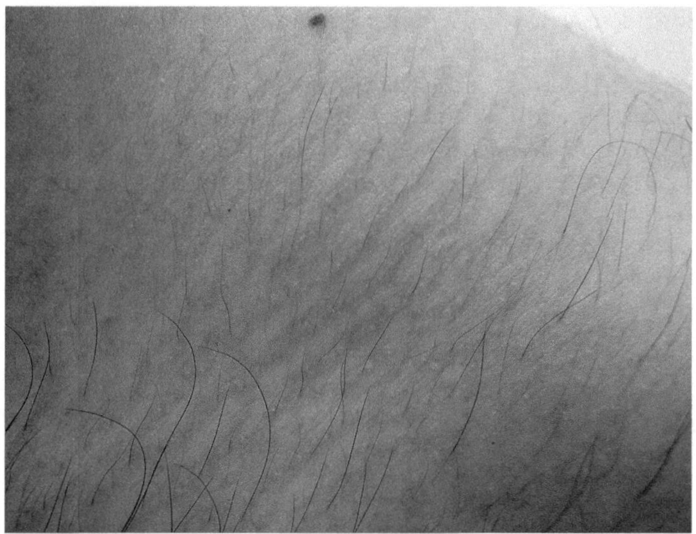

Fig. 23.1 Curvilinear pink or flesh-toned papules that follow Blashko Lines

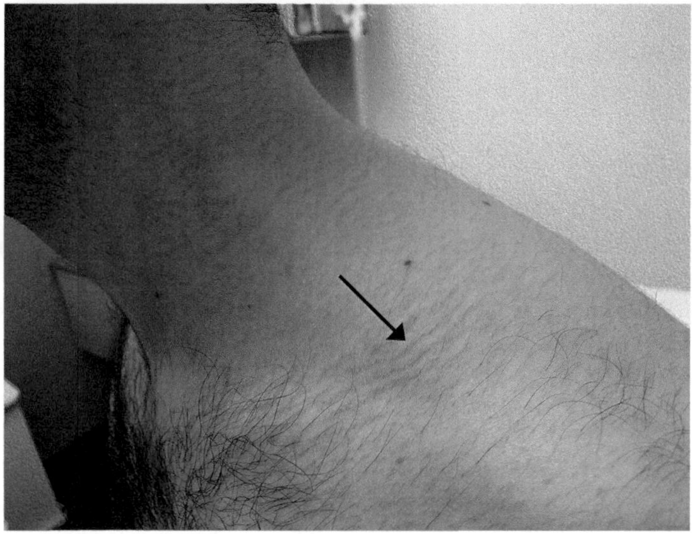

Fig. 23.2 This benign finding must be asymptomatic or look for another diagnosis

D. Reich et al., *Top 50 Dermatology Case Studies for Primary Care*,
DOI 10.1007/978-3-319-18627-6_23

Primary Care Visit Report

A 26-year-old male with no past medical history presented with "lines" around his neck that he had had for a few weeks. They were not itchy and he was otherwise feeling well.

Vital were normal. On exam, his bilateral lateral neck and supraclavicular area featured a very fine linear yellow papular rash with normal skin in between the linear lines of rash. There was no scale and no erythema.

Unsure what this was, I prescribed a trial of topical mometasone 0.1 % daily and asked the patient to follow up in 1 week.

One week later, there was no change in the rash. I switched the patient to topical clotrimazole 1 % twice daily.

Four weeks later, the patient reported no change in the rash. I advised the patient to try 40 % urea cream and/or to get a dermatology evaluation. The rash did not bother the patient, and he declined further treatment.

Discussion from Dermatology Clinic

Differential Dx

- Juxtaclavicular beaded lines
- Pseudoxanthoma elasticum
- Papular mucinosis
- Flat warts
- Molluscum contagiosum

Favored Dx

Juxtaclavicular beaded lines are favored in this case. The linear arrangement and yellow color of the papules are indicators. Additionally, treatment with topical steroid and antifungal had no effect, which weakens the case for an inflammatory, or a fungal condition.

Overview

Juxtaclavicular beaded lines (JCBL) are a rare form of sebaceous gland hyperplasia that occurs adjacent to the clavicle. The condition is characterized by small yellow papules arranged in parallel lines, resembling strands of beads.

JCBLs generally appear in the second to fifth decades of life, and they are more common among African Americans [1]. There is a slight female predominance [2]. Etiological factors linked to the condition include hormones, corticosteroid use, and eruptions resembling acne. JCBLs often appear during puberty when increased androgen production begins [2]. Long-term topical or systemic corticosteroid use has been associated with the lesions, as the steroids have an effect on androgen levels [2].

Presentation

JCBLs appear as a linear, papular eruption involving the neck and supraclavicular areas. They are usually asymptomatic. The papules are flesh-colored or slightly yellow, approximately 1–2 mm in size, and lack scale. A small, fine, light-colored (vellus) hair may be seen piercing through the papules.

Workup

JCBLs may be diagnosed visually, according to the appearance and location of the lesions. A 4-mm punch biopsy would confirm diagnosis. Histopathology would reveal sebaceous gland lobules that account for the dome-shaped epidermal papules. The overlying epidermis becomes slightly thinned while the adjacent epidermis can be hyperkeratotic and hyperplastic [2]. Tissue cut parallel to the rows of papules shows multiple pilosebaceous follicles that contain cellular debris [3].

Treatment

JCBLs are a benign condition considered to be a normal anatomical variant. No treatment is necessary, but patients may be bothered by the cosmetic appearance of JCBL. The options for treatment include electrodesiccation [4], oral and topical retinoid use [5, 6], and treatment with CO_2 lasers [6, 7].

Electrodesiccation, a method of surgical destruction using high frequency electric current, can remove individual lesions and CO_2 lasers can shrink them, but neither can control for recurrence. Maintenance doses of oral [5, 6] (e.g., 20 mg every other day, or 10 mg daily for 1 year) and topical [5] (e.g., 0.05 % daily) isotretinoin doses have been shown to prevent future recurrence. Topical isotretinoin alone may be effective in reducing the appearance of lesions.

Follow-Up

Follow-up for JCBLs depends on the approach to therapy. No follow-up is needed if patients are not bothered by the lesions. Electrodesiccation and CO_2 laser treatment would warrant a follow-up to ensure proper healing. Monthly follow-up is necessary if oral isotretinoin is prescribed, in order to monitor blood levels for cumulative dosage and potential systemic side effects. All courses of therapy should be periodically monitored for improvement and possible remission.

Questions for the Dermatologist

- *Are JCBL contagious, and do they spread from initial presentation?*

JCBL are not contagious. There is thought to be a genetic component to their development. They do not spread beyond the juxtaclavicular region, but more papules can develop over time.

- *Is there any danger in not treating them?*

There is no danger in leaving them untreated as they are benign; however, patients may be bothered by their appearance. Topical retinoids can be prescribed to reduce appearance, and hyfrecation, a type of electrosurgery, may be used to remove individual lesions. CO_2 lasers have also been successful in treating JCBL.

- *Do they go away on their own? If so, do they often recur?*

JCBL do not spontaneously go away. Patients are likely to get more papules as the condition develops.

- *Would there have been any utility in the patient trying urea cream, which I suggested after the steroid and anti-fungal treatments failed?*

Urea cream is a keratolytic, which would not really have an expected effect on JCBL. Topical retinoids would be more likely to have a mild shrinking effect on JCBL.

References

1. Eisen DB, Michael DJ. Sebaceous lesions and their associated syndromes: Part I. J Am Acad Dermatol. 2009;61(4):549–60.
2. Finan MC, Apgar JT. Juxta-clavicular beaded lines: a subepidermal proliferation of sebaceous gland elements. J Cutan Pathol. 1991;18(6):464–8.
3. Butterworth T, Johnson WC. Juxta-clavicular beaded lines. Arch Dermatol. 1974;110:891–3.
4. Bader RS, Scarborough DA. Surgical pearl: intralesional electrodesiccation of sebaceous hyperplasia. J Am Acad Dermatol. 2000;42(1 Pt 1):127–8.
5. Grimalt R, Ferrando J, Mascaro JM. Premature familiar sebaceous gland hyperplasia: successful response to oral isotretinoin in three patients. J Am Acad Dermatol. 1997;37(6):996–8.
6. Noh S, Shin JU, Jung JY, Lee JH. A case of sebaceous hyperplasia maintained on low-dose isotretinoin after carbon dioxide laser treatment. Int J Dermatol. 2014;53(3):e151.
7. Kim SK, Do JE, Kang HY, et al. Combination of topical 5-aminolevulinic acid-photodynamic therapy with carbon dioxide laser for sebaceous hyperplasia. J Am Acad Dermatol. 2007; 56(3):523–4.

Chapter 24
Folliculitis

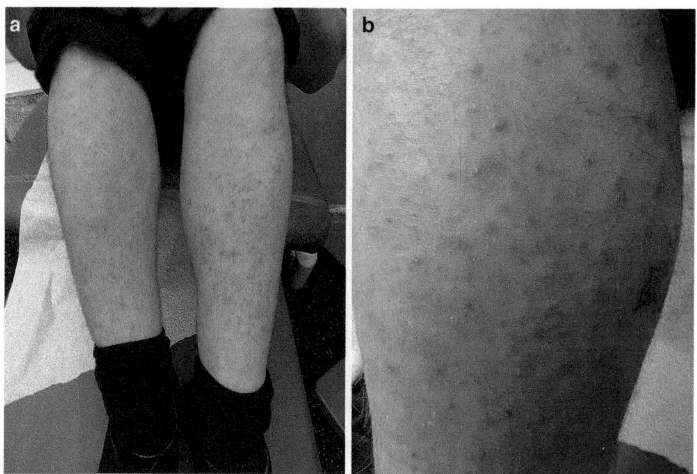

Fig. 24.1 (**a** and **b**) Pretibial legs with innumerable perifollicular papules and pustules

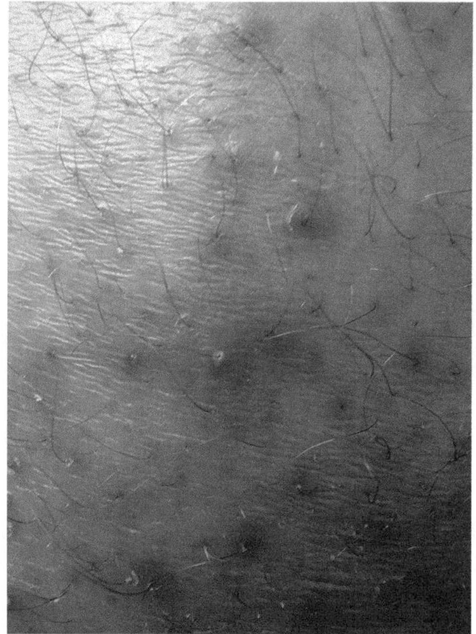

Fig. 24.2 Perifollicular pustules on erythematous base

D. Reich et al., *Top 50 Dermatology Case Studies for Primary Care*,
DOI 10.1007/978-3-319-18627-6_24

Primary Care Visit Report

A 33-year-old male with no past medical history presented with itchy bumps on his legs, torso and arms, present for over 1 year. He had seen a primary care doctor the prior year, where he was diagnosed with folliculitis and given 2 weeks of oral antibiotics (he could not recall which one). He said the treatment made the whiteheads go away but that the bumps remained. The patient reported improvement in cooler weather and almost complete resolution in winter. With humid weather, the rash returned. He noted the rash got worse immediately after showering. Over the past few weeks, he'd noticed that each morning he was waking up with more lesions on his legs. He ran, played tennis, and surfed 2–3 times per week. He had been using over-the-counter hydrocortisone 1 % cream with little effect.

Vitals were normal. On exam, there were multiple 4–5 mm erythematous papules, some with pustules, scattered diffusely over the bilateral anterior lower extremities, and less diffusely on the posterior lower extremities. There were scattered 4–5 mm erythematous papules on the lower forearms and abdomen as well.

This appeared to be folliculitis. Given the severity, duration, and failure to resolve on 2 weeks of oral antibiotics, the patient was referred to dermatology for further evaluation.

Discussion from Dermatology Clinic

Differential Dx

- Bacterial folliculitis
- Fungal folliculitis
- Pityrosporum folliculitis
- *Pseudomonas* folliculitis (AKA "hot tub" folliculitis)
- Eosinophilic folliculitis of HIV
- Acne
- Keratosis pilaris

Favored Dx

Erythematous papules and pustules that occur at the openings of hair follicles are consistent with common bacterial folliculitis. This particular patient's history, with no recent exposure to whirlpools or hot tubs and no predisposing conditions, and the appearance of his lesions also indicate common bacterial folliculitis.

Overview

Folliculitis describes a common inflammation of the pilosebaceous unit—which includes the hair shaft, hair follicle, sebaceous gland, and erector pili muscle. It can occur due to infection (bacterial, fungal, viral, parasitic), irritation, trauma, some medications, and certain diseases. Folliculitis is classified as superficial or deep depending on which parts of the hair follicle are affected. The most common type of folliculitis is superficial bacterial folliculitis caused by *Staphylococcus aureus* [1–3]. *S. epidermidis* and *Streptococcus* species have also been implicated [3].

There are several variants of folliculitis, each associated with different pathogens or predisposing conditions. Approximately 4% of patients on long-term antibiotic treatment for acne may develop peri-oral gram-negative folliculitis, frequently caused by *Pseudomonas aeruginosa* [1, 4]. *P. aeruginosa* is also involved in "hot tub" folliculitis [2, 4]. Other gram-negative bacteria involved in the pathogenesis of folliculitis are *Klebsiella, Proteus, Escherichia, Enterobacter*, and *Citrobacter* species [1, 4, 5]. Fungal folliculitis may be caused by dermatophytes (most frequently *Malassezia* and *T. rubrum*), pityrosporum yeasts, and *Candida* [4]. *Candida* species are implicated in folliculitis of immunocompromised people and heroin abusers [2, 3]. Herpes simplex virus and herpes zoster virus are two common causes of viral folliculitis.

Noninfectious causes of folliculitis may be due to trauma to, or occlusion of, the hair follicle. This can occur due to friction, from wearing tight clothing. Other risk factors for folliculitis are HIV (eosinophilic folliculitis), diabetes mellitus, and nutritional deficiency [1, 3]. Trauma and friction from facial shaving is a predisposing factor to pseudofolliculitis barbae, a sterile folliculitis, also called non-infectious folliculitis of the beard area [1].

Presentation

Superficial folliculitis presents as small, raised, erythematous papules and pustules that occur at the hair orifices. The lesions occur in clusters. Folliculitis is often accompanied by pruritus and a burning sensation. The most commonly affected areas are the face, scalp, upper back, axilla, thighs, and groin [2, 4]. Superficial folliculitis can advance to deep folliculitis. Deep folliculitis typically presents with pain. Lesions may appear as boils or furuncles, and can cause scarring.

Workup

Folliculitis is diagnosed on clinical examination. The history of how the rash developed may be helpful in determining the correct causative agent. A culture of exudate from a pustule should be performed to determine associated pathogens. "Hot tub" folliculitis may be diagnosed when there is a history of extensive hot tub use. Eosinophilic folliculitis of HIV may require a biopsy. Histopathology would reveal infiltration of the pilosebaceous unit by eosinophils and neutrophils.

Treatment

The treatment of folliculitis depends on its cause, anatomical location, and degree of severity. Topical medications are often sufficient to treat superficial folliculitis. Deep folliculitis and eosinophilic folliculitis are more difficult to treat, and warrant a referral to dermatology.

Superficial bacterial folliculitis may be treated with topical mupirocin (Bactroban), bacitracin, clindamycin, or erythromycin three times daily for 5–7 days [1–3]. Adjunctive therapy with intranasal mupirocin ointment can clear any nasal reservoirs of bacteria, which could prevent recurrence [1]. Folliculitis with extensive surface area of involvement, or which does not demonstrate a sufficient response to topical treatment, warrants treatment with an oral antibiotic. Antibiotics may be chosen empirically, taking into account community prevalence of MRSA. A 10–14 day course of dicloxacillin or cephalexin 500 mg four times daily, or 5 day course of azithromycin 250 mg daily is appropriate for folliculitis caused by *S. aureus* [3, 5]. In areas with high prevalence of MRSA, a 10–14 day course of trimethoprim-sulfamethoxazole twice daily, or clindamycin 300–450 mg three times daily, is the recommended regimen [6]. The patient in this case would be treated for a presumed staph or strep bacterial folliculitis with a first generation cephalosporin like cephalexin 500 mg four times a day for 10–14 days. If we were concerned for MRSA, we would instead use trimethoprim-sulfamethoxazole or clindamycin for 10–14 days.

Folliculitis caused by *P. aeruginosa* and other gram-negative bacteria may be treated with oral ciprofloxacin 500 mg twice daily for 5 days [5]. Dermatophyte and pityrosporum folliculitis may be treated with topical antifungals (e.g., ketoconazole) twice daily, or oral itraconazole 200 mg daily for 1–2 weeks. Oral itraconazole treatment is also recommended for folliculitis caused by *Candida.* Herpetic folliculitis responds to treatment with oral antivirals. Aciclovir 200 mg five times daily for 5 days is recommended.

Follow-Up

Culturing at the time of the first visit is important in identifying the correct offending pathogen in order to ensure appropriate treatment. Even with correct medication, patients sometimes experience persistence and recurrence of folliculitis that can require prolonged antibiotic courses [5]. The main complication of folliculitis that does not respond to treatment is abscess formation (in which case an incision and drainage might be necessary). Resistant and recalcitrant cases may be referred to dermatology for follow-up treatment.

For patients who have successfully achieved clearance, prophylactic steps may be taken to prevent recurrence. *S. aureus* folliculitis may be prevented with nasal mupirocin ointment applied twice daily for 5 days [5]. Antibacterial washes, and warm compresses may be used in affected areas [1]. Properly controlling diabetes and immune function can help prevent folliculitis with systemic causes.

Questions for the Dermatologist

– *Patient history indicated variation associated with humidity and water contact. Is that a phenomenon associated with folliculitis?*

Any warm, moist, humid area mimics the conditions of a petri dish and gives bacteria a chance to grow.

– *Is it possible for folliculitis to be exacerbated by surfing? Does being in the water make folliculitis worse?*

Being in the water does not make folliculitis worse; however, getting out with a wet bathing suit, and being in a humid environment can. Any sport in tight spandex can result in folliculitis. This irritant form of folliculitis from tight clothing is easy to distinguish because there are no pustules, just papules with hairs coming out of them.

– *Is folliculitis treated empirically, or is it worthwhile to see which bacteria are causing the folliculitis and whether there is any associated antibiotic resistance?*

The vast majority of bacterial folliculitis is caused by staph and strep. Antibiotic treatment should start with a first generation cephalosporin, unless MRSA is suspected. If MRSA is suspected, start with Bactrim or clindamycin. I would not wait on culture results to start the patient on oral antibiotics.

References

1. Laureano AC, Schwartz RA, Cohen PJ. Facial bacterial infections: folliculitis. Clin Dermatol. 2014;32(6):711–4.
2. Kelly EW, Magilner D. Chapter 147. Soft tissue infections. In: Tintinalli JE, Stapczynski J, Ma O, Cline DM, Cydulka RK, Meckler GD, editors. Tintinalli's emergency medicine: a comprehensive study guide. 7th ed. New York: McGraw-Hill; 2011. Available from: http://accessmedicine.mhmedical.com.ezproxy.cul.columbia.edu/content.aspx?bookid=348&Sectionid=40381624. Accessed 24 Feb 2015.
3. Luelmo-Aguilar J, Santandreu MS. Folliculitis: recognition and management. Am J Clin Dermatol. 2004;5(5):301–10.

4. Durdu M, Ilkit M. First step in the differential diagnosis of folliculitis: cytology. Crit Rev Microbiol. 2013;39(1):9–25.
5. Berger TG. Dermatologic disorders. In: Papadakis MA, McPhee SJ, Rabow MW, editors. Current medical diagnosis & treatment 2015. New York: McGraw-Hill; 2014. Available from: http://accessmedicine.mhmedical.com.ezproxy.cul.columbia.edu/content.aspx?bookid=1019&Sectionid=57668598. Accessed 24 Feb 2015.
6. Liu C, Bayer A, Cosgrove SE, Daum RS, Fridkin SK, Gorwitz RJ, Kaplan SL, Karchmer AW, Levine DP, Murray BE, J Rybak M, Talan DA, Chambers HF, Infectious Diseases Society of America. Clinical practice guidelines by the infectious diseases society of America for the treatment of methicillin-resistant Staphylococcus aureus infections in adults and children. Clin Infect Dis. 2011;52(3):e18–55.

Chapter 25
Pityriasis Rosea

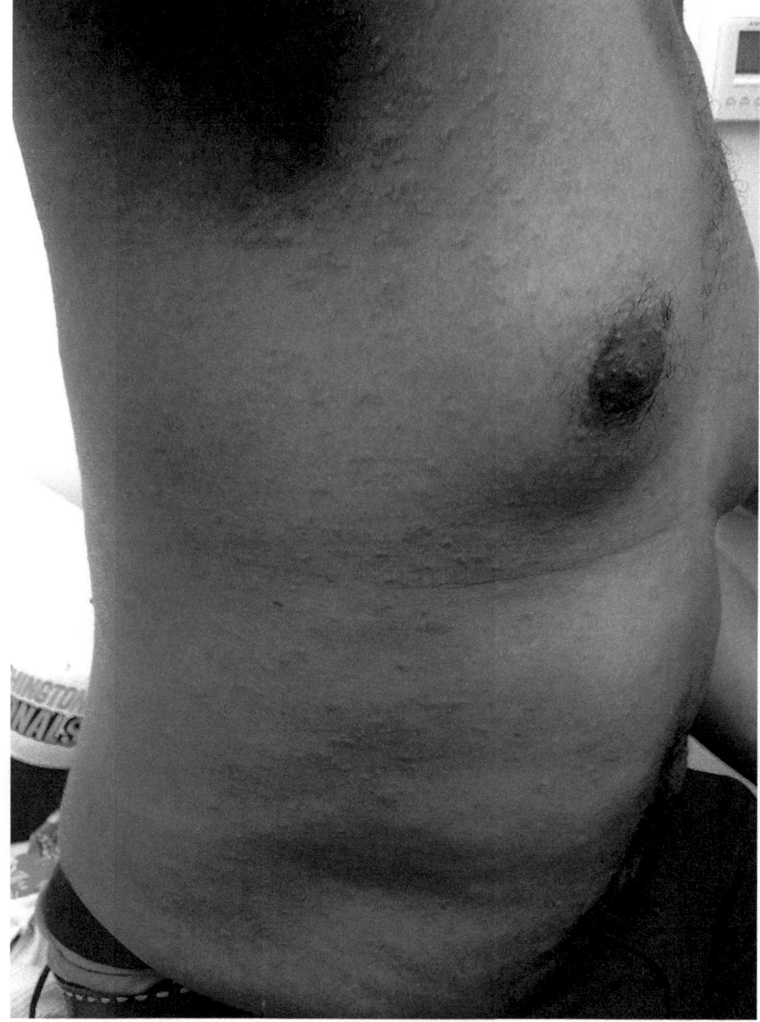

Fig. 25.1 Innumerable guttate papulo-plaques with fine scale predominate on the trunk

D. Reich et al., *Top 50 Dermatology Case Studies for Primary Care*,
DOI 10.1007/978-3-319-18627-6_25

Fig. 25.2 Variably itchy, these lesions often follow a mild upper respiratory illness

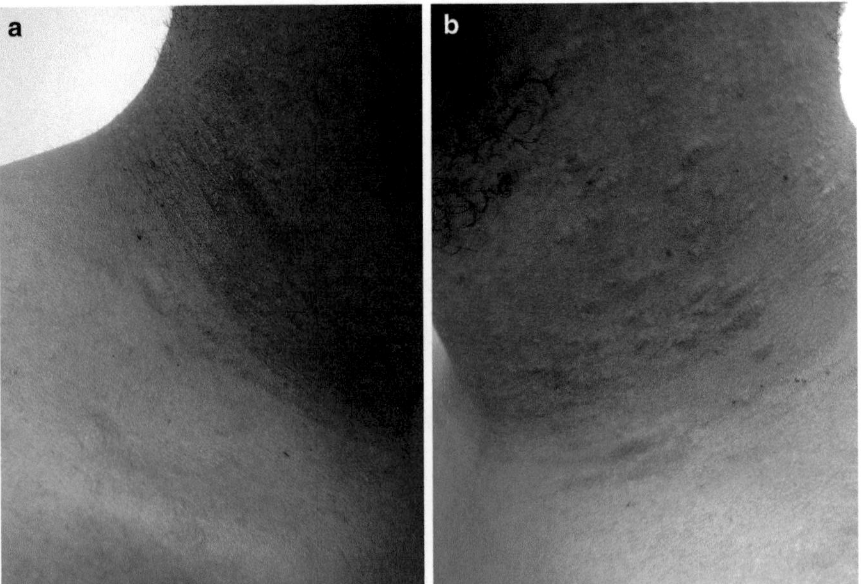

Fig. 25.3 (**a** and **b**) Lesions also extend to the neck

Primary Care Visit Report

A 31-year-old male with past medical history of hypertension, treated with amlodipine, presented with an itchy rash over his torso and buttocks which started 5 days prior. The patient reported exacerbation with a hot shower, and improvement when he used moisturizing lotion.

Vitals were normal. On exam, scattered on his abdomen, torso, bilateral flanks and neck, there were many diffuse, slightly scaly, erythematous papules.

This was presumed to be pityriasis rosea and the patient was told it would resolve on its own.

Discussion from Dermatology Clinic

Differential Dx

- Pityriasis rosea
- Drug eruption
- Tinea versicolor
- Guttate psoriasis

Favored Dx

Definitive diagnosis would benefit from thorough history of the development of the rash. Pityriasis rosea often begins with a single, "herald patch" although this is not present in all cases. Pityriasis rosea is the favored diagnosis in this case due to the eczematous papular appearance of lesions.

Overview

Pityriasis rosea is an acute, exanthematous (a skin rash occurring as a symptom of an infection or disease) eruption which is thought to be brought on by an infectious agent. Although bacteria, fungi, and viruses have all been implicated, the literature most strongly supports an association with reactivations of human herpesvirus (HHV) types 6 and 7 [1–3]. The exact etiology is unknown. The incidence in dermatology patients is estimated to be 0.68 %, and annual incidence is thought to be 0.16 % [1, 3]. Pityriasis rosea typically occurs in ages 10–35 years, and affects women more commonly than men [3]. A high proportion of women who develop pityriasis rosea during the first 20 weeks of gestation experience premature delivery, miscarriage, and spontaneous abortion [4].

Presentation

Pityriasis rosea presents as an acute, exanthematous papular rash. Fifty to 90 % of patients report a primary plaque, called a "herald patch," that is most commonly located on the trunk, and typically precedes the generalized eruption by 2 weeks [3]. Lesions are often described as salmon colored, they are oval or round, erythematous, and may feature scale. Distribution may occur in a "Christmas tree" pattern, with plaques appearing on the trunk and extending laterally and down the back. Pityriasis rosea may be accompanied by pruritus and systemic, flu-like symptoms.

Workup

Pityriasis rosea is usually diagnosed on clinical examination. KOH test may be performed to rule out fungal infections. If a biopsy is performed, histopathology would reveal spongiosis, erythrocyte extravasation, and lymphocytic infiltrate.

Treatment

Pityriasis rosea is a self-limiting eruption that does not require treatment. Patients experiencing severe pruritus may require symptomatic relief. Antihistamines such as hydroxyzine or diphenhydramine, or topical corticosteroids may be prescribed to relieve pruritus. Patients may also experience relief from over-the-counter antipruritic moisturizers, and oatmeal baths [3]. Oatmeal baths can be prepared by using store-bought oatmeal bath packets, or by putting about ½ cup of plain oatmeal into a coffee filter or cheese cloth, tying off, and adding to bathwater.

Patients experiencing a severe eruption may benefit from treatment with acyclovir, especially if treatment is initiated within the first week of onset. Oral acyclovir 800 mg may be given five times daily for 7 days to adults. Children should be dosed at 20 mg/kg four times daily for 7 days. Use of antiviral medication is a relatively new approach to treatment, and it is associated with significant regression of the eruption within 2 weeks [5, 6].

Follow-Up

The course of pityriasis rosea is unpredictable; however, it may spontaneously resolve in as few as 2 weeks, and more typically within 6–8 weeks [1]. Follow-up is open for patients who decline treatment; however, they should return to the office if there is no resolution after 2 months. Patients treated with acyclovir should be seen again after 1 week of treatment. Relapse of the condition is very uncommon with a rate of 3.8 % [7].

Questions for the Dermatologist

– *What can the patient do to relieve symptomatic itching while he waits for the condition to resolve?*

The condition will usually resolve on its own within 4–6 weeks. Topical steroids, light therapy, and antihistamines can help provide symptomatic relief.

– *What triggers pityriasis rosea?*

We believe it is related to HHV-6 and -7. These viruses are not related to the sexually transmitted form of herpes.

– *Is there a way to make a definitive diagnosis, or is it made based on clinical examination?*

The diagnosis is clinical. It has distinct features under a microscope, like lymphocytic infiltrate and dyskeratosis, but it is not necessary to biopsy.

– *This patient did not exhibit the classic Christmas tree distribution of pityriasis rosea. In what proportion of cases is that distribution present?*

The Christmas tree distribution is not seen often; perhaps it is present in 10 % of cases. It usually presents as scattered, randomly positioned, small guttate (drop-shaped) plaques. The herald patch is more commonly seen, in more than half of cases. The herald patch is a single, larger patch that appears 5–7 days before all the others.

References

1. Drago F, Broccolo F, Ciccarese G, Rebora A, Parodi A. Persistent pityriasis rosea: an unusual form of pityriasis rosea with persistent active HHV-6 and HHV-7 infection. Dermatology. 2015;230(1):23–6.
2. Broccolo F, Drago F, Careddu AM, Foglieni C, Turbino L, Cocuzza CE, Gelmetti C, Lusso P, Rebora AE, Malnati MS. Additional evidence that pityriasis rosea is associated with reactivation of human herpesvirus-6 and -7. J Invest Dermatol. 2005;124(6):1234–40.
3. Blauvelt A. Chapter 42. Pityriasis rosea. In: Goldsmith LA, Katz SI, Gilchrest BA, Paller AS, Leffell DJ, Wolff K, editors. Fitzpatrick's dermatology in general medicine. 8th ed. New York: McGraw-Hill; 2012. Available from: http://accessmedicine.mhmedical.com.ezproxy.cul.columbia.edu/content.aspx?bookid=392&Sectionid=41138739. Accessed 27 Feb 2015.
4. Drago F, Broccolo F, Zaccaria E, Malnati M, Cocuzza C, Lusso P, Rebora A. Pregnancy outcome in patients with pityriasis rosea. J Am Acad Dermatol. 2008;58(5 Suppl 1): S78–83.
5. Ganguly S. A randomized, double-blind, placebo-controlled study of efficacy of oral acyclovir in the treatment of pityriasis rosea. J Clin Diagn Res. 2014;8(5):YC01–4.
6. Drago F, Vecchio F, Rebora A. Use of high-dose acyclovir in pityriasis rosea. J Am Acad Dermatol. 2006;54(1):82–5.
7. Drago F, Ciccarese G, Rebora A, Parodi A. Relapsing pityriasis rosea. Dermatology. 2014; 229(4):316–8.

Chapter 26
Seborrheic Keratosis

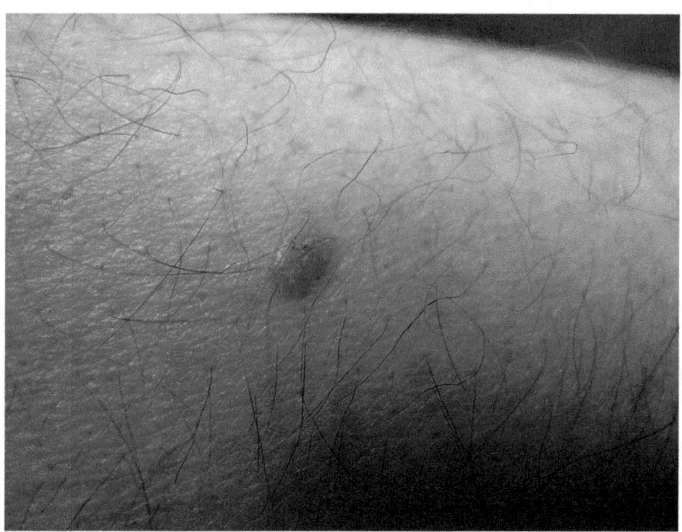

Fig. 26.1 Stuck-on pink papule with hyperkeratotic surface

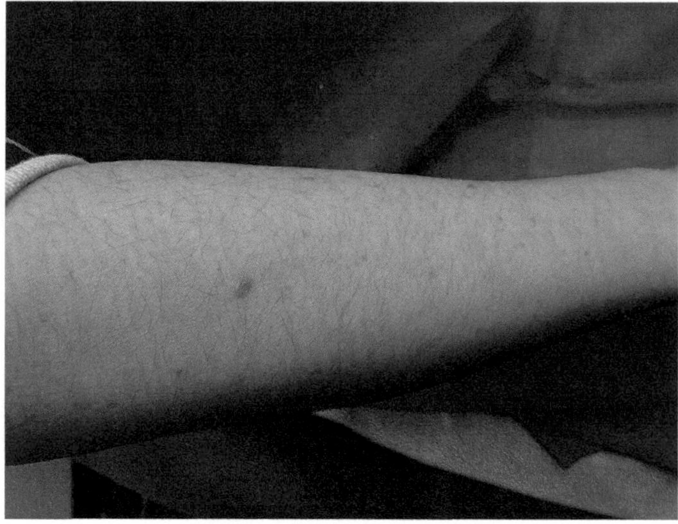

Fig. 26.2 Roughened papule 0.8 cm—these lesions are more commonly brown in color

D. Reich et al., *Top 50 Dermatology Case Studies for Primary Care*,
DOI 10.1007/978-3-319-18627-6_26

Primary Care Visit Report

A 39-year-old female with past medical history of migraines presented with a new mole on her right upper arm that "just popped up," per the patient. She noticed it about 6 months prior, and noted that it had changed in size since it appeared and bled occasionally.

Vitals were normal. On exam, there was a 4 mm×4 mm erythematous, soft, fleshy papule on the patient's right lateral forearm.

Because this was a new mole that was changing in size, the patient was referred to dermatology for further evaluation. The dermatologist biopsied the lesion and found it was seborrheic keratosis.

Discussion from Dermatology Clinic

Differential Dx

- Seborrheic keratosis
- Melanoma
- Pigmented basal cell carcinoma
- Verruca plana
- Common acquired nevus
- Acrochordon (skin tag)

Favored Dx

Malignant skin transformations should always be part of a differential that includes rapid growth and recent changes to a lesion. On clinical examination, this lesion appears to be a benign seborrheic keratosis.

Overview

Seborrheic keratoses (SK) are very common, benign epidermal tumors. They can occur at any age, though they more commonly occur in people above the age of 50, and tend to increase in number with age. There is no gender preference [1, 2].

Inheritance may play a role in their development, as they tend to run in families in an autosomal dominant fashion. Sun exposure has also been associated with SKs [2, 3]. Malignant transformations of SKs are extremely rare; however, there have been some cases of melanoma and basal cell carcinoma arising out of SK lesions [3–6].

Presentation

Seborrheic keratoses tend to be oval or circular, sharply demarcated lesions that are brown, tan, pink, or flesh-colored. Their surface may appear rough, verrucous (wart-like), or waxy. They are often described as having a "stuck on" appearance. Individual SKs tend to grow quickly until reaching a static size. They tend to be raised, leaving them more susceptible to trauma and bleeding from friction. They are usually asymptomatic, although they can sometimes be pruritic, which may also lead to scratching and bleeding. They appear on any surfaces except mucous membranes, palms, and soles of feet.

An individual may have anywhere between one and hundreds of SKs. Any explosive onset of multiple SKs should raise suspicion for internal malignancy. This is referred to as the Leser–Trélat sign and is most frequently associated with gastrointestinal adenocarcinomas [3].

Workup

Seborrheic keratoses can usually be diagnosed on clinical examination. If any malignant transformation is suspected, the lesion should be biopsied. Typical histological findings of seborrheic keratosis include hyperkeratosis (thickened stratum corneum), papillomatosis (finger-like projections), acanthosis (diffuse epidermal thickening), and horn-like cysts representing obstructed hair follicles.

SKs have several histological variants, including reticulated (or adenoid), acanthotic, hyperkeratotic, clonal, irritated, and pigmented. They each have some variation in their predominant characteristics. Dermatosis papulosa nigra (DPN) is histologically indistinguishable from SK. It presents as small brown or black papules that commonly appear on Fitzpatrick scale type IV (moderate brown skin), V (dark brown skin), and VI (deeply pigmented brown to black skin). All variants are treated in the same manner.

Treatment

Seborrheic keratoses are benign and therefore do not require any treatment. If the lesions become symptomatic or irritated, or patients are bothered by their cosmetic appearance, SKs may be removed by cryosurgery, electrodesiccation, or laser therapy by a dermatologist [3, 6, 7]. Recurrence of lesions may occur, and there is no way to prevent the growth of new SKs.

Follow-Up

No follow-up is required unless a procedure is done. Following procedure, patients of darker skin types should be monitored for post-inflammatory hyperpigmentation.

Questions for the Dermatologist

– *Is this a dangerous lesion with malignant potential?*

No, seborrheic keratoses are not considered dangerous, and never have malignant potential.

– *What is its natural course if left alone? Does it continue to grow?*

It may grow very slightly, for example by 1–2 mm, but SKs usually stay approximately the same size. They usually do not spontaneously fall off, but they are sometimes inadvertently picked off by patients.

– *Is there more cause for concern if the lesion bleeds occasionally?*

Bleeding alone in a classic SK is not cause for concern as the lesions can be traumatized. If the lesion does not have a typical presentation, bleeding would warrant questioning whether SK is the correct diagnosis.

References

1. Phulari RG, Buddhdev K, Rathore R, Patel S. Seborrheic keratosis. J Oral Maxillofac Pathol. 2014;18(2):327–30.
2. Yeatman JM. The prevalence of seborrhoeic keratoses in an Australian population: does exposure to sunlight play a part in their frequency? Br J Dermatol. 1997;137(3):411–4.
3. Thomas VD, Snavely NR, Lee KK, Swanson NA. Chapter 118. Benign epithelial tumors, hamartomas, and hyperplasias. In: Goldsmith LA, Katz SI, Gilchrest BA, Paller AS, Leffell DJ,

Wolff K, editors. Fitzpatrick's dermatology in general medicine. 8th ed. New York: McGraw-Hill; 2012. p. 1319–23.
4. Bedir R, Yurdakul C, Güçer H, Sehitoglu I. Basal cell carcinoma arising within seborrheic keratosis. J Clin Diagn Res. 2014;8(7):YD06–7.
5. Salerni G, Alonso C, Gorosito M, Fernández-Bussy R. Seborrheic keratosis-like melanoma. J Am Acad Dermatol. 2015;72(1 Suppl):S53–5.
6. Tay YK, Tan SK. A study comparing the efficacy and risk of adverse events using two techniques of electrocautery for the treatment of seborrheic keratoses. Dermatol Surg. 2003;39(5):810–3.
7. Herron MD, Bowen AR, Krueger GG. Seborrheic keratoses: a study comparing the standard cryosurgery with topical calcipotriene, topical tazarotene, and topical imiquimod. Int J Dermatol. 2004;43(4):300–2.

Chapter 27
Nummular Eczema

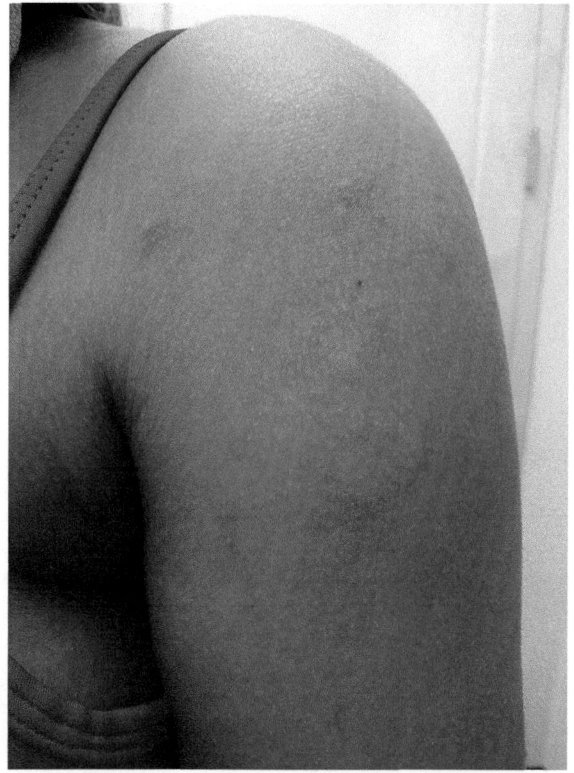

Fig. 27.1 Often misdiagnosed as ringworm, this circular plaque is less pruritic and has scale throughout

D. Reich et al., *Top 50 Dermatology Case Studies for Primary Care*,
DOI 10.1007/978-3-319-18627-6_27

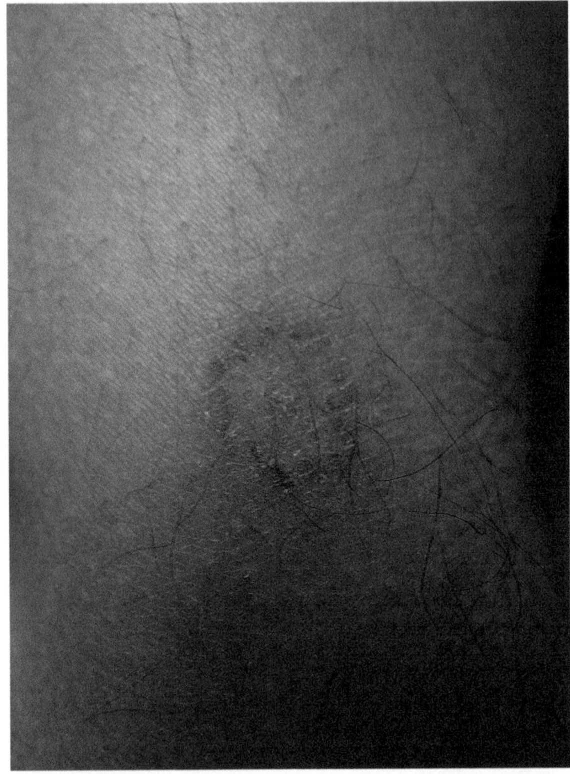

Fig. 27.2 This coin-shaped lesion has a chapped appearance and is exceedingly common

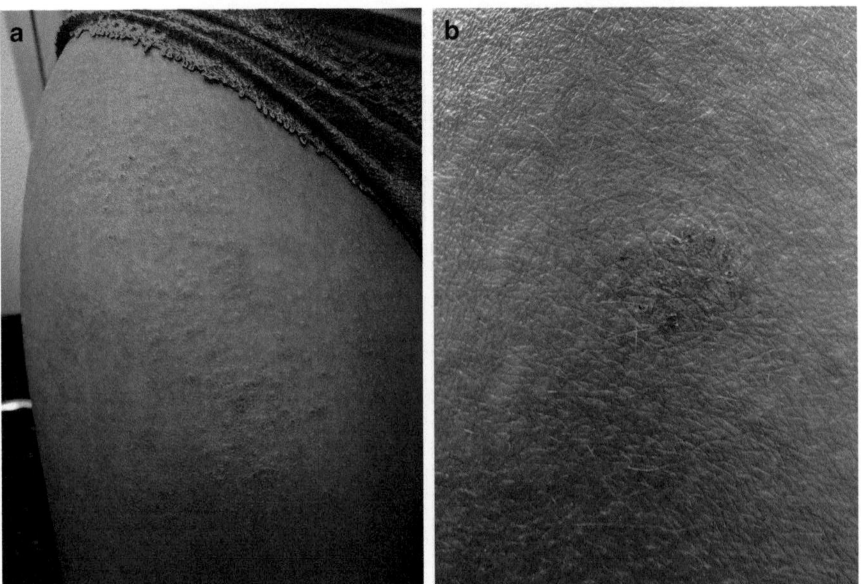

Fig. 27.3 (**a** and **b**) Follicular prominence is the first sign of xerosis, a clue to your diagnosis

Primary Care Visit Report

A 23-year-old female with past medical history of recurrent vaginal yeast infections, treated with weekly fluconazole 100 mg, presented with a pruritic rash. The rash started 2 weeks prior to this visit, with lesions on her right cheek (mostly resolved at visit), two round lesions on her right upper arm, a single lesion on her left shoulder area, and a rash on her upper thighs and abdomen. All lesions were pruritic and the patient reported a "burning, irritated" feeling on her legs. She had started using Tom's soap for the first time about 1 month prior. Otherwise, no new skin products were reported.

Vitals were normal. On exam, there was a 5 mm × 5 mm round papular lesion with hyperpigmented border on her right upper arm, and a 1 cm × 1 cm scaly dry plaque with central clearing on her left upper arm. Her abdomen and bilateral thighs featured rough, papular, scaly dry plaques.

The considered differential was eczema versus a fungal infection. The patient was initially treated for eczema, and was prescribed topical desonide 0.05 % cream (Class VI) twice daily for 14 days. The patient was advised to discontinue use if the rash was not resolving with desonide, and instead try clotrimazole 1 % cream twice daily.

Discussion from Dermatology Clinic

Differential Dx

- Nummular eczema
- Contact dermatitis (allergic or irritant)
- Tinea corporis
- Psoriasis
- Majocchi's granuloma
- Lichen simplex chronicus

Favored Dx

The favored diagnosis as classified by dermatology is nummular eczema, due to the annular (circular) shape, xerotic (dry) appearance, and distribution of the lesions.

Overview

Nummular eczema, also called discoid dermatitis or discoid eczema, is a clinical entity characterized by distinct, coin-shaped, pruritic lesions [1]. It shows a male predominance and primarily affects adults between the ages of 50 and 65 years [2, 3]. There is a second peak incidence in women between the ages of 15 and 25 years [3]. Unlike classic eczema, nummular eczema is rarely associated with a predisposition to intrinsic allergic hypersensitivity as is often seen with atopic eczema or asthma [2, 3]. There is an increased incidence of contact allergy in nummular eczema and lesions of nummular eczema may be a manifestation of contact allergy [2].

The exact cause of nummular eczema is not known, and its pathogenesis is thought to be multifactorial, involving environmental, allergic, emotional, infective, and nutritional factors [1, 2]. It can be exacerbated by dry skin, hot showers, harsh soaps, and cold weather and is most commonly due to environmental factors like dry air [1]. Nummular eczema is most often a descriptive term used to indicate the round shape of lesions—it is a term used to classify a rash with this classic appearance whether or not the cause is known. For example, if subsequent patch testing identifies an allergic cause of the nummular eczema rash, the condition could then be reclassified as contact dermatitis.

Presentation

Nummular eczema presents with round, well-demarcated, erythematous plaques. They may be pruritic. Lesions may initially manifest as papules or vesicles, which can coalesce, and ooze or crust. Plaques of nummular eczema may feature central clearing. Chronic plaques may feature lichenification (thickened skin from scratching). Lesions most frequently appear on the extensor aspects of extremities, with dorsa of the hands frequently affected in women [1–3].

Workup

Patch testing can be useful in identifying underlying contact allergy [4, 5]. Nickel, potassium dichromate, cobalt chloride, perfume mix, neomycin, rubber chemicals, and formaldehyde have been identified as frequently associated irritants [2, 4, 5]. Bacterial culture should be performed on any exudate material if there is evidence of infection. If there is strong suspicion of tinea corporis, a KOH test may be performed.

Treatment

Nummular eczema is treated with topical corticosteroids. Extensor surfaces of the extremities, where most lesions appear, can be treated with mid- to high-potency steroids. Triamcinolone 0.1 % ointment (Class III) twice daily for up to 2 weeks is recommended. Moisturizers and emollients (such as over-the-counter products like, Vaseline) may be used as adjunctive therapy for abnormally dry skin. Any secondary bacterial infection should be treated empirically with oral antibiotics.

Follow-Up

Nummular eczema tends to be a chronic, recurrent condition [3]. The most effective way to limit its recurrence is by identifying and eliminating the trigger. If patients declined patch testing at the initial visit, recurrence is an indication for allergic patch testing.

Questions for the Dermatologist

– *How can nummular eczema be differentiated from fungal rashes?*

Fungal rashes have a very prominent, serpiginous border, and can be fiercely pruritic. Nummular eczema shows greater variance in itchiness, with a fine scale throughout the affected area. In this case, the ring-like shape, xerotic (dry) appearance, and the distribution of the lesions are what help to rule out a fungal condition.

– *Does nummular eczema respond to the same treatment as regular eczema?*

Yes, it does. Topical corticosteroids are the treatment of choice.

– *Is nummular eczema exacerbated by the same environmental triggers that exacerbate regular eczema?*

Yes, it is. The same triggers should be avoided. Patients should be advised to use lukewarm instead of hot water when bathing, avoid long baths and showers, avoid wearing synthetic materials or wools, limit contact with rugs, and use moisturizers and soaps without dyes or fragrances.

References

1. Halberg M. Nummular eczema. J Emerg Med. 2012;43(5):e327–8.
2. Bonamonte D, Foti C, Vestita M, Ranieri LD, Angelini G. Nummular eczema and contact allergy: a retrospective study. Dermatitis. 2012;23(4):153–7.
3. Burgin S. Chapter 15. Nummular eczema, lichen simplex chronicus, and prurigo nodularis. In: Goldsmith LA, Katz SI, Gilchrest BA, Paller AS, Leffell DJ, Wolff K, editors. Fitzpatrick's dermatology in general medicine. 8th ed. New York: McGraw-Hill; 2012. Available from: http://accessmedicine.mhmedical.com.ezproxy.cul.columbia.edu/content.aspx?bookid=392&Sectionid=41138710. Accessed 26 Feb 2015.
4. Krupa Shankar DS, Shrestha S. Relevance of patch testing in patients with nummular dermatitis. Indian J Dermatol Venereol Leprol. 2005;71(6):406–8.
5. Fleming C, Parry E, Forsyth A, Kemmett D. Patch testing in discoid eczema. Contact Dermatitis. 1997;36(5):261–4.

Chapter 28
Inflamed Epidermal Inclusion Cyst

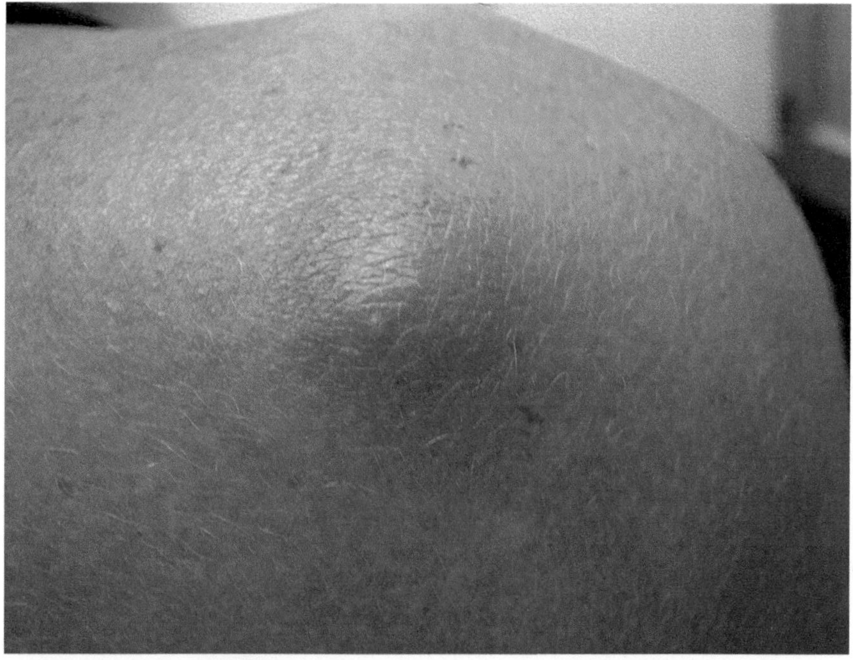

Fig. 28.1 These lesions are often misdiagnosed as infectious, but the inflammation seen here is a foreign body reaction to keratin

D. Reich et al., *Top 50 Dermatology Case Studies for Primary Care*,
DOI 10.1007/978-3-319-18627-6_28

Primary Care Visit Report

A 36-year-old female with no past medical history presented with a bump on her right shoulder, which had been present and unchanged for years. However, a few days prior to this visit, it became red, tender, and painful. She felt well otherwise.

Vitals were normal. On exam, on her right posterior shoulder, there was a 1 cm × 1 cm erythematous papule that was tender to palpation and indurated.

The diagnosis was uncertain, and the patient was referred to dermatology for further evaluation.

Discussion from Dermatology Clinic

Differential Dx

- Epidermal inclusion cyst (EIC)
- Lipoma
- Pilomatricoma
- Abscess

Favored Dx

Patient history is suggestive of a ruptured and inflamed EIC.

Overview

Epidermal inclusion cysts (EIC), also called epidermoid cysts, are epithelial-lined cysts filled with keratin and lipid-rich debris. The term sebaceous cyst is also commonly used; however, it is inaccurate, as the cysts neither involve sebaceous glands nor contain sebum.

EICs can occur at any age and on any part of the body, although they are more likely to appear in adults [1]. They frequently appear on the chest, back, face, neck, and scalp. The most common cause is occlusion of the pilosebaceous unit. They may also be caused by trauma, when penetration by an object may cause implantation of epidermal cells into deeper tissue of the dermis, or by congenital sequestration of a collection of epidermal cells. Hereditary diseases such as Gardner syndrome, pachyonychia congenita, and Gorlin syndrome all feature multiple EICs.

EICs can remain stable or can grow in size. They can also become spontaneously inflamed and rupture. It is difficult to predict which EICs will remain stable and which will grow or rupture.

Presentation

EICs are dome-shaped dermal or subcutaneous nodules that often have a small central punctum. They are firm and freely movable on palpation. They usually present as skin-colored or white cysts. Sometimes cheesy, odorous debris can be expressed from them. Unruptured cysts should have well-defined borders. If they have ruptured, they may be irregular with red and tender surrounding areas.

Workup

EICs may be diagnosed on clinical examination. Physicians should look for a small, pore-like opening. Applying pressure may cause expression of debris, which can be cultured if there is any suspicion of secondary infection. Inflammation is generally due to foreign-body reaction when cysts rupture and their contents spill into surrounding tissue. The unlikely secondary infections are most commonly caused by *Staphylococcus aureus*, group A *Streptococcus*, *E. coli*, *Peptostreptococcus* species, and *Bacteroides* species. Infections tend to be polymicrobial [1]. Genetic conditions should be considered for patients presenting with multiple cysts and family history of EICs.

Treatment

EICs that are inflamed but not infected can resolve on their own, though they do tend to recur. It is only necessary to treat these if the patient desires it. Excision surgery is the most definitive treatment approach though it is best performed when the EIC is not inflamed. When inflamed, the cyst wall is very friable and difficult to completely remove by excising thus risking recurrence. Therefore, inflamed cysts may be injected with a 10 mg/ml concentration of intralesional steroid such as kenalog a few days prior to excision. If the EIC is fluctuant, rather than injecting steroids, an incision and drainage procedure should be performed.

For excising the lesion, punch, elliptical, and minimal incision techniques can be used, depending on the nature and location of the cyst. A study comparing punch and elliptical excisions found punch excision to produce better cosmetic outcomes, smaller size of wound, shorter surgery time, and comparably low recurrence rates at 3.2 %. These results were most notable in cysts under 2 cm in diameter [2]. Another study found recurrence rates by punch incision to be highest for cysts removed from the back (13.8 %) and ear (13 %) [3]. During surgery, the entire cyst wall should be removed to minimize chances of recurrence. Minimal incision techniques have demonstrated some success for cysts under 1 cm in diameter, and are most useful for areas of cosmetic concern as the 3 mm incision can be left to heal without sutures [4].

For patients who prefer a non-surgical approach to treatment, injection with intralesional kenalog with adjunctive oral antibiotic therapy is an option. There are no controlled studies investigating the efficacy of this treatment; however, it is part of clinical practice, and the contents of inflamed cysts do demonstrate colonization by aerobic and anaerobic bacteria, including *S. aureus*, *Peptostreptococcus*, and *Bacteroides* species [5]. If oral antibiotics are considered, the choice of a specific regimen should be empirically chosen to cover those organisms mentioned or to cover MRSA if clinically indicated.

Follow-Up

Patients will need to follow up for suture removal if those were placed. The incision should be monitored for any inflammation or infection. Patients should be instructed to follow up in the unlikely event of cyst recurrence.

Questions for the Dermatologist

– *What is an epidermal inclusion cyst?*

EICs are benign lesions; however, they can become inflamed. Inflammation is not evidence of an infection usually, rather it represents a foreign body reaction to dead skin that escapes the cyst and penetrates surrounding tissue. It is possible for a cyst to become infected, but less likely.

– *How is it treated or removed?*

EICs can be removed by excision. Puncturing and draining tends not to be a successful therapy as the cyst is likely to reform; however, many providers still treat it that way. If the cyst is inflamed, it can be injected with intralesional steroids a few days prior to excision. There is no indication for oral antibiotics unless culturing reveals a secondary infection. Although it is part of common practice, our office avoids oral antibiotic use for EICs due to concerns about increasing bacterial resistance and costs.

References

1. Thomas VS, Snavely NR, Lee KK, Swanson NA. Chapter 118. Benign epithelial tumors, hamartomas, and hyperplasias. In: Goldsmith LA, Katz SI, Gilchrest BA, Paller AS, Leffell DJ, Wolff K, editors. Fitzpatrick's dermatology in general medicine. 8th ed. New York: McGraw-Hill; 2012. p. 1333–4.

2. Lee HE, Yang CH, Chen CH, Hong HS, Kuan YZ. Comparison of the surgical outcomes of punch incision and elliptical excision in treating epidermal inclusion cysts: a prospective randomized study. Dermatol Surg. 2006;32(4):520–5.
3. Mehrabi D, Leonhardt JM, Brodell RT. Removal and keratinous and pilar cysts with the punch incision technique: analysis of surgical outcomes. Dermatol Surg. 2002;28(8):673–7.
4. Yang HJ, Yang KC. A new method for facial epidermoid cyst removal with minimal incision. J Eur Acad Dermatol Venereol. 2009;23(8):887–90.
5. Diven DG, Dozier SE, Meyer DJ, Smith EB. Bacteriology of inflamed and uninflamed epidermal inclusion cysts. Arch Dermatol. 1998;134(1):49–51.

Part VI
Anogenital

Chapter 29
Tinea Cruris

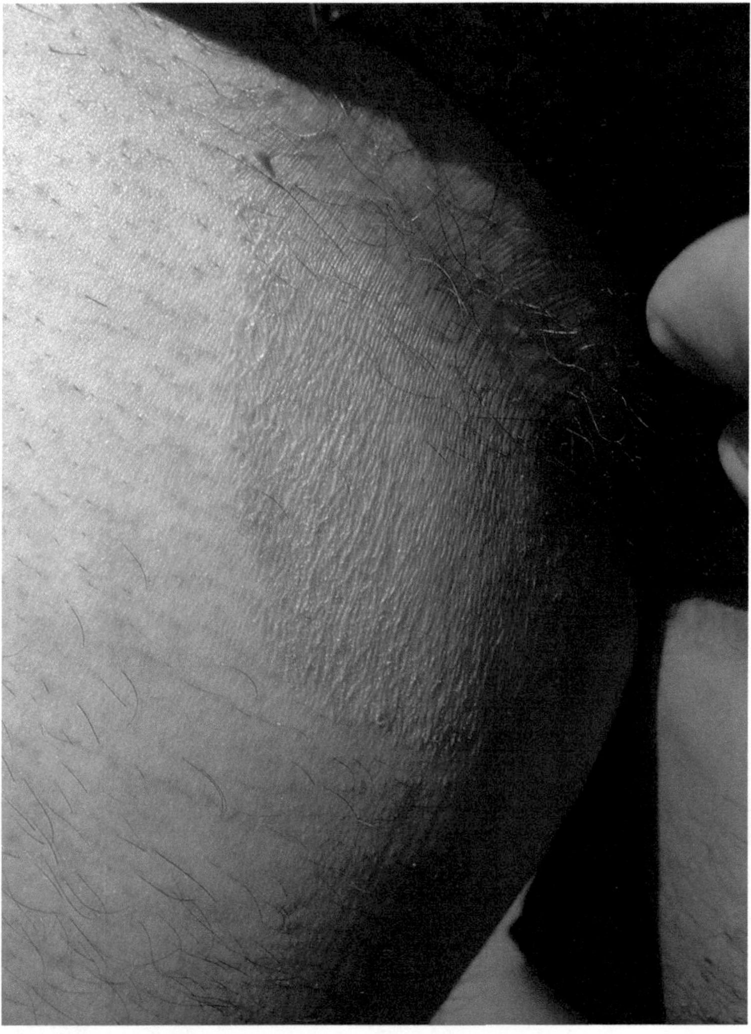

Fig. 29.1 Heavy itch and most commonly seen in more sedentary individuals with a higher body mass index (BMI)

D. Reich et al., *Top 50 Dermatology Case Studies for Primary Care*,
DOI 10.1007/978-3-319-18627-6_29

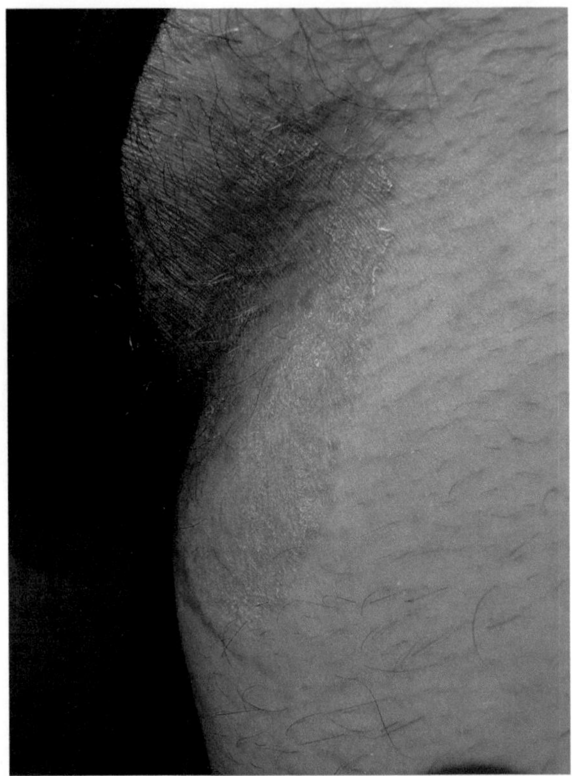

Fig. 29.2 May be bilateral as in this patient or unilateral. Maceration may be present if perspiration is heavy

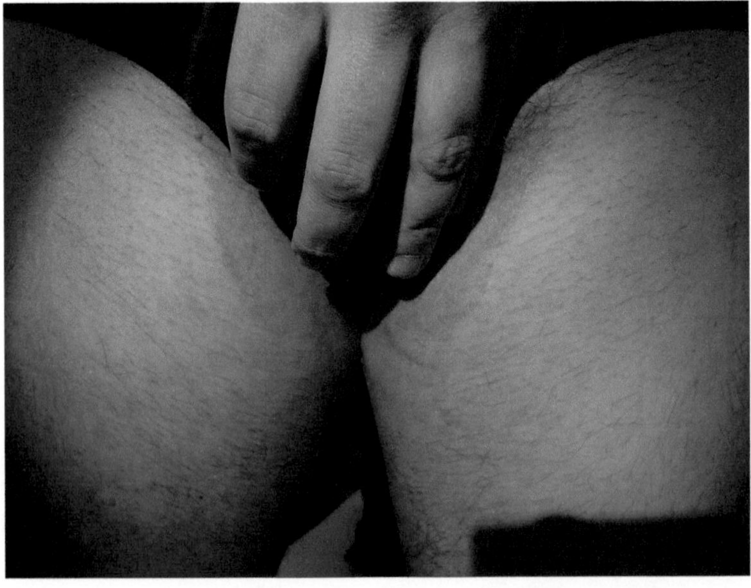

Fig. 29.3 The wavy border seen in this condition helps differentiate it from inverse psoriasis

Primary Care Visit Report

A 33-year-old male with no prior medical history presented with a rash in his inguinal creases. The patient described the rash as itchy, and said it felt irritated and had a rough texture. He had a similar rash 3 years prior for 3 weeks but it resolved on its own. Over the prior 1½ years, the rash had recurred and abated, sometimes lasting for 6 months at a time. During that time, the patient used over-the-counter hydrocortisone cream, which helped with the itchiness and irritation, but the discoloration and texture-change remained. The present rash recurred 3 months prior to this visit. The patient reported exacerbation with exercise or warm weather. The patient tried changing to a different detergent, which had no effect.

Vitals were normal. On exam, in the bilateral inguinal creases, there were erythematous scaly patches with well-delineated borders extending inferiorly to the medial thighs and extending medially about 1 cm medial to the inguinal crease. Woods lamp exam revealed orange fluorescence in a 2 cm × 1 cm area in the left inguinal crease. The remainder of the rash did not fluoresce.

The differential diagnosis considered was erythrasma vs. tinea cruris vs. contact dermatitis. Since the rash did not fluoresce red overall (as would be expected with erythrasma), it was treated as tinea cruris with 2 % ketoconazole cream twice daily for 21 days. The patient was advised to change out of sweaty gym clothes immediately after exercising.

Discussion from Dermatology Clinic

Differential Dx

- Tinea cruris
- Erythrasma
- Contact dermatitis
- Intertrigo
- Inverse psoriasis
- Langerhans' cell histiocytosis (rare)

Favored Dx

Tinea cruris thrives in warm, humid conditions. The patient history of symptoms getting worse with exercise and warm weather is suggestive of tinea cruris. Pruritus is a requisite in making this diagnosis.

Overview

Tinea cruris is a fungal infection of the thighs, groin, and pubic region commonly referred to as "jock itch." It is a superficial cutaneous subacute or chronic dermatophytosis most often caused by the *Trichophyton rubrum* fungus. The infection typically occurs in adulthood and is more common in males [1]. Infection can be passed from person to person via skin-on-skin contact; however, it is not a common cause of contagion. It may also be passed through shared unwashed clothing [2] or other objects that carry the infected scales [3]. Contact sports may be associated with tinea because of frequent or prolonged skin-on-skin contact, or other factors such as contact with wrestling mats, time spent in sweaty clothes, and use of shared shower facilities.

Autoinfection can occur when foot fungus is passed to the groin [3] (for example while pulling on underpants), and thus tinea pedis is often seen in tinea cruris patients [1]. In addition to tinea pedis, patient history can include immunocompromised state, previous occurrences of tinea cruris, use of sports facilities, family members with dermatophyte infections, and sharing clothing [2].

Presentation

Tinea cruris is characterized by a confluent, erythematous, scaling, well-demarcated rash. It occurs in the groin, proximal medial thighs, and pubic area, and it may also be seen in the perianal skin. Scrotum and penis, or labia majora are typically spared. Patches appear red, tan, or brown in color with central clearing. If patients have already initiated over-the-counter antifungal therapies, lesions may lack scale. If hyphae have invaded the hair shaft (Majocchi granuloma), pustules may also appear. If there is a secondary infection or maceration of skin, patients may also experience pain.

Workup

KOH examination can be performed by scraping the lesions, placing the scraped scale on to a microscope slide, covering it in 10 % KOH solution, waiting 10–15 min, and then looking at the slide under a microscope. All non-fungal cells will be destroyed, allowing for easier identification of fungal hyphae. A fungal culture from the scrapings may also be sent to lab for analysis if the diagnosis is still uncertain; however, cultures usually take about 2 weeks to grow. If there is a high clinical suspicion of tinea cruris, treatment should be initiated in the interim.

Treatment

Recommended first-line treatment for tinea cruris are topical antifungal creams. Drugs from the imidazole (e.g., ketoconazole, clotrimazole, econazole) and the allylamine (e.g., terbinafine) families are both effective in treating tinea cruris; however, there is evidence to suggest allylamine topicals help the condition resolve more quickly [4–6]. Terbinafine 1 % (available as over-the-counter Lamisil) can be used twice daily for 1 week or ketoconazole 2 % twice daily for 2 weeks.

Systemic antifungals may be used if the infection is recurrent, covers a large surface area, involves the hair follicles, or is recalcitrant to topical therapy. Both terbinafine 250 mg/day for 2 weeks, and fluconazole 150 mg/day for 1 week have been shown to be successful in eradicating tinea cruris [3]. No bloodwork is routinely recommended when using oral antifungals for less than 2 weeks.

Follow-Up

Patients should follow up 2 weeks after therapy is initiated to ensure the infection is resolving. If the condition is resolving but not fully cleared, the treatment may be continued for another week. Mycologic cure rates depend largely on patient compliance. If patients stop treating when they see lesions improving, it is possible residual hyphae and spores can cause recurrence. For that reason, a second follow-up 4–6 weeks later is beneficial for monitoring relapse. Patients should be advised to practice good hygiene, keep the area dry, and use antifungal powders, like Zeasorb, Lotrimin, or any over-the-counter antifungal powder for jock itch, as prophylactic therapies.

Questions for the Dermatologist

– *Do I treat tinea cruris any differently than tinea corporis? Do you recommend powders or creams?*

Tinea cruris and tinea corporis are treated in the same way, with topical antifungals. Creams should be used as the first line of treatment. After the infection resolves, powders such as the ones listed above may be used prophylactically to keep tinea cruris from returning. The groin area should be kept dry whenever possible.

– *Is it true that applying steroids to fungal lesions will make them worse? In this case, the patient reported that steroids helped treat the itchiness.*

It is true that fungal lesions treated with steroids may get worse. In fact, patients may initially report improvement as the anti-inflammatory eases attendant redness.

However, this untreated infection will recur if not addressed. There is no harm in treating fungal infections with steroids for a week or 2. It is a common mistake to make given the differential we have reviewed, and fungal rashes are often initially misdiagnosed. A problem arises when topical steroids with several refills are prescribed and patients do not return for follow-up. Untreated tinea can lead to Majocchi Granuloma, a dermatophyte infection deep in the follicle that generally requires a 6-week oral antifungal treatment course.

– *What precautions can patients take to avoid future infection?*

Keeping the area dry and using prophylactic antifungal powders like over-the-counter Zeasorb or Lotrimin are great ways to prevent recurrence. People who are prone to sweating and sit a lot for their jobs, like truck drivers, should get up and move around throughout the day. Contagion can also be avoided by washing clothes and towels in hot water, cleaning exercise mats after use, and wearing flip-flops in communal showers.

– *Are oral antifungals ever needed to treat tinea cruris?*

Tinea cruris can be more successfully treated with oral antifungals, and would certainly respond safely and quickly to an oral course of therapy. Although safe, side effects with oral therapy, such as fever, headache, nausea, and hives, are possible. Unless the infection is very severe, as in Majocchi Granuloma, for garden variety tinea cruris, a course of topical antifungals should be sufficient.

References

1. Wolff K, Johnson RA, Suurmond D. Chapter 23, Cutaneous fungal infections. In: Wolff K, editor. Fitzpatrick's color atlas & synopsis of clinical dermatology. 5th ed. New York: McGraw-Hill; 2005. p. 699–700.
2. Drake LA, Dinehart SM, Farmer ER, Goltz RW, Graham GF, Hardinsky MK, Lewis CW, Pariser DM, Skouge JW, Webster SB, Whitaker DC, Butler B, Lowery BJ, Elewski BE, Elgart ML, Jacobs PH, Lesher Jr JL, Scher RK. Guidelines of care for superficial mycotic infections of the skin: tinea corporis, tinea cruris, tinea faciei, tinea manuum, and tinea pedis. J Am Acad Dermatol. 1996;34(2 Pt 1):282–6.
3. Gupta AK, Chaudhry M, Elewski B. Tinea corporis, tinea cruris, tinea nigra, and piedra. Dermatol Clin. 2003;21(3):395–400.
4. Singal A, Pandhi D, Agrawal S, Das S. Comparative efficacy of topical 1% butenafine and 1% clotrimazole in tinea cruris and tinea corporis: a randomized, double-blind trial. J Dermatol Treat. 2005;16(5/6):331–5.
5. Gupta AK, Tu LQ. Dermatophytes: diagnosis and treatment. J Am Acad Dermatol. 2006;54(6):1050–5.
6. Smith EB. Topical antifungal drugs in the treatment of tinea pedis, tinea cruris, and tinea corporis. J Am Acad Dermatol. 1993;28(5):S24–8.

Chapter 30
Psoriasis of the Penis

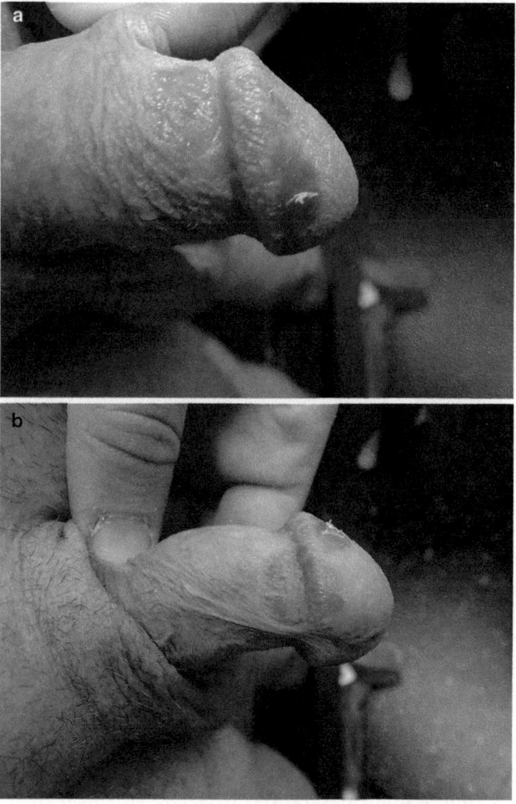

Fig. 30.1 (**a** and **b**) Scaly erythematous plaques on the penile coronal

Primary Care Visit Report

A 31-year-old male with no past medical history presented with a rash on his penis that had been present for 1 week. There was no pain, no discharge, and no dysuria. The patient had multiple sexual partners and said he had never had STD testing.

Vitals were normal. On exam, there were multiple 2–3 cm erythematous raised plaques over the meatus and glans with irregular borders and scaling. There was no pus, and no penile discharge. The penis was circumcised. The patient had no other rashes on his body.

D. Reich et al., *Top 50 Dermatology Case Studies for Primary Care*,
DOI 10.1007/978-3-319-18627-6_30

The patient was tested for HIV, syphilis, and gonorrhea/chlamydia. The patient was advised to use bacitracin ointment on the penile lesions and, if no improvement, to then try over-the-counter lotrimin cream and aquaphor lotion.

The patient was found to be positive for Chlamydia and was treated with 1 g azithromycin.

Four weeks later, the lesions on his penis persisted despite lotrimin and aquaphor. A mild Class VI steroid cream was started (desonide 0.05 % twice daily) to treat for potential psoriasis on his penis.

Discussion from Dermatology Clinic

Differential Dx

- Penile psoriasis
- Lichen planus
- Candida
- Seborrheic dermatitis
- Contact dermatitis
- Squamous cell carcinoma
- Zoon's balanitis

Favored Dx

Family history, and the examination of extensor surfaces of elbows and knees, scalp, lumbosacral region, and nails for signs of psoriatic plaques and nail pitting can help in making a diagnosis of psoriasis. Psoriatic plaques can present in isolation, however, and the penis may sometimes be the first site of onset of psoriasis. The red, scaly appearance of the lesions in this patient suggests psoriasis.

Overview

Psoriasis is a chronic, immune-mediated inflammatory skin condition characterized by red, or salmon-colored scaly plaques. Psoriasis is the most common noninfectious dermatosis that occurs on the glans penis [1]. Chronic plaque psoriasis affects approximately 2 % of the population [2, 3] with up to 40 % of those patients experiencing genital involvement [3]. Psoriasis can occur at any age. There are two peak ages of onset observed, at 16–22 years, and 57–60 years old [3]. It is most common in Caucasians [4].

The thick plaques of psoriasis are attributed to hyperproliferation of epidermal keratinocytes. Genetic, environmental, and immunological factors have been implicated in the disease's pathogenesis [2, 4].

Presentation

Penile psoriasis presents with erythematous plaques that have overlying white or silvery scales. They are often accompanied by small depressions or dents in the nails, referred to as nail pitting, and lesions on other sites of the body, commonly the extensor surfaces of knees and elbows, scalp, and intergluteal cleft [3]; however, the penis can be the initial location of psoriasis onset [1]. The plaques can be thick, thin, large, or small, and are well delineated from the surrounding normal skin. Patients usually complain of pruritus.

Workup

Penile psoriasis is diagnosed on physical examination, based on presentation and patient history. Biopsy is only recommended if the diagnosis is unclear, or if neoplasm is a consideration [3].

Treatment

Because psoriasis is chronic, treatment should focus both on resolution of active flares, as well as long-term management.

The first line of treatment for localized psoriasis is topical corticosteroids. For the genital region, mild corticosteroids, such as desonide 0.05 % (Class VI), should be prescribed, as the skin is already delicate and there is a risk of atrophy. Any accompanying lesions on sites like the trunk, arms, or legs, may be treated with stronger topical steroids. Application to the genital area twice daily for 1 week should be sufficient because the skin is readily permeable [3].

Follow-Up

Patients should follow up 2 weeks after their initial visit to ensure plaques are resolving. From there, long term management plans vary from patient to patient. Some are able to keep their condition under control with use of nonsteroidal Protopic and Elidel creams. Those with more persistent localized flares may require intermittent topical corticosteroid use in conjunction with prescription emollients, or a regimen of steroid use every other day, or only on weekends.

Other options for topical maintenance treatments include Vitamin D derivatives like calcipotriene, or tazarotene [2, 5]. It may not be feasible for patients with widespread or severe psoriasis to treat only with topical medications. There are several other treatment options available, including UVB phototherapy, cyclosporine, and biologics [2, 5]. These should be reserved for severe and recalcitrant cases, and implemented after thorough discussion of risks and benefits.

Questions for the Dermatologist

– *How do I spot psoriasis in unlikely places?*

A scaly penis is immediately suggestive of either seborrheic dermatitis or psoriasis. In the case of psoriasis, look for its features in other places, like the elbows and knees. Both can be treated with intermittent use of mild topical steroids, such as desonide 0.05 %.

– *How do I differentiate psoriasis from other lesions?*

It can be difficult to differentiate. Things that point to psoriasis would be a family history of psoriasis, and other lesions in typical locations, like the scalp, elbows, and knees.

– *Should this patient expect to have recurrent lesions now that he has had his first psoriatic lesion? Or could this just happen once and not again?*

Psoriasis is a lifetime diagnosis. It can be controlled easily, and it can be mild for some patients; however, it is likely that it will recur. It may not spread diffusely or increase in severity, but in his lifetime there will likely be other episodes of psoriatic outbreaks.

References

1. Wolff K, Johnson RA, Suurmond D. Chapter 32, Disorders of the genitalia, perineum, and anus. In: Fitzpatrick's color atlas & synopsis of clinical dermatology. 5th ed. New York: McGraw-Hill; 2005. p. 1038–9.
2. Menter A, Korman NJ, Elmets CA, Feldman SR, Gelfand JM, Gordon KB, Gottlieb A, Koo JYM, Lebwohl M, Leonardi CL, Lim HW, Van Voorhees AS, Beutner KR, Ryan C, Bhushan R. Guidelines of care for the management of psoriasis and psoriatic arthritis: Section 6. Guidelines of care for the management of psoriasis and psoriatic arthritis: case-based presentations and evidence-based conclusions. J Am Acad Dermatol. 2011;65(1):137–74.
3. Teichman JM, Sea J, Thompson IM, Elston DM. Noninfectious penile lesions. Am Fam Physician. 2010;81(2):167–74.
4. Griffiths CE, Barker JN. Pathogenesis and clinical features of psoriasis. Lancet. 2007;370(9583): 263–71.
5. Menter A, Griffiths CE. Current and future management of psoriasis. Lancet. 2007;370(9583): 272–84.

Chapter 31
Diaper Dermatitis

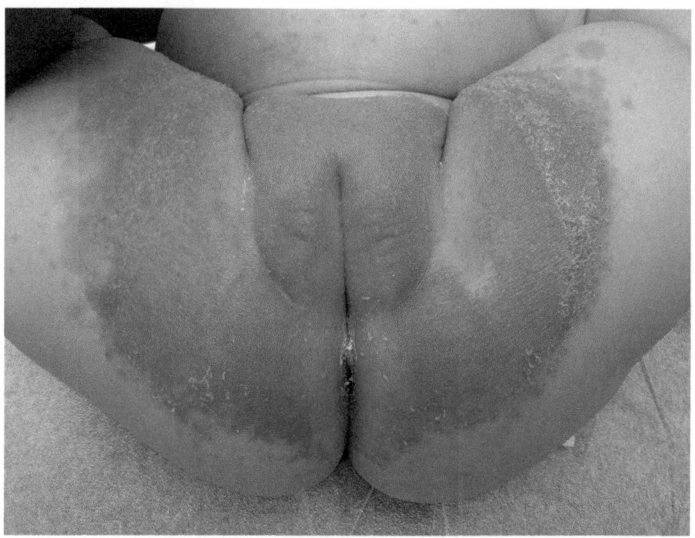

Fig. 31.1 Note relative sparing of inguinal and intergluteal areas protected from exposure

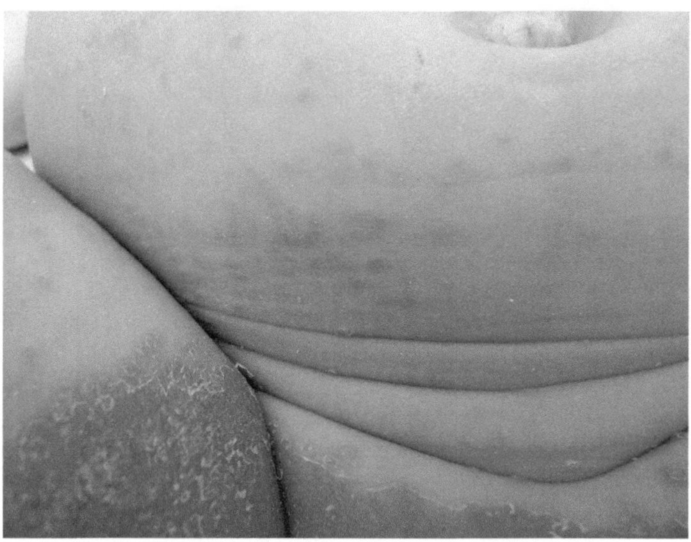

Fig. 31.2 Satellite lesions on abdomen indicate a different process than the confluent beefy red rash

D. Reich et al., *Top 50 Dermatology Case Studies for Primary Care*,
DOI 10.1007/978-3-319-18627-6_31

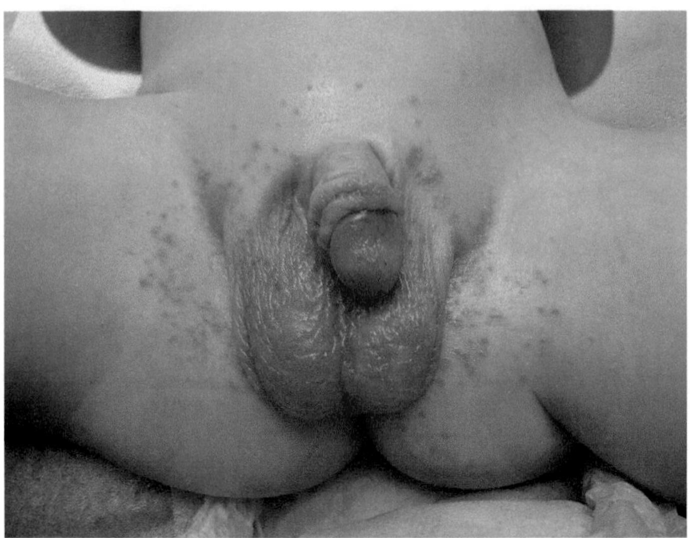

Fig. 31.3 Erythematous beefy-red satellite papules in bilateral groin

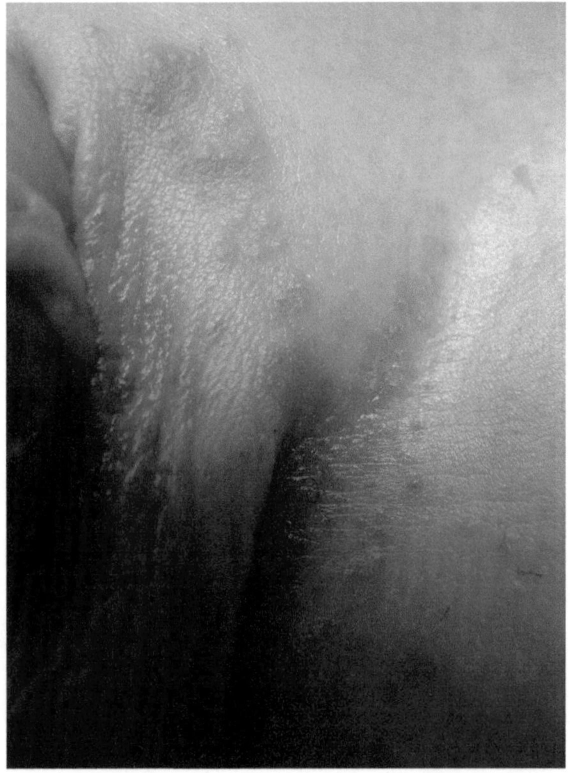

Fig. 31.4 Grouped erythematous papules in the inguinal crease

Primary Care Visit Report

The first patient was an 11-month-old female with no past medical history who presented with a diaper rash. The rash had started 6 days prior, and her parents had applied Desitin diaper rash treatment and gave her plenty of diaper-free time. They said the rash had started to spread outside the diaper area and that the patient had started scratching it. She also had a small rash in her neck fold and on her face.

Her vitals were normal. On exam, in her genital area there was a confluent 10 cm × 15 cm erythematous macular patch with scaling at the edges, with some individual erythematous satellite papular lesions on the periphery of the confluent area. Her inguinal folds had some excoriated areas. Her lower abdomen and chest had scattered 2–3 mm erythematous papular lesions.

This was treated as both irritant contact dermatitis as well as a fungal infection. The patient was prescribed over-the-counter hydrocortisone 1 % cream (Class VII) twice daily for 7 days and nystatin cream 100,000 unit/g three times daily or with every diaper change. The parents were advised to use a barrier cream such as Desitin, A&D, Vaseline, or zinc on top of the steroid cream and the nystatin. They were advised to apply the creams in this order: hydrocortisone cream first, then nystatin, and finally barrier cream.

The second patient was a 1 year-old male with no past medical history who presented with a cough, fever, and diaper rash. The patient had been seen 1 week prior for his 1-year well visit and had the diaper rash then. At that point, he was instructed to use bacitracin ointment on the rash, and to let the area air-dry after each bath. He returned 1 week later for a cough and fever that had developed 2 days after his well visit, and for a persistent diaper rash. He was urinating normally but was having loose stool.

The patient was febrile at 102.4, and his vitals were otherwise normal. On exam, there were erythematous papules and plaques on his penis, scrotum, suprapubic area, and inguinal folds. The rash was confluent on his scrotum with scattered individual papules elsewhere.

He tested positive for influenza A and was treated with Tamiflu for his cough and fever. The rash appeared to be unrelated to the flu as it preceded the flu by 2–3 days. It was treated as a fungal diaper rash with clotrimazole 1 % twice daily and as much diaper-free time as the parents could give him.

Discussion from Dermatology Clinic

Differential Dx

- Candidiasis
- Irritant dermatitis
- Atopic dermatitis

- Seborrheic dermatitis
- Allergic contact dermatitis
- Psoriasis
- Granuloma gluteale infantum
- Langerhans cell histiocytosis
- Acrodermatitis enteropathica (zinc deficiency)

Favored Dx

The female patient has a confluent, erythematous rash typical of irritant diaper dermatitis, as well as satellite papules suggestive of superimposed candidiasis. The male patient's rash is prominent in the inguinal skin folds and features papules consistent with candidal diaper rash.

Overview

Diaper dermatitis (also called napkin dermatitis or diaper rash) is a nonspecific term used to describe any inflammatory eruption of the skin in the diaper area. Although there are several causes of diaper dermatitis, the general term of diaper dermatitis is most often considered a form of irritant contact dermatitis that presents as a result of prolonged contact with urine and feces. Excessive hydration leads to maceration of the skin, which compromises its barrier function. Additionally, feces and urine increase the pH of the skin, leading to increased fecal enzyme activity and reduced protection from natural skin flora [1]. The area then becomes more susceptible to damage from friction against the diaper and cleansing wipes, as well as damage from increased contact with irritants, such as fecal proteases and lipases, ammonia, and pathogens such as bacteria and yeasts [2]. If irritant diaper dermatitis is not treated, after 3 days, it can then become secondarily infected. *Candida albicans* is the most common pathogen complicating diaper rash, which leads to candidal diaper dermatitis.

Diaper dermatitis is a very common condition, affecting one in four children under the age of 2 [1, 2]. Peak prevalence occurs between 9 and 12 months of age. The genders and races are equally affected [3]. Although diaper dermatitis is more common in children, the condition can affect people of any age who wear diapers [4].

Presentation

The presentation of diaper dermatitis depends greatly on severity. Mild cases may be asymptomatic and feature limited involvement and mild erythema. Moderate irritant diaper dermatitis presents as confluent, erythematous macules on the convex skin surfaces in direct contact with the diaper—i.e., the buttocks, upper thighs, lower abdomen, and genitalia. The skin folds, which are generally not in direct contact with the diaper, are typically spared. In more severe cases, the skin may be painful, elevated, scaly, eroded, peeling, or weeping.

Candidal diaper dermatitis presents as a beefy-red rash with papules and pustules. There may be satellite pustules outside of the main rash's border. In contrast to irritant diaper dermatitis, candidal diaper dermatitis commonly involves the skin folds. Patients with candidal diaper dermatitis have often recently taken oral antibiotics [2].

Workup

Diagnosis is made based on clinical examination. Fungal culture or KOH slide prep from skin scrapings may be done if confirmation of candidiasis is needed.

Treatment

Mild cases of irritant diaper dermatitis are often self-limiting with resolution within 2–3 days, and can simply be treated with some diaper-free time and barrier creams or ointments (such as Desitin or A&D) [3, 5]. More severe cases may warrant further treatment. Irritant diaper dermatitis is treated with mild topical corticosteroids. Prescription-strength hydrocortisone 2.5 % (Class VII) is appropriate for mild or moderate cases. Mild topical corticosteroids can be used twice daily sparingly on affected areas until the rash resolves, for up to 2 weeks under physician supervision [3, 5]. Combination products like nystatin/triamcinolone and clotrimazole/betamethasone are contraindicated due to excessive steroid potency for young children [3, 6]. Use of these products can lead to Cushing syndrome, as well as skin atrophy and telangiectasias.

Candidal diaper dermatitis is treated with topical antifungal creams. Ketoconazole and econazole are effective against *Candida*. These creams may be used 2–3 times daily until the rash resolves. Irritant diaper dermatitis with superimposed bacterial infection should be treated with topical mupirocin 3 times daily until the rash resolves [3].

Follow-Up

Over-hydration of the diaper area leads to increased absorption of corticosteroid creams, thus patients treated with topical corticosteroids should be closely monitored. Topical corticosteroids should be discontinued once the rash resolves. After diaper dermatitis has resolved, it may require long-term management. Recurrence is common as diaper dermatitis tends to be an episodic condition; however, certain preventative measures may be helpful.

When possible, periodically exposing the diaper area to air can help dry it out and restore the skin barrier [5, 6]. Powders, such as cornstarch medicated with zinc, can also help keep the area dry. They should be applied with care to avoid inhalation. Thick applications of barrier creams or ointments with zinc oxide (such as Desitin or A&D) can help reduce irritation by physically blocking the skin from contact with irritants and moisture. They may be applied with every diaper change and can be covered with petroleum jelly to avoid sticking to the diaper. Skin products with preservatives, dyes, or fragrances should be avoided [2, 3].

Diapers should be changed frequently to minimize contact with urine and feces. Cleaning with warm water and mild soap, rather than using wipes, is recommended [3, 5]. Parents may pat the area dry rather than wiping, or allow the area to air dry if possible. There is some evidence to suggest disposable diapers are more effective against diaper dermatitis than cloth diapers, although a recent Cochrane review found there was not enough evidence to support either conclusion [1, 3, 6]. Educating parents on the above recommendations, and providing support are essential to preventing recurrence of diaper dermatitis.

Questions for the Dermatologist

– *How can a fungal diaper rash be distinguished from an irritant diaper rash? Are there tell-tale signs?*

There are some clues to help distinguish between the two. Intertriginous skin surfaces of a pudgy baby's groin will typically be spared in irritant diaper dermatitis, because causative urine feces and that cause the irritation will not come into contact with those areas. Candidiasis features pustules. A candidal rash is a beefier, darker red color, classically with no sparing of skin folds, and may feature satellite pustules outside of the border of the rash. There are no such pustules in irritant diaper dermatitis.

– *Is there a difference between contact dermatitis and irritant dermatitis?*

Contact dermatitis describes an inflammatory rash that occurs as a result of exposure to a trigger. That trigger could be a chemical or physical irritant (which classifies the rash as irritant dermatitis, or irritant contact dermatitis) or an allergen (allergic dermatitis, or allergic contact dermatitis). Examples of common irritants are bleach, benzoyl peroxide, alcohol, dry air or wind, repeated or prolonged exposure to water, or mechanical friction. Common allergens include poison ivy, nickel, gold, bacitracin, neomycin, and fragrances.

– *Is it possible to have both forms of diaper rash, irritant and fungal, at the same time? Does one develop before the other? Does one form make the area more susceptible to the other?*

It can be both. If you have irritant dermatitis, you get a compromised skin barrier. At that point, a bacterial or fungal infection becomes more likely.

– *In the case above of the male with candidal diaper dermatitis, is it presumed he also had irritant dermatitis that preceded this? Or is it possible to just get candidal diaper dermatitis as a primary infection?*

It is possible to get candida diaper dermatitis without an obvious case of irritant dermatitis preceding the infection. *Candida* can invade the skin and cause an infection as long as there is a break in the continuity of the skin barrier allowing it to do so. Increased moisture in the diaper area could lead to some local maceration, which would provide an entry point for a yeast infection.

– *If both a steroid cream and a topical antifungal are prescribed, does it matter in which order they are applied?*

Ideally, as in other cases that involve a differential diagnosis of an eczematous process vs. tinea, you would pick one class of medication and try it for 1–2 weeks to help determine the nature of the rash. However, there are instances like this one when you would want to use a low potency steroid together with an antifungal. The low potency steroid will address the inflammatory component of diaper dermatitis, and should not promulgate any fungal infection. It does not really matter in what order they are applied. If a barrier cream is also being applied, it should be put on last.

– *What steroid potency is okay to use on the genital area? What is the duration of treatment?*

A low potency (Class V–VII) steroid, such as hydrocortisone 2.5 % (Class VII) for up to 2 weeks is appropriate.

– *Should the fungal cream be applied with every diaper change?*

If an azole cream is given, it should be applied twice daily. We do not recommend its use, but if the patient is using nystatin, it may be applied with every diaper change for a few days. However, if no improvement is noted, they should switch to an azole antifungal.

– *How do you know when to prescribe nystatin cream and when to use clotrimazole?*

Our practice does not prescribe a lot of nystatin, or clotrimazole. Clotrimazole and nystatin have decent coverage against yeasts, but I start with a prescription-strength azole medication for yeast infections. Econazole and ketoconazole 2 % are good options, but most azoles have similar effects.

– *When is it also necessary to apply a barrier cream—with the fungal form, or only with the irritant form?*

A barrier cream can be helpful for both. It will help protect the skin from any additional irritants and pathogens in the area.

– *Does it help to have diaper free time?*

Yes, it might be helpful but it could also be impractical. It would help dry out the irritated area. I would measure this recommendation against the potential hassle. Diaper dermatitis can be treated without diaper free time.

– *Is there something the parents can do when they first notice the rash developing to keep it from progressing?*

Parents can start with over-the-counter treatments: clotrimazole for darker red rashes with pustules, or hydrocortisone 1 % for irritant diaper dermatitis. Alternatively they can try both until they get to their doctor.

References

1. Baer EL, Davies MW, Easterbrook KJ. Disposable nappies for preventing napkin dermatitis in infants. Cochrane Database Syst Rev. 2006;3, CD004262.
2. Atherton DJ. A review of the pathophysiology, prevention and treatment of irritant diaper dermatitis. Curr Med Res Opin. 2004;20(5):645–9.
3. Shin HT. Diagnosis and management of diaper dermatitis. Pediatr Clin North Am. 2014;61(2):367–82.
4. Ward DB, Fleischer Jr AB, Feldman SR, Krowchuk DP. Characterization of diaper dermatitis in the United States. Arch Pediatr Adolesc Med. 2000;154(9):943–6.
5. Kane KS, Lio PA, Stratigos A, Johnson RA. Section 3, Diaper dermatitis and rashes in the diaper area. In: Color atlas and synopsis of pediatric dermatology. 2nd ed. New York: McGraw-Hill Professional Publishing; 2009. p. 54–6.
6. Klunk C, Domingues E, Wiss K. An update on diaper dermatitis. Clin Dermatol. 2014;32(4): 477–87.

Chapter 32
Genital Lesions: Molluscum Contagiosum and Warts

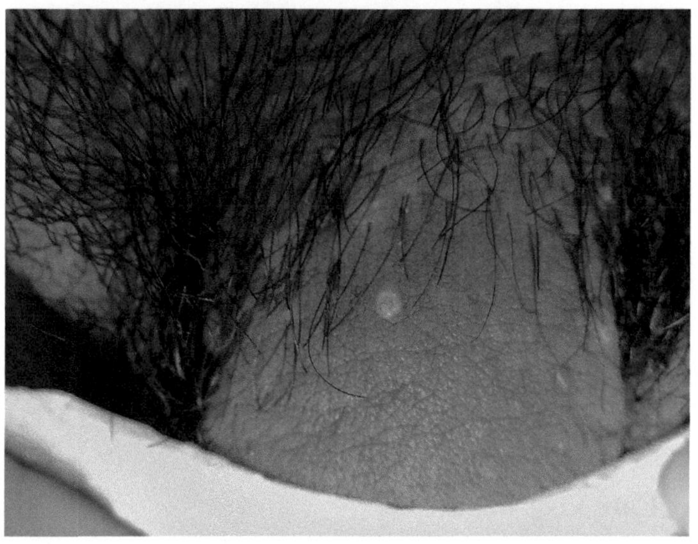

Fig. 32.1 Variably umbilicated pink shiny 3–4 mm papules on penile shaft

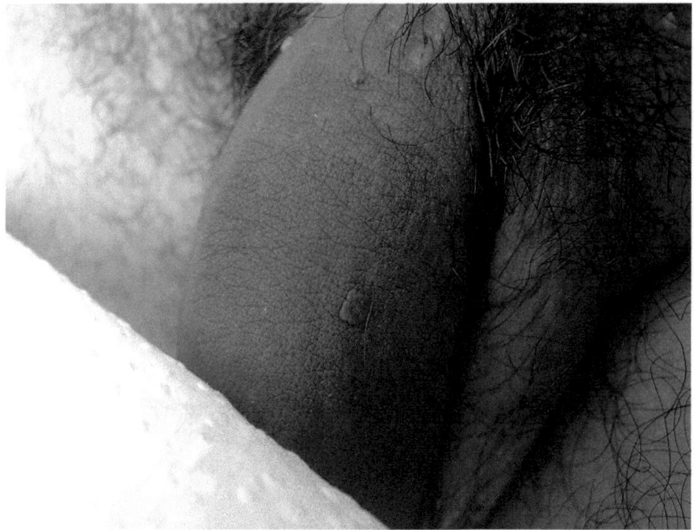

Fig. 32.2 Flesh-toned flat topped verrucous papules on penile shaft

D. Reich et al., *Top 50 Dermatology Case Studies for Primary Care*,
DOI 10.1007/978-3-319-18627-6_32

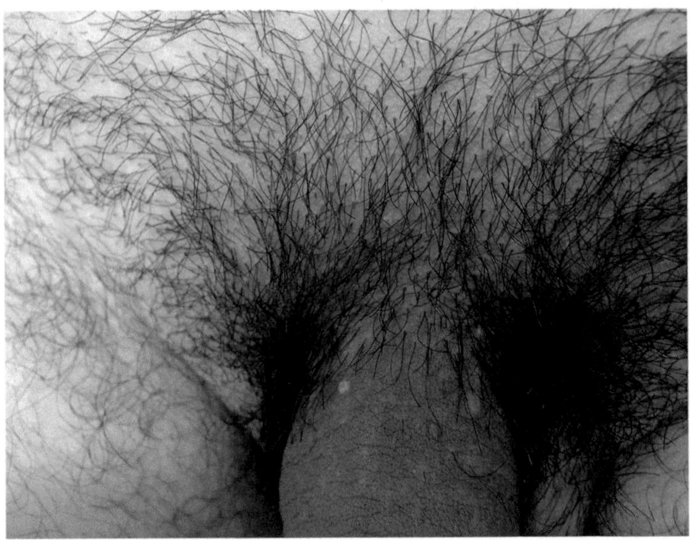

Fig. 32.3 Note here the difference between molluscum and warts found here concurrently on penile shaft

Primary Care Visit Report

A 27-year-old male with past medical history of genital warts presented with new lesions in his genital area. The wart-like lesions had been present for about 1 year. The smaller pink lesions had been present for 2–3 weeks. All were non-itchy. The patient had been to a urologist 3 weeks prior, who advised the lesions were both molluscum contagiosum and genital warts. The urologist gave the patient a prescription for cryo sticks to use at home, but he had not been able to find these in any pharmacy.

Vitals were normal. On examination, there were approximately 20 lesions scattered on his pubic mound, shaft of penis and medial thighs. The smallest lesion was 1–2 mm, the largest was about 7–8 mm. Some lesions were irregularly textured flesh-colored papules, and other lesions were smooth, erythematous papules with central umbilication.

About 20 lesions were treated with cryotherapy, treating with two sets of 30 s of iceball formation per lesion (with complete thawing in between each set). The patient was also given Aldara (imiquimod) 5 % cream to use three times per week after the lesions had healed from cryotherapy.

The patient returned 2 weeks later and said all lesions that were frozen with cryotherapy had fallen off but he also noticed that some new lesions had formed. Cryotherapy was again performed on all remaining lesions. The patient never used the Aldara cream.

Discussion from Dermatology Clinic

Dermatology was in agreement with the urologist that the penis featured both molluscum contagiosum and genital warts. Both conditions are discussed separately below.

Molluscum Contagiosum

Differential Dx

- Molluscum contagiosum
- Verruca

Favored Dx

The lesions at the base and proximal shaft of the penis have a smooth, pearly appearance consistent with molluscum contagiosum.

Overview

Molluscum contagiosum (MC) is a skin infection caused by the Molluscum Contagiosum virus (MCV), a type of poxvirus. It is spread by person-to-person contact. MC is a common infection in children, with incidence rates estimated between 5.6 and 7.4 %, and much higher during outbreaks in closed communities [1]. Children with atopic dermatitis are more susceptible to MC, and have a higher likelihood of developing multiple lesions and a prolonged course of illness [1–3]. Adulthood MC primarily affects the genital region and is considered a sexually transmitted disease [4].

MC is usually benign and self-limiting in healthy individuals; however, it may take 6–12 months to resolve [1]. Immunocompromised persons, including HIV-infected individuals, can develop very large lesions (>15 mm), overlaying bacterial superinfections, and a prolonged and more severe course of disease [2]. The prevalence in HIV-infected people may be as high as 18 % [1]. Patients with HIV/AIDS are more likely to develop lesions on extragenital sites.

Presentation

MC lesions typically present as multiple, skin-colored or pearly-white dome-shaped papules that are 2–5 mm in size. Lesions often feature a central depression, referred to in the literature as an umbilication. There may be surrounding erythema and eczematous patches, sometimes called molluscum dermatitis [3]. Typically 1–20 lesions present on a healthy patient; however, hundreds can appear in some cases. Children can develop lesions anywhere, while adults typically present with lesions on the genitals, perineum, inner thighs, mons pubis, and lower abdomen. MC lesions may appear in a linear arrangement if patients have scratched and spread them. Scratching can also cause vulnerability to secondary infections, which may be noted.

Workup

MC is typically a clinical diagnosis. A biopsy is indicated if a deep fungal infection such as histoplasmosis is on the list of differential diagnoses for any severely immunocompromised people.

Treatment

MC is typically a self-limiting infection; however, aesthetic and contagion concerns, or prolonged presence of lesions may prompt individuals to seek treatment. Immunocompromised patients with MC should be referred to dermatology or an infectious disease specialist.

MC lesions are treated by physical destruction. This may be achieved by applying cantharidin, salicylic acid, or retinoids. Physical destruction may also be achieved by cryosurgery, or curettage; however, there are considerations for associated pain and a slight risk of scarring with those procedures [2]. A recent Cochrane Database review did not find enough evidence to support any single therapy against molluscum, and treatment is not necessary due to the benign, self-limiting nature in most cases [1]. Treatment options should be thoroughly discussed with the patient.

For pediatric patients, cantharidin 0.7 % may be used to treat individual lesions. This is often applied using the wood end of a cotton-tipped applicator. It must be carefully applied only to lesions and not to healthy skin, and rinsed off after 4 h. Cantharidin causes blistering within 1–2 days, and the lesion typically resolves within 1 week [5]. Clearance has been reported in up to 90 % of patients [6]. Rarely it may cause severe blistering that results in scarring [3]. It is not recommended for use on the face or genital area [4]. Imiquimod 5 % cream is an immune response modifier that may be used to treat MC in adults; however, it is not approved as a treatment for MC in children. Clearance in 50 % of adult genital MC lesions has been noted [7]. It may cause erythema and pruritus in some patients.

The preferred treatment for adult genital MC is curettage or cryotherapy [2]. Topical anesthetic should be used prior to curettage as it can be painful. One study found that use of imiquimod combined with destruction led to lower recurrence rates [7]. Cryosurgery is a reliable mode of lesion destruction; however, it may be uncomfortable for patients with many lesions, and it may involve multiple treatments due to the appearance of new lesions. Both curettage and cryotherapy may cause scarring.

Follow-Up

If patients choose to treat MC, they may require multiple visits. Lesions should be reevaluated after 1–2 weeks to monitor healing, and patients should be examined for new lesions. Scratching the lesions should be avoided, as it makes the skin more susceptible to secondary bacterial infection. MC can spread by autoinoculation so patients should avoid touching lesions. There is no need to keep children away from school if they have MC. If there is concern of spreading the virus, the lesions may be covered with bandages. This also aids in avoiding touching the lesions. Adults should avoid intimate contact until the genital lesions have resolved.

Genital Warts

Differential Dx

- Genital warts (AKA condylomata acuminata)
- Molluscum contagiosum
- Pearly penile papules
- Condylomata lata of secondary syphilis
- Premalignant or malignant tumor (e.g., squamous cell carcinoma, penile carcinoma in situ, Bowen disease of the penis)

Favored Dx

The lesion on the shaft of the patient's penis has a fleshy, verrucous appearance consistent with a genital wart.

Overview

Anogenital warts—also called condyloma acuminata—are a common sexually transmitted infection (STI) that causes superficial skin lesions in the anogenital area. The lesions are caused by the dsDNA human papillomavirus (HPV). While there are over 70 unique strains of HPV, about 35 of these subtypes are specific for the anogenital epithelium. Of those, the low-risk subtypes 6 and 11 are the most common cause of anogenital warts and are present in up to 95 % of lesions [8–10].

Anogenital warts are highly contagious through skin-to-skin contact, with transmission rates of up to 65 % [10, 11]. Viral particles infect the skin epithelium and mucosa by entering the skin in areas where the epithelial barrier is compromised, especially where there is maceration or trauma from sexual intercourse.

After inoculation, the virus has a typical incubation period of 3 weeks to 8 months, with warts usually appearing within 2–3 months [11, 12]. Viral particles shed—and therefore are contagious—while warts are visible, as well as during subclinical infection when lesions may not be visible (i.e., asymptomatic carriers with lesions that can not be detected by inspection alone but might be detectable by aceto-white or other methods). However, viral particles are not shed during latent infection which occurs after someone acquires HPV but before presenting with any lesions. This latent period can last up to 8 months and some people remain in latency indefinitely and never go on to develop lesions [11, 12]. When genital warts are adequately treated, the median time to complete clearance is about 6 months. Up to 90 % of people with high- or low-risk HPV clear the infection within 2 years.

HPV is the most common viral STI in the USA, with an estimated incidence of 1–3 % in sexually active adults and adolescents. It is slightly more common in women than men. Women primarily contract genital warts through vaginal intercourse [11]. For men, lesions on the penile shaft and foreskin can occur through heterosexual sex; however, most perianal lesions are seen in men who have anal-receptive sex with men. There is an increased incidence of HPV infection in both sexes among individuals who have multiple sexual partners, or whose partner has had multiple sexual partners. Peak incidence of HPV occurs in the 15–30-year-old age group. Twenty to 30 % of patients with anogenital warts have another STI present, so consultation should include recent sexual history to identify risk factors for HIV and other infections, as well as discussion of STI screening [8].

While the majority of anogenital warts are benign, it is possible for lesions to be coinfected with high-risk subtypes, such as subtype 16, a strain that carries a higher risk of malignant transformation. Coinfection with high-risk strains is somewhat common, occurring in up to one third of HPV infections [13]. Infections with high-risk strains may resolve spontaneously. However, if the lesions are ulcerated, are recalcitrant to treatment, or fail to resolve after 6 months, they are at higher risk of progressing to malignancy and biopsy is indicated.

Given their frequency, likelihood of recurrence, and potential for disfigurement, genital warts represent a significant economic and psychosocial burden. Patients should be reassured the lesions are common and relatively harmless, and counseled on ways to practice safe sex and prevent transmission to partners.

Presentation

Genital warts are diagnosed clinically. Lesions may appear in isolation; however, it is more common for 5–15 discrete lesions to occur. The lesions are typically a few millimeters in diameter and rarely coalesce, except in immunocompromised hosts. Lesions may be flat, smooth, papular, verrucous, or cauliflower-like. They may feature underlying erythema. Patients may report pain or itching in the affected area. In men genital warts typically appear on the glans and shaft of the penis. They often appear under the foreskin of uncircumcised men. In women the lesions appear in the vulvovaginal and cervical areas. Lesions can also affect the urethra and perianal area of either sex.

Workup

Genital warts are diagnosed on clinical appearance. Biopsy is not always necessary. Indications for biopsy include uncertain diagnosis, and lesions that are unresponsive to treatment and suspected to be caused by high-risk subtypes. Consider screening for additional STIs (e.g., gonorrhea, chlamydia, syphilis, Hepatitis B or C, HIV) depending on the patient history, as they frequently occur with genital warts. A Papanicolaou smear would be indicated for females with cervical lesions to rule out any coinfection of the lesions with high-risk strains [9, 14]. Partner screening may be offered.

Treatment

Treatment of genital warts is guided by the size, number, and morphology of warts, their anatomical location, and patient preference. Warts close to the urethral meatus warrant a referral to a urologist, and cervical warts should be managed by a gynecologist. Warts in the anal canal should be referred to a colorectal surgeon.

For external warts, the available treatment options are provider-administered tissue destruction and excision techniques. These are cryotherapy with liquid nitrogen, electrodessication, application of trichloroacetic acid, and excision by curettage. Viable patient-administered therapy is by immune-modulating topical medication such as imiquimod (Aldara) 5 % cream, or podophyllotoxin (Condylox) 0.5 % gel. Topical medications are recommended as an adjunct rather than alternative treatment.

First-line treatment for patients with a small number of papular warts on the shaft of the penis or vulva is cryotherapy with liquid nitrogen. Two freeze–thaw cycles are recommended, done by spraying liquid nitrogen onto the lesions for 5–10 s to achieve frost, waiting about 30 s and then repeating the procedure. Clearance rates are estimated to be up to 88 % within three treatments [10, 11]. There may be some blistering or irritation in the treated area for up to 3 weeks after treatment. Cryotherapy may be performed in isolation, or in combination with a patient-administered topical medication.

As an adjunct to provider-administered therapy, patients with clusters of external soft warts may also self-administer topical podophyllotoxin 0.5 % gel. Treatment occurs in cycles, with 3 days of twice-daily treatment followed by 4 days off. This treatment cycle is repeated 4–5 times. Podophyllotoxin can cause local erythema and irritation, and it is contraindicated in pregnancy. Reported clearance rates are in the range of 40–70 % [10, 11].

External warts may also be treated with topical imiquimod 5 %. Imiquimod is applied three times per week at night and washed off in the morning. Treatment should continue until warts resolve, for a maximum of 16 weeks. Clearance rates are similar to those of podophyllotoxin. Imiquimod should not be used on internal lesions and it is contraindicated in pregnancy. Along with treating visible lesions, topical medications such as imiquimod have the additional advantage of potentially treating any subclinical lesions that have not yet become visible on examination, and would therefore not be treated with a physician-administered tissue destruction method.

The only treatment with clearance rate close to 100 % is surgery [10]. Surgical excision also carries the advantage of removing most lesions quickly, during a single office visit. Surgical excision is recommended for a small number of hardened or coalesced warts. The procedure may cause scarring.

If no treatment is pursued, genital warts can spontaneously resolve, remain the same, or grow in number or size [14].

Follow-Up

Most genital warts resolve within 3 months for patients with competent immune systems who comply with their treatment regimen. Treatments target symptomatic lesions; however, they do not eradicate the virus, which can remain latent in infected individuals for the duration of their lifetime. For this reason, all treatment modalities carry about a 20 % risk of wart recurrence within 3 months of treatment and a 30–70 % chance of recurrence after 6 months. Spontaneous regression of lesions can also occur in 20–30 % of condyloma cases [8, 10]. Following up with patients within 2–3 weeks ensures their response to treatment can be monitored and any new lesions can be addressed. It also permits clarification of patient-administered treatment regimen so that they may potentially treat any recurrence.

It is recommended that patients avoid sexual intercourse while irritation or any wounds from therapeutic intervention are healing. Sexual contact should be avoided while warts are present in order to decrease transmission rates. While they have no effect on individuals who have already been infected by these strains of HPV, the quadrivalent recombinant HPV vaccine (Gardasil), which protects against HPV types 6, 11, 16, and 18, may be considered for young men and women in order to help prevent HPV infection rates.

Questions for the Dermatologist

– *How can you tell the difference between MC and genital warts?*

Molluscum contagiosum lesions are umbilicated, translucent, flesh-toned papules with a smooth top. Warts are pink, brown, or flesh toned, verrucous, rough papules.

– *Is MC treated differently, or can cryotherapy be used for both MC and genital warts?*

Cryotherapy is appropriate for both MC and genital warts. You could also hyfrecate both, or scrape both types of lesions with a curette. Most of the treatments for the two conditions overlap. However, cantharidin, a compound derived from blister beetles, is primarily used for MC and not warts. The virus that causes warts (HPV) lives in basal epithelial cells that tend to be too deep for cantharidin to penetrate. MC is a more superficial process.

– *Is there an optimal amount of time the liquid nitrogen should be sprayed? Is this amount of time constant spraying? Or spray as needed to keep the skin white? How long do you thaw for? How many freeze–thaw cycles are appropriate?*

You typically want to achieve about 8–10 s of frost. That does not mean constant spraying for 8–10 s. It should take close to 3 s of spraying for the lesion to stay frosty for about 5 more seconds. We typically perform 2–3 freeze–thaw cycles, depending on what the patient can tolerate.

– *How often should cryotherapy be performed? How many cryo treatments are recommended and how much time should elapse between them?*

Cryotherapy should be performed every 2 weeks. Our practice averages three sessions for common warts; however, the number of treatments will depend on how many warts are present and the host's immunity.

– *Are there different results between cryo vs. aldara vs. acid treatments? Which is preferred?*

A destruction method like cryotherapy or curettage is preferable for adult genital MC. Otherwise any irritant would work well. Salicylic acid (for non-genital MC), and the retinoid tazarotene (not for children under 12) irritate the skin and send inflammatory cells to the area, which notice and respond to the virus. Until recently, Aldara (imiquimod) was a component of pediatric MC treatment. However, in trials with almost 700 children, imiquimod performed as well as placebo, so we no longer use it to treat childhood MC [15].

– *Are there any home remedies or self-cryo that can be done?*

Some patients use apple cider vinegar, or Dr. Scholl's cryotherapy. Anecdotally, there have been mixed results. The cryotherapy tends not to be cold enough to destroy some warts. Vinegar can be a decent irritator of the skin. Pharmacological agents have better irritants that provoke the immune system to attack viral particles.

– *Does bacitracin have to be applied after treatment with cryo?*

No, there is no skin disruption after cryotherapy so bacitracin is not necessary. If the MC lesions, or warts, have been aggressively frozen and an ulcer forms, then yes, bacitracin may be needed. However if there is no skin barrier rupture, and normally there should not be, then bacitracin is not needed.

– *Does Aldara work on both MC and warts?*

Aldara works against warts; however, it is not useful in treating MC.

References

1. van der Wouden JC, Menke J, Gajadin S, Koning S, Tasche MJ, van Suijlekom-Smit LW, Berger MY, Butler CC. Interventions for cutaneous molluscum contagiosum. Cochrane Database Syst Rev. 2006;2, CD004767.
2. Hughes CM, Damon IK, Reynolds MG. Understanding U.S. healthcare providers' practices and experiences with molluscum contagiosum. PLoS One. 2013;8(10):e76948.
3. Piggott C, Friedlander S, Tom W. Chapter 195. Poxvirus infections. In: Goldsmith LA, Katz SI, Gilchrest BA, Paller AS, Leffell DJ, Wolff K, editors. Fitzpatrick's dermatology in general medicine. 8th ed. New York: McGraw-Hill; 2012. Available from: http://accessmedicine.mhmedical.com.ezproxy.cul.columbia.edu/content.aspx?bookid=392&Sectionid=41138924. Accessed 4 Mar 2015.
4. Basta-Juzbašić A, Čeović R. Chancroid, lymphogranuloma venereum, granuloma inguinale, genital herpes simplex infection, and molluscum contagiosum. Clin Dermatol. 2014;32(2):290–8.
5. Moed L, Shwayder TA, Chang M. Cantharidin revisited: a blistering defense of an ancient medicine. Arch Dermatol. 2001;137(10):1357–60.
6. Skinner Jr RB. Treatment of molluscum contagiosum with imiquimod 5% cream. J Am Acad Dermatol. 2002;47(4 Suppl):S221–4.
7. Hengge UR, Cusini M. Topical immunomodulators for the treatment of external genital warts, cutaneous warts and molluscum contagiosum. Br J Dermatol. 2003;149 Suppl 66:15–9.
8. Delaney EK, Baguley S. Genital warts. BMJ. 2008;337:a1171.
9. Androphy EJ, Kirnbauer R. Chapter 196. Human papilloma virus infections. In: Goldsmith LA, Katz SI, Gilchrest BA, Paller AS, Leffell DJ, Wolff K, editors. Fitzpatrick's dermatology in general medicine. 8th ed. New York: McGraw-Hill; 2012. Available from: http://access-

medicine.mhmedical.com.ezproxy.cul.columbia.edu/Content.aspx?bookid=392&Sectionid=41138925. Accessed 13 Mar 2016.

10. Lacey CJ, Woodhall SC, Wikstrom A, Ross J. 2012 European guideline for the management of anogenital warts. J Eur Acad Dermatol Venereol. 2013;27(3):e263–70.
11. Fathi R, Tsoukas MM. Genital warts and other HPV infections: established and novel therapies. Clin Dermatol. 2014;32(2):299–306.
12. Anic GM, Giuliano AR. Genital HPV infection and related lesions in men. Prev Med. 2011;53 Suppl 1:S36–41.
13. Garland SM, Steben M, Sings HL, James M, Lu S, Railkar R, Barr E, Haupt RM, Joura EA. Natural history of genital warts: analysis of the placebo arm of 2 randomized phase III trials of a quadrivalent human papillomavirus (types 6, 11, 16, and 18) vaccine. J Infect Dis. 2009;199(6):805–14.
14. Anogenital Warts—2015 STD Treatment Guidelines [Internet]. Cdc.gov. 2016 [cited 7 April 2016]. Available from: http://www.cdc.gov/std/tg2015/warts.htm
15. Katz KA. Dermatologists, imiquimod, and treatment of molluscum contagiosum in children: righting wrongs. JAMA Dermatol. 2015;151(2):125–6.

Part VII
Lesions Affecting Multiple Areas

Chapter 33
Thermal Scald Burn

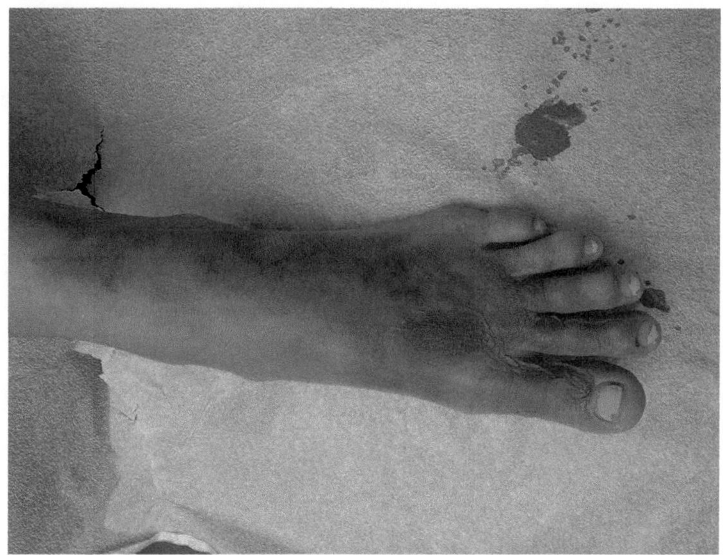

Fig. 33.1 Areas of erythema proximal to blistered areas represent more superficial injury

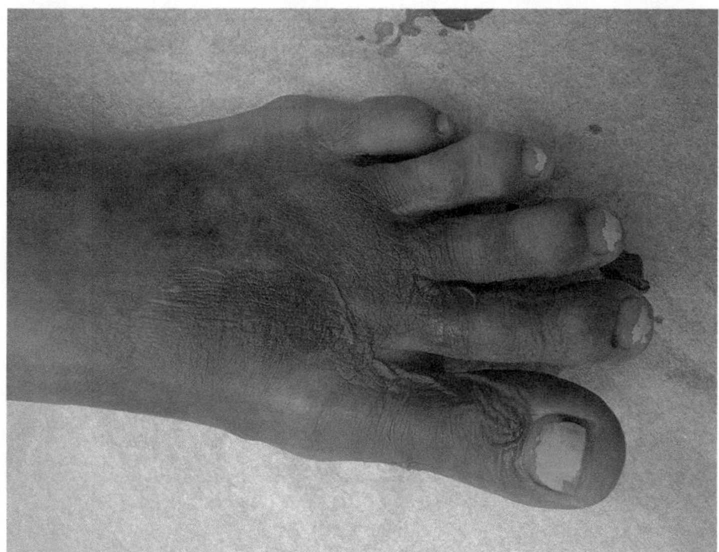

Fig. 33.2 Figurate bullae with serous drainage dorsal foot

D. Reich et al., *Top 50 Dermatology Case Studies for Primary Care*,
DOI 10.1007/978-3-319-18627-6_33

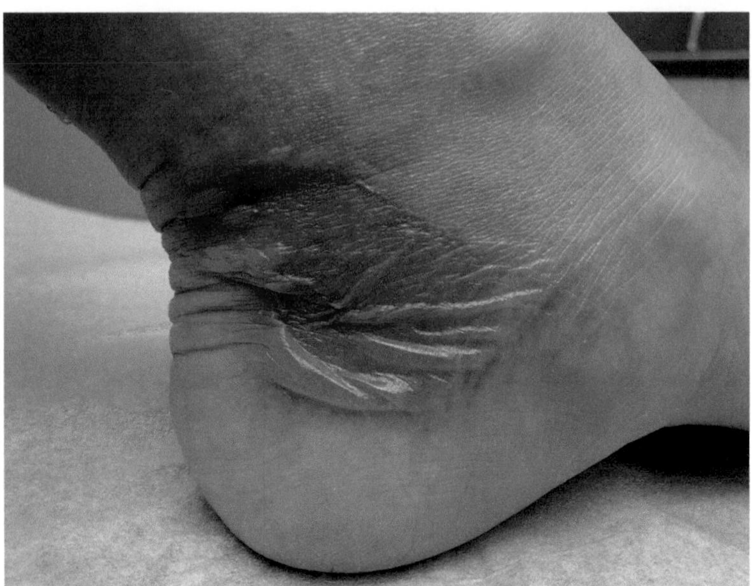

Fig. 33.3 Flaccid bullae at left ankle

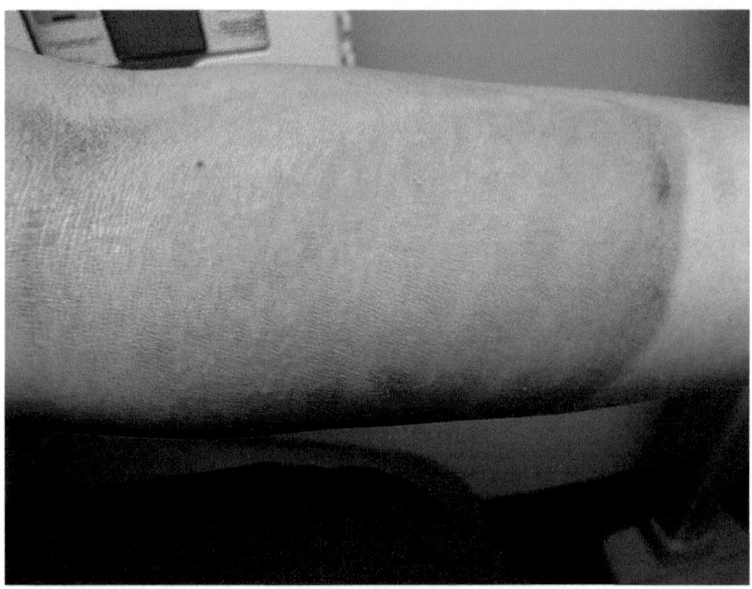

Fig. 33.4 Note sharp cutoff most consistent with an external source

Primary Care Visit Report

A 39-year-old female presented with burns to her foot, ankle, and forearm. Five days prior, she had been carrying a pot of boiling water when it slipped out of her hand and scalded her left foot and her left forearm. Immediately after the incident, the skin of the left foot and ankle blistered. She had been putting Neosporin on the burns, wrapping them in gauze, and wearing her clogs to continue working as a professional cook. She had been taking 400–600 mg ibuprofen every 6 h as needed for the pain. She came in to be seen because the pain was becoming intolerable.

Vitals were normal. On exam, the left dorsal aspect of her left foot and toes had a 12 cm × 17 cm erythematous base with an overlying intact roof from burst bullae (with no remaining fluid inside). The left medial heel area had a 4 cm × 6 cm erythematous base with intact bullae, and the left forearm had an 11 cm × 7 cm erythematous macular area, with no blisters or bullae.

The patient's burn was treated with silver sulfadiazene and the area was wrapped in gauze, with instructions to change the dressing twice daily. The patient was also referred to a burn clinic given the involvement of her toes and ankle. The patient was given a prescription for 50 mg tramadol every 6 h as needed to help with pain control. Her tetanus immunization was up to date.

Discussion from Dermatology Clinic

Differential Dx

- Thermal scald burn
- Chemical burn
- Cellulitis

Favored Dx

Patient history and examination indicate a partial-thickness thermal scald burn.

Overview

Burn injuries can occur after exposure to flames, heat, chemicals, or electricity. Several vital functions of the skin can be compromised after injury, including its protective barrier, fluid homeostasis, thermoregulation, immunologic, and neurosensory functions.

The American Burn Association estimates that almost half a million people receive medical treatment for burns each year in the USA [1]. Male burn victims outnumber females in all age groups except patients above the age of 80, in which women show a slight predominance. The age group with the highest prevalence of burns is between 20 and 60, although children below the age of 16 account for a substantial proportion at 30 % [2]. The majority of children who experience burn injuries are under 3 years of age [3]. Almost three quarters of burns affect less than 10 % of total body surface area (TBSA). The most common causes of burn injury are fire and scalding accidents, accounting for 80 % of cases [2]. Scald burns (which are caused by heated liquids or steam) account for the majority of pediatric burn injuries [3, 4]. Most of these data come from hospitalization studies, thus representing more severe burn injuries. However, of the over one million burn injuries that occur in the USA annually, the majority are minor burns and can be managed on an outpatient basis.

Burns have a wide range of severity, with the most severe associated with an increased risk in morbidity and mortality. Populations especially vulnerable to infections, delayed healing, and increased morbidity from burns include diabetics and immunocompromised populations. Children with burn wounds should be evaluated for the possibility of child abuse.

Presentation

Burns can be grouped into three categories depending on severity. Superficial or epidermal (first degree) burns involve only the epidermis. Partial thickness (second degree) burns involve the epidermis and part of the dermis. The degree of damage to the dermis further classifies burns as superficial partial thickness, or deep partial thickness where blood vessels, nerves, and hair follicles may be involved. Full thickness (third degree) burns involve the entirety of the epidermis and dermis, and may include involvement of bones and muscles. The term fourth degree is sometimes used to describe the most severe burns that extend into bone, muscles, and joints.

Superficial burns tend to be painful, dry, and erythematous. They do not blister and they blanch with pressure. Two to three days after the initial burn, the pain and erythema usually subside. Four days after the initial burn, the injured epidermis begins to peel revealing the newly healed epidermis. Full healing generally occurs in about 6 days. This is commonly seen with sunburns.

Partial thickness burns are blistered, red, and very painful. Superficial partial thickness burns will generally form blisters between the epidermis and dermis within 24 h of the initial burn, thus what might appear at first to be an epidermal burn may reveal itself to be partial thickness 24 h later. These burns are moist, often weep, they blanch with pressure, and generally heal in 7–21 days. Scarring is rare but pigment changes can be seen.

Deep partial thickness burns involve more of the dermis, including hair follicles and glandular tissue. They are painful only to pressure, appear wet or waxy dry, have blisters that are easily unroofed, can have a mottled color (patchy white to red) and do not blanch with pressure. These burns will generally heal in 3–9 weeks.

Patients with full thickness burns may present without complaints of pain. These burns can feature any number of colors—white, red, charred, pink, or burgundy. Vessels will be visibly burnt under the dead skin and hairs can be pulled easily from follicles. The skin is dry (there are no blisters), inelastic and the burnt area does not blanch with pressure. Full thickness burns are more likely to feature systemic consequences, such as fever, osmotic shock, and hypovolemia. They should be referred to a burn center as they may require fluid replacement, nutritional therapy, and surgical intervention.

Workup

Patient history and physical examination provide the basis for diagnosing burns. Physical examination should assess the severity of the injury by evaluating the depth of burn, and taking into account the age of the patient, the anatomical location of the burn, potential injury to any other vital organs, and TBSA involvement. Based on that assessment, burns can be classified as minor, moderate, or major according to the American Burn Association's burn injury severity grading system. ECGs should be performed for any patients reporting electrical injuries.

TBSA involvement for partial- and full-thickness burns only (superficial burns are not included in TBSA) can be estimated using either a Lund–Browder chart or the "Rule of Nines." Lund–Browder is best used for children (and adults as well) and assigns relative percentage of body surface area based on age. For adults, a quicker method is to use the "Rule of Nines" which assigns each leg 18 % TBSA, each arm 9 % TBSA, anterior and posterior trunk each 18 % TBSA, and the head 9 % TBSA.

Treatment

Treatment of burn injuries depends on location, depth, and severity, and ranges from self-treatment to surgical interventions. Management of superficial and partial thickness burns should aim for promoting healing and minimizing bacterial infection. This can be done with topical antimicrobials and dressings.

The treatment of burn blisters is not unanimously agreed upon. For ruptured blisters, many argue for keeping the ruptured blister roof intact for natural wound protection and others argue that ruptured blisters should be debrided. For intact blisters, there is similar division with some arguing for leaving the blisters intact and others arguing for unroofing the intact blisters. There are no well-designed studies that offer conclusive answers.

Similarly, there is no consensus on which specific topical agent or which dressing is best for burn wound management. However, since burns are at risk of bacterial colonization and infection, a topical antibiotic should be put on any non-superficial burn. Polysporin ointment (a combination of bacitracin zinc and polymyxin B sulfate) is often used as the chosen antimicrobial and then covered with a nonadherent dressing. For deeper wounds or if there is concern for MRSA, mupirocin can be used instead. Superficial burns and superficial partial-thickness burns with an intact epidermis do not need topical antibiotics—instead a bismuth-impregnated petroleum based gauze (i.e., xeroform) can be used and then covered with a bulky dressing. Xeroform can also be used as a non-adherent dressing on clean partial-thickness burns (without intact epidermis).

The author's preferred dressings for superficial and partial-thickness burns are ones containing hydrogel. Hydrogel dressings lead to strong healing outcomes and reduce pain by hydrating the wound. They consist of up to 90 % water or glycerin, which creates an ideal, moist environment for wound healing and autolytic debridement. Hydrogel is available over the counter as an amorphous gel in a tube, impregnated onto gauze, or on a sheet. The gel form (e.g., Tegaderm or DuoDERM) is ideal for burn wounds that are large in surface area or irregularly shaped. The gel can be applied to the wound with nonstick gauze and then wrapped with a secondary dressing. Hydrogel in sheet form (e.g., Aquasorb, AquaDerm, or Derma-gel) has the hydrogel suspended inside a thin mesh and can be cut to fit the burn's shape. The hydrogel dressings can be applied on top of any topical antibiotic. Hydrogel dressings are not appropriate for burns with heavy exudate as they have limited absorptive capacity. They should be changed at minimum every 4 days, or when the wound seems abundantly moist.

Wrapping the wound, after applying the initial treatment of choice (topical antibiotic, hydrogel and/or xeroform), is best done with a first layer of non-adherent gauze, then a second layer of fluffed dry gauze and an outer layer of an elastic gauze roll (i.e., Kerlix). If fingers and toes are involved, they need to be individually wrapped and separated with fluffed gauze to keep them from adhering to each other.

Although silver sulfadiazene cream is still commonly used, there is some evidence that it increases risk of bacterial infection and wound healing time due to toxic effects on developing keratinocytes [5–7]. Some traditional gauze dressings adhere to the newly forming epithelium and traumatize it when they are changed. Consequently they have fallen out of favor and non-adherent gauze is preferred.

There is little evidence to support use of prophylactic systemic antibiotics in burn wound management except with smoke inhalation burns which can increase the risk of developing pneumonia [6]. Patients may be given over-the-counter or prescription-strength analgesics to treat pain as necessary.

It is important to ask the patient about their tetanus status and if due or unknown, to give a tetanus shot, especially for any burns deeper than superficial-thickness.

Follow-Up

Superficial wounds tend to heal within 1–2 weeks. More severe wounds may take months to heal. Patients with superficial and partial thickness burns should be evaluated again after 1 week to ensure the healing process is under way and to look for any scarring or contracture. They should be monitored for infections and cellulitis. If the wounds begin to smell, ooze lots of fluid, become more painful, or edematous, they should be instructed to follow up immediately.

Scarring tends to be minimal in superficial burns. Patients can prevent scarring by applying emollient creams and ointments once skin is intact. Examples include unscented Cetaphil, Cerave, Aveeno, or Aquafor. They should also avoid sun exposure as it can make scars more prominent, and apply sun block to any previously burnt areas exposed to the sun. If any hypertrophic scarring is seen, the patient should be referred to a burn center.

Epithelialization—which consists of tiny opalescent islands of epithelium visible throughout the wound—should be seen by 10–14 days in black individuals and young children or 14–21 days in all other ages and races. Once this is seen, a non-perfumed moisturizing cream (i.e., Vaseline Intensive Care, Eucerin, Nivea, mineral oil, or cocoa butter) can be applied to the burn site until the skin's natural lubrication returns. If epithelialization is not seen by 3–4 weeks after the burn, the patient should be referred to a burn center.

Questions for the Dermatologist

– *Literature indicates that a burn on the foot warrants referral to a burn clinic. Is this correct, or is referral to dermatology adequate? Or treating the burn as it was in primary care?*

Burn care strongly depends on location and severity. First degree burns are manageable in primary care or dermatology settings. Second degree or more severe burns, or burns on anatomically critical areas like the face, should be referred to a burn clinic. There are areas of the body more susceptible to infection, such as the feet, genitalia, and perianal area. The American Burn Association recommends patients with burns in those areas should also be referred to a burn clinic.

– *Should the blister tops be debrided off during the office visit?*

Keeping flaccid dead skin over the burn is very important for healing. It also acts as an occlusive dressing. If there is necrosis, debridement may be necessary as well as referral to a burn clinic. Otherwise, it is our practice's approach that flaccid dead skin should be left alone.

– *What should the patient use to clean the wound and how often? Every time the dressings are changed?*

The answer depends on location and activity. Using a gentle cleanser like Cetaphil or unscented Dove 1–2 times per day is adequate. If the patient is immobile, or the area is difficult to clean twice per day, cleaner areas (not including the axilla, groin, perianal area, or feet) can be managed by gently cleansing, covering with a dressing, and changing the dressings every 2–3 days.

– *How often should dressings be changed?*

Dressings on cleaner parts of the body can be changed every 2–3 days. Otherwise, the areas should be monitored more carefully. Areas with higher density of bacteria, such as the axilla, groin, perianal area, and feet, should be checked daily. If the wound is pink or tender which are indications of impending infection, the dressing should be changed.

– *What should be done when the blister tops start coming off on their own?*

Our practice advises that blisters should not be actively removed. If they start coming off on their own, there is no reason for concern if the patient is keeping the area clean. New skin will re-epithelialize beneath it.

References

1. Burn incidence and treatment in the United States: 2013 Fact Sheet [Internet]. 2014 [cited 2015 Jan 20]. Available from: http://www.ameriburn.org/resources_factsheet.php
2. Bessey PQ, Phillips BD, Lentz CW, Edelman LS, Faraklas I, Finocchiaro MA, Kemalyan NA, Klein MB, Miller SF, Mosier MJ, Potenza BM, Reigart CL, Browning SM, Kiley MT, Krichbaum JA. Synopsis of the 2013 annual report of the National Burn Repository. J Burn Care Res. 2014;35(2):S218–34.
3. Gabbe BJ, Watterson DM, Singer Y, Darton A. Outpatient presentations to burn centers: data from the Burns Registry of Australia and New Zealand outpatient pilot project. Burns. 2014;pii: S0305-4179(14)00416-1.
4. Riedlinger DI, Jennings PA, Edgar DW, Harvey JG, Cleland MH, Wood FM, Cameron PA. Scald burns in children aged 14 and younger in Australia and New Zealand—an analysis based on the burn registry of Australia and New Zealand (BRANZ). Burns. 2014;pii: S0305-4179(14)00255-1.
5. Wasiak J, Cleland H, Campbell F, Spinks A. Dressings for superficial and partial thickness burns (Review). Cochrane Database Syst Rev. 2013;3, CD002106.
6. Barajas-Nava LA, López-Alcalde J, Roqué i Figuls M, Solà I, Bonfill Cosp X. Antibiotic prophylaxis for preventing burn wound infection. Cochrane Database Syst Rev. 2013;6, CD008738.
7. Vloemans AF, Hermans MH, van der Wal MB, Liebregts J, Middelkoop E. Optimal treatment for partial thickness burns in children: a systematic review. Burns. 2014;40(2):177–90.

Chapter 34
Lichen Simplex Chronicus

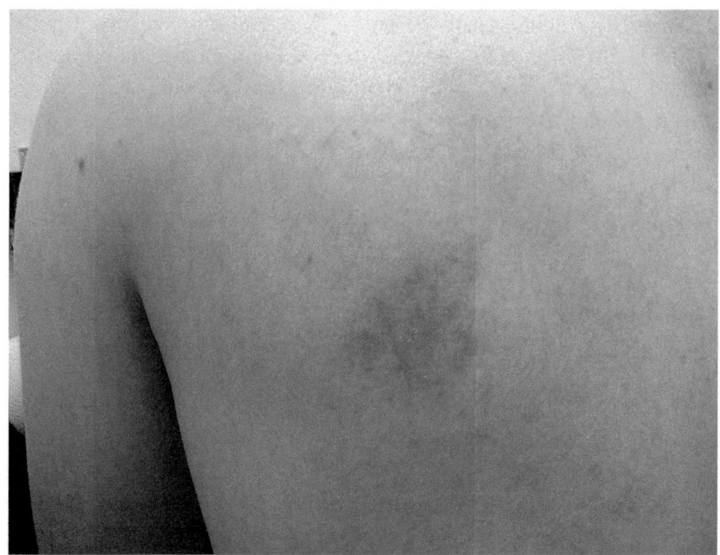

Fig. 34.1 Eczematous plaque with poorly defined margins at left upper back

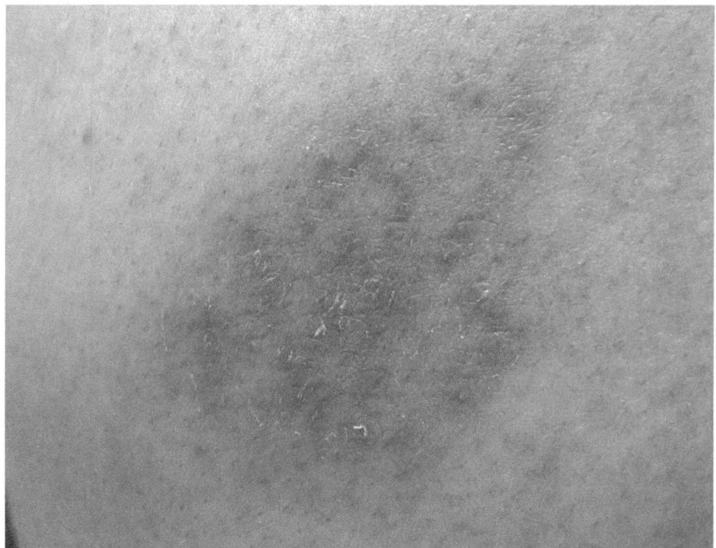

Fig. 34.2 Accentuated skin markings overlying an eczematous plaque

D. Reich et al., *Top 50 Dermatology Case Studies for Primary Care*,
DOI 10.1007/978-3-319-18627-6_34

Primary Care Visit Report

A 26-year-old male with no past medical history presented with an erythematous rash on his left upper back that had been present for 3 weeks. When it first appeared, the rash was raised and the patient's entire back, beyond the site of the rash, was extremely itchy. The itchiness of the entire back had since resolved but the rash itself remained itchy. The patient treated the rash with mupirocin ointment for 3–4 days but it didn't seem to help. The patient felt otherwise well.

Vitals were normal. On exam, on his left scapular area, there was a 4 cm × 2.5 cm erythematous papular rash with some scaling and some discrete 1–2 mm erythematous papules.

Although the diagnosis was uncertain, the rash was treated with a steroid cream due to its dryness and scale. The patient was advised to first try an over-the-counter hydrocortisone cream on the rash twice daily to see if that helped. If there was no improvement after 2 days, the patient was advised to switch to the mid-strength (Class IV) prescription steroid mometasone furoate cream 0.1 % once daily.

Discussion from Dermatology Clinic

Differential Dx

- Lichen simplex chronicus
- Atopic dermatitis
- Contact dermatitis
- Psoriasis
- Discoid lupus
- Hypertrophic lichen planus

Favored Dx

Lichen simplex chronicus is favored because of the elevated, thickened appearance of the lesion, and the history of local itchiness.

Overview

Lichen simplex chronicus, also known as neurodermatitis, is a secondary skin disorder that results from excessive scratching. The primary condition that starts the cycle is severe pruritus—which can be due to any number of underlying reasons—and the excessive scratching that results from the severe pruritus produces the thickened, leathery (lichenified) plaques of lichen simplex chronicus. Chronic scratching perpetuates the pruritus, leading to an itch–scratch cycle. Lesions can only occur in sites that are accessible for scratching. Underlying causes of pruritus have been associated with a variety of conditions, including atopy, renal insufficiency, liver failure, hypothyroidism and hyperthyroidism, HIV, and lymphoma [1, 2]. It has also been linked with increased psychopathology, particularly depression, anxiety, and obsessive-compulsive disorder although the direction of that relationship is uncertain [1, 3]. Increased heat and humidity in the environment are associated with exacerbation and increased irritation of lesions [4]. Lichen simplex chronicus is more prevalent in women than men, and tends to occur between the ages of 30–50 [1].

Presentation

Individuals with lichen simplex chronicus present with pruritic, well-demarcated plaques of thickened, leathery texture. Plaques can be erythematous, scaly, and hypopigmented or hyperpigmented. The plaques are induced by rubbing, picking, and scratching highly pruritic areas. Scratching can occur during sleep. Lesions of lichen simplex chronicus are within the individual's reach, and are most commonly found on the scalp, posterior neck, wrists, elbows, ankles, and anogenital region [1]. Excoriations and prurigo nodules (hard crusty lumps that itch intensely) may appear within the plaque, and can sometimes become secondarily infected.

Workup

Diagnosis can be made on clinical findings; however, lichenification occurs secondary to itching, and the underlying cause of pruritus is important to identify. If there is suspicion of a systemic cause, complete blood count with differential, renal, kidney, and thyroid function tests may be useful. Skin biopsies can confirm diagnosis. Tinea cruris should be ruled out in the anogenital region.

Treatment

Treatment should focus on identifying any underlying disease, improving skin barrier function, reducing inflammation, and breaking the itch–scratch cycle [4]. Treating the underlying disease will reduce the pruritus driving the itch–scratch cycle. If no cause can be identified, physicians should focus on treating symptoms, and emphasize the importance of avoiding scratching.

Choices of topical treatment include steroids and calcineurin inhibitors. Mid and high potency topical steroids (classes I–IV) are first-line treatment for relieving pruritus and inflammation associated with lichen simplex chronicus. These would include triamcinolone 0.1 % (class IV—mid-strength) or fluocinonide 0.05 % (class II—high-potency). Steroids can be applied twice daily for up to 2 weeks (or less if resolved), and under occlusion of a dressing or bandage to help prevent further scratching. Calcineurin inhibitors are recommended for treating intertriginous areas where strong steroids would be inappropriate. Tacrolimus 0.1 % ointment and pimecrolimus 1 % have both demonstrated efficacy [1, 5, 6]. If topical corticosteroids fail, oral prednisone tapers or intralesional cortisone may be considered [4].

There is some evidence to support use of capsaicin 0.025 % cream for symptom relief [7]. Sleep-inducing antihistamines, such as hydroxyzine or diphenhydramine, can be given to individuals whose pruritus is disrupting sleep, or who are nocturnal scratchers [1, 4]. Persistent and recalcitrant lichen simplex chronicus can be referred to dermatology for a trial of UV phototherapy [1].

Follow-Up

If potent steroids are given, follow-up within 2 weeks is prudent to ensure resolution and to prevent any steroid-induced atrophy related to long-term steroid use. Atrophy presents as thinned skin with prominent vasculature known as telangiectasia. Lichen simplex chronicus should respond to potent steroid treatment within a week. If the lesion does not improve in a 2-week timeframe, steroids should be discontinued, and an alternate diagnosis should be considered. Patients who respond to treatment should be advised to continue avoiding any identified itch triggers. Patients may continue applying over-the-counter moisturizers or emollients to help maintain a competent skin barrier.

Questions for the Dermatologist

– *When the etiology of a rash is unclear, are there any clues to aid in the decision of whether to treat with topical steroids versus antifungals?*

Eczematous rashes tend to be less distinct and more poorly demarcated than fungal rashes. Eczematous rashes also tend to occur bilaterally, demonstrating a symmetry that is not typically seen with fungal rashes. If the etiology is unclear, there is no danger in trying either topical steroids or topical antifungals for 1 week. If the incorrect class is chosen, after 1 week with no resolution, have the patient switch to the other medication. One week of a mid-to-strong potency steroid would improve or clear an eczematous process but not a fungal one.

– *How many days' worth of over-the-counter hydrocortisone treatment are appropriate to know if a condition requires steroid, as most prescription strength steroids are expensive even with insurance?*

Over-the-counter hydrocortisone 1 % is not a fair test of whether topical steroids will work. It is not strong enough to clear out eczematous processes of any cause. Not all prescription strength steroids are expensive. Generic triamcinolone 0.1 %, which is a mid-potency steroid, can cost $5–10 without insurance coverage.

– *What determines the duration of treatment with steroid creams? Should patients discontinue as soon as the rash resolves or continue beyond that time?*

Our office usually writes topical steroid prescriptions for a 2-week course. Depending on the medication strength, 2 weeks is plenty of time to assess improvement. If there is uncertainty over the infectious nature of a rash or lesion, we ask to see patients back in 1 week to assess progress. Otherwise, patients may discontinue topical steroid use once their rash has resolved.

– *What determines the appropriate potency and preparation (ointment, cream, lotion) of steroid prescription? How do you choose the particular steroid medication within a potency class? Which body parts warrant separate consideration?*

There are two considerations for the choice of potency: location of lesions and severity of inflammatory process. The face, genitals, and intertriginous areas warrant mild steroids (see steroid potency chart). Ointment preparations tend to be the most effective but some patients may not like the greasiness. We also occasionally use specific compounding materials—for example, one preparation with anecdotal success in our practice is prescription Locoid lipocream (hydrocortisone butyrate in emollient base). Any specific medication within the same potency class will serve a similar purpose, and sometimes the decision is unfortunately based on insurance coverage.

– *Is lichen simplex chronicus basically created from over-scratching? (i.e., the itching started from something else but the scratching created the lesion?)*

Yes, it is an itch–scratch cycle. Scratching creates irritation and itchiness, which leads to further scratching.

References

1. Burgin S. Chapter 15. Nummular eczema, lichen simplex chronicus, and prurigo nodularis. In: Goldsmith LA, Katz SI, Gilchrest BA, Paller AS, Leffell DJ, Wolff K, editors. Fitzpatrick's dermatology in general medicine. 8th ed. New York: McGraw-Hill; 2012.
2. Aschoff R, Wozel G. Topical tacrolimus for the treatment of lichen simplex chronicus. J Dermatolog Treat. 2007;18(2):115–7.
3. Konuk N, Koca R, Atik L, Muhtar S, Atasoy N, Bostanci B. Psychopathology, depression and dissociative experiences in patients with lichen simplex chronicus. Gen Hosp Psychiatry. 2007;29(3):232–5.
4. Lynch PJ. Lichen simplex chronicus (atopic/neurodermatitis) of the anogenital region. Dermatol Ther. 2004;17(1):8–19.

5. Tan ES, Tan AS, Tey HL. Effective treatment of scrotal lichen simplex chronicus with 0.1% tacrolimus ointment: an observational study. J Eur Acad Dermatol Venereol. 2014. doi:10.1111/jdv.12500.
6. Goldstein AT, Parneix-Spake A, McCormick CL, Burrows LJ. Pimecrolimus cream 1% for treatment of vulvar lichen simplex chronicus: an open-label, preliminary trial. Gynecol Obstet Invest. 2007;64(4):180–6.
7. Boyd K, Shea SM, Patterson JW. The role of capsaicin in dermatology. In: Abdel-Salam OME, editor. Capsaicin as a therapeutic molecule. Basel, Switzerland: Springer Basel; 2014. p. 293–306.

Chapter 35
Atopic Eczema

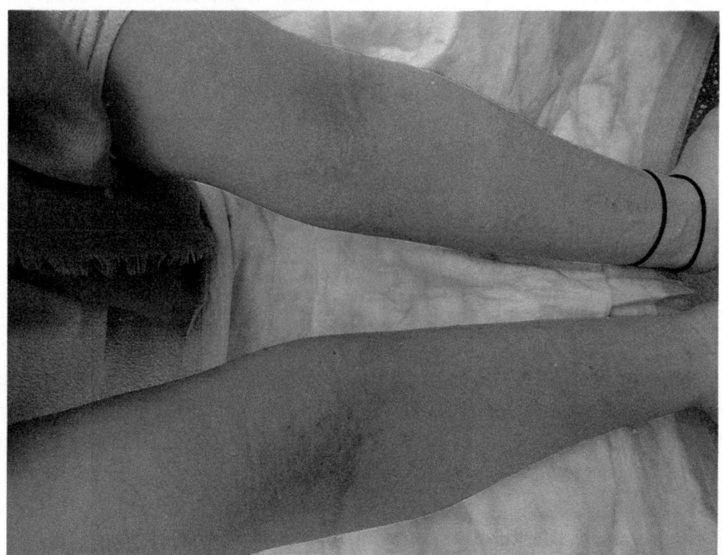

Fig. 35.1 Antecubital poorly marginated erythematous, excoriated plaques

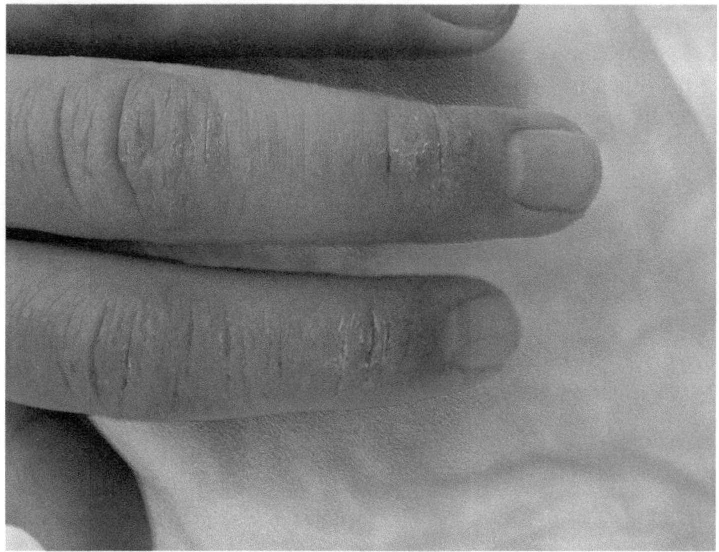

Fig. 35.2 Lichenified, scaly, erythematous plaques dorsal fingers

D. Reich et al., *Top 50 Dermatology Case Studies for Primary Care*,
DOI 10.1007/978-3-319-18627-6_35

Primary Care Visit Report

A 29-year-old female with past medical history of asthma, atopic eczema, and sesame/peanut allergies presented with an atopic eczema flare. The patient had atopic eczema and asthma since childhood and experienced frequent flares. She had recently started taking high dose probiotics—75 billion cfu/day—for 3 weeks and while taking them she experienced no atopic eczema flares. One week after stopping the probiotics, she had an acute flare on her fingers, elbows, face, and neck. She initially started getting the rash on her fingers and hands about 15 years ago. The eczema on her face started about 5 years prior when she first started to wear makeup. The eczema on her neck started about 2 years prior. She had run out of higher potency steroid cream so she tried applying polysporin antibiotic ointment as she found the lower potency steroid cream she had made the rash itchier.

The patient's last severe eczema flare was about 3 months prior and at that time, she was treated with Hydrocortisone Butyrate Ointment (Class V) 0.1 % as well as an oral prednisone 10-day taper.

The patient reported that her asthma had flared as well and she needed to use her albuterol inhaler at least twice daily during this time.

The patient had tried to cut gluten out of her diet but only succeeded in doing this for 1 week and did not notice any improvement.

Vitals were normal. On examination, the dorsum of her hands and fingers featured an erythematous, textured papular rash with some open shallow ulcers on her fingers bilaterally; her antecubital fossae had erythematous plaques bilaterally; her anterior neck had erythematous macules; and her face had erythematous macules on the left cheek, left infraorbital area and across the bridge of her nose extending to her right cheek.

This was treated as an atopic eczema flare and she was prescribed topical hydrocortisone butyrate ointment 0.1 % (Class V) twice daily for 14 days as well as oral prednisone, given the severity. The prednisone was prescribed as a 10-day taper starting with 80 mg daily × 3 days, 60 mg/day × 3 days, 40 mg/day × 3 days, and 20 mg/day × 1 day.

Discussion from Dermatology Clinic

Differential Dx

- Atopic eczema
- Allergic contact dermatitis
- Irritant dermatitis
- Scabies

- Tinea corporis
- Seborrheic dermatitis
- Psoriasis

Favored Dx

The xerotic (abnormally dry) and fissured presentation of the patient's hands is consistent with atopic eczema.

Overview

Atopic eczema (AE) is a non-contagious, chronic, and relapsing highly pruritic inflammatory skin disease. It is very common, with an estimated 15–30 % lifetime prevalence in children and 8–10 % lifetime prevalence in adults [1]. It is often considered a disease of childhood, as up to 85 % of cases are diagnosed before the age of 5; however, it is not uncommon in adults. AE is slightly more prevalent in females.

The overall incidence of AE has increased significantly over the last several decades, especially in developed countries and urban areas [1, 2]. Some have explained this phenomenon in relation to the hygiene hypothesis, which is the idea that decreased exposure to infections and allergens has prompted a rise in allergic diseases; however, this association only appears to be true in affluent countries [1, 3]. In fact, the pathogenesis of AE is complex and influenced by multiple genetic, social, and environmental factors.

Mutations in the filaggrin gene *FLG*, which encodes a structural protein that contributes to water retention in the skin and maintaining the skin's barrier function, and dysregulated type 2 T helper cells (Th2) are known to have a strong association with AE [1, 4, 5]. The role of genetic factors is further demonstrated by increased risk of developing AE when there is positive parental history of eczema, asthma, or allergic rhinitis (hayfever), and higher concordance rates in monozygotic compared to dizygotic twins [1, 6–9]. Having AE in childhood predisposes individuals to developing asthma and allergic rhinitis later in life, which is sometimes referred to as the allergic or atopic march [5, 10].

In addition to genetics, social and environmental factors play a role in the pathogenesis of AE. The prevalence of AE is higher among people of black or mixed race, and in metropolitan areas [2]. Emotional stress and infections are associated with acute flares [1]. Having multiple siblings, childhood pet dogs, parents who were born outside the USA, and living in a rural area demonstrate a protective effect against developing AE [2, 11, 12].

Presentation

The presentation of AE varies depending on the age of the patient, and the duration and severity of the disease. In infants, the condition tends to appear on the scalp and face, particularly in the cheek area, and on extensor surfaces of the arms and legs. The rash looks highly erythematous and may be weeping. Childhood AE most commonly appears on flexor surfaces of the extremities, specifically the antecubital and popliteal fossa, and the neck, wrists, and ankles. Adults also tend to experience AE in the antecubital and popliteal fossa, as well as the neck and face, especially in the periorbital area.

AE presents as a xerotic, erythematous rash. For all age groups, it is a highly pruritic condition that can be severe enough to interrupt sleep. Some patients experience pruritus intermittently, corresponding with acute flares, while others experience the sensation at all times. As such, AE lesions may feature excoriations caused by scratching, as well as papules, scaling, and fissures. Symptoms may get worse in the winter months, when air tends to be more dry. Patients who have experienced atopic eczema for years may present with dyspigmented, lichenified (thickened) skin. The dry, cracked skin typical of AE allows pathogens to penetrate and makes individuals more susceptible to infections.

Workup

AE is typically a clinical diagnosis, with appearance of lesions, report of pruritus, history of recurrence, family history of AE, and associated atopic conditions all providing evidence to support the diagnosis. Allergy patch testing can be performed if patient history suggests a specific allergen which triggers a flare, or if contact dermatitis needs to be ruled out. IgE levels are elevated in a large proportion of individuals with AE; however, this parameter is non-specific as IgE can be elevated in other atopic conditions.

Treatment

Treatment of AE aims to reduce inflammation, restore the skin's barrier function, and control any exacerbating factors to prevent future flares. Topical corticosteroids, sedating antihistamines, and emollients are the mainstays of treatment. The condition's severity should help to determine the exact treatment regimen. Several validated tools are available to aid in making a severity assessment, including The Eczema Area and Severity Index (EASI) and Scoring of Atopic Dermatitis (SCORAD), but these are not commonly used in clinical practice [1, 4, 13]. Severity calculators can be found online, or via a number of different smartphone applications.

Infants may be treated with a lower potency class of corticosteroids, such as hydrocortisone 2.5 % (Class VII) [1]. If the rash has not adequately improved within 7 days, a slightly stronger (Class V or VI) steroid may be used. Children may be treated with a mid-strength corticosteroid such as hydrocortisone valerate (Westcort 0.2 %—Class V). Intertriginous areas (where skin touches skin) and the face should be treated with milder topical corticosteroids, such as Desonide (Class VI). Children over 12 years of age and adults can be treated with more potent (Class II or III) corticosteroids for lesions on the trunk and extremities. For lesions on the hands, as in this case, superpotent or potent topical steroids (Class I or II) would be indicated. It is recommended that topical steroids be used twice daily for up to 2 weeks, and discontinued before that time if the rash resolves. When higher potency corticosteroids are used, AE flares tend to resolve within 4–5 days. Special care should be taken when treating AE around the eyes, as topical steroids can increase intraocular pressure.

A short (2-week) tapered course of systemic corticosteroids may be useful in controlling a severe flare of AE. This should be reserved for extreme cases as oral steroids are associated with significant rebound flares [1, 14].

Antihistamines are not effective as a monotherapy for AE; however, they are useful in decreasing the impact of pruritus. First generation sedating H_1 blockers such as hydroxyzine (Atarax) are most effective for this purpose, and can be especially helpful in patients whose sleep is disrupted [13, 14].

Topical emollients are an integral part of AE therapy as they help reestablish the skin's barrier function. Many emollients are available, such as Cutemol, Aquaphor, Aveeno, CeraVe, Curél, and Cetaphil, and individuals are best suited to determine their preferred brand. These should be used liberally and frequently (at least twice daily) as part of a maintenance regimen. During flares, emollients may be used as adjunct therapy alongside topical corticosteroids. Ideally emollients should be free from any allergens or irritants, such as perfumes or dyes.

AE that does not respond to topical corticosteroids may be referred to a dermatologist for further treatment. Topical calcineurin inhibitors, phototherapy, and disease-modifying agents such as cyclosporine have all demonstrated efficacy in treating AE, and may be trialed under specialist care [1, 13, 14].

Follow-Up

Acute flares of AE should be monitored closely to ensure topical corticosteroids are used correctly and to determine whether any adjustments to steroid potency are needed. Although 60–70 % of infant and child AE cases resolve before the age of 15 years, the condition is chronic and relapsing for many individuals [10]. Several office visits and changes to the treatment regimen may be required before finding one that works. Different preparations (cream, gel, ointment), potencies, and combinations of treatment may be trialed in order to find one that is successful. For patients with more severe presentations of AE, it may be beneficial to use corticosteroids on weekends only, with over-the-counter emollients during the week, as a preventative treatment.

In addition to emollients and preventative corticosteroids, a number of recommendations can be made to help prevent flares. Use of hot water should be avoided in baths and showers, bathing and showering should be limited to 5 min if possible, and gentle cleansers without harsh dyes or fragrances are favored [13]. When taking baths, using bath oils can help prevent skin dehydration. Wool clothes, itchy fabrics, and contact with carpeting or rugs should be avoided as they may exacerbate AE. There is very little evidence to indicate a relationship between diet and AE; however, if a certain food is identified as a trigger, it should be avoided [13].

Questions for the Dermatologist

– *What class of steroids is best for treating atopic eczema flares?*

There is not a specific potency of steroid that is appropriate for all AE flares. The body surface area affected, anatomical location, severity of lesions, and size of the affected person are the considerations for determining steroid potency.

– *When are oral steroids necessary for treating AE?*

Oral steroids are only required for treating AE in rare instances. If someone is experiencing a severe flare and I am trying to bring it under rapid control, I will occasionally reach for oral steroids. It is a tempting solution to turn to but there is high potential for rebound, so oral steroids should be reserved for very severe cases with extensive body surface area involvement.

– *Is a 10-day prednisone taper adequate or is a longer course preferable?*

Our office would recommend a 2-week taper starting at 1 mg per kilogram per day.

– *Is it common to see an asthma exacerbation simultaneously present with an AE flare?*

While the two conditions track together, it is not particularly common to see flares of asthma and AE at the same time. Both are indicative of a hyperreactive immune system, generally referred to as "atopy"; however, I do not tend to see asthma exacerbations at the same time as AE flares.

– *Does gluten free diet play a role in controlling AE flares?*

We do not have excellent data on the role of diet in AE. I have not seen gluten free regimens help control flares. That being said, there is more we do not know about diet and AE than we do know. There is some light evidence to suggest lower glycemic index diets can be somewhat helpful.

– *Are there any foods that are common triggers?*

No, not that we know of from studies. Unhealthy diets are triggers but that is not a sophisticated descriptor. A more balanced diet can be beneficial, but there are no specific food triggers we know of.

– *Can high dose probiotics help stop AE recurrences?*

Unfortunately we do not have great data on diet's effect on AE. We would need double-blinded, placebo-controlled, randomized studies to be able to draw good conclusions, and it is very difficult to control for other dietary aspects in such a study. Are participants taking probiotics and eating an otherwise unhealthy diet? Without putting participants in a controlled, inpatient setting, it would be very difficult to tell if probiotics have any effect. There is some evidence that probiotics have a protective effect against developing AE at the start of life [12, 15, 16]. According to a 2008 Cochrane review, there is no evidence to suggest probiotics have a role in adult AE treatment [10]. Having said that, probiotics can certainly be beneficial to health in general, we just cannot cite good data to support their use in AE.

– *Can wearing makeup exacerbate facial AE?*

Certain makeup can exacerbate symptoms, for example alcohol-based products can paradoxically dry out the skin and encourage a flare. It is more so binding agents and preservatives in some makeup rather than color itself causing problems. Preservatives can cause contact dermatitis, and patients with AE have a higher incidence of contact dermatitis. Propylene glycol, which is commonly found in makeup, is another common cause of contact dermatitis. Wearing natural, fragrance-free makeup and removing it at the end of the day may help reduce the potential for irritation.

References

1. Bieber T. Atopic dermatitis. Ann Dermatol. 2010;22(2):125–37.
2. Shaw TE, Currie GP, Koudelka CW, Simpson EL. Eczema prevalence in the United States: data from the 2003 National Survey of Children's Health. J Invest Dermatol. 2011;131(1):67–73.
3. Strachan DP, Aït-Khaled N, Foliaki S, Mallol J, Odhiambo J, Pearce N, Williams HC, ISAAC Phase Three Study Group. Siblings, asthma, rhinoconjunctivitis and eczema: a worldwide perspective from the International Study of Asthma and Allergies in Childhood. Clin Exp Allergy. 2015;45(1):126–36.
4. Madhok V, Futamura M, Thomas KS, Barbarot S. What's new in atopic eczema? An analysis of systematic reviews published in 2012 and 2013. Part 1. Epidemiology, mechanisms of disease and methodological issues. Clin Exp Dermatol. 2015;40(3):238–42.
5. Irvine AD, McLean WH, Leung DY. Filaggrin mutations associated with skin and allergic diseases. N Engl J Med. 2011;365(14):1315–27.
6. Larsen FS, Holm NV, Henningsen K. Atopic dermatitis. A genetic-epidemiologic study in a population-based twin sample. J Am Acad Dermatol. 1986;15(3):487–94.

7. Schultz Larsen F. Atopic dermatitis: a genetic-epidemiologic study in a population-based twin sample. J Am Acad Dermatol. 1993;28(5 Pt 1):719–23.
8. Barnes KC. An update on the genetics of atopic dermatitis: scratching the surface in 2009. J Allergy Clin Immunol. 2010;125(1):16–29.e1–11. quiz 30–1.
9. Darsow U, Eyerich K, Ring J. Eczema (E), atopic eczema (AE) and atopic dermatitis (AD). Munich: World Allergy Organization; 2014. Available from: http://www.worldallergy.org/professional/allergic_diseases_center/atopiceczema/.
10. Boyle RJ, Bath-Hextall FJ, Leonardi-Bee J, Murrell DF, Tang MLK. Probiotics for treating eczema. Cochrane Database Syst Rev. 2008;4, CD006135.
11. Schram ME, Tedja AM, Spijker R, Bos JD, Williams HC, Spuls PI. Is there a rural/urban gradient in the prevalence of eczema? A systematic review. Br J Dermatol. 2010;162(5):964–73.
12. Madhok V, Futamura M, Thomas KS, Barbarot S. What's new in atopic eczema? An analysis of systematic reviews published in 2012 and 2013. Part 2. Treatment and prevention. Clin Exp Dermatol. 2015;40(4):349–54. quiz 354–5.
13. Ring J, Alomar A, Bieber T, Deleuran M, Fink-Wagner A, Gelmetti C, Gieler U, Lipozencic J, Luger T, Oranje AP, Schäfer T, Schwennesen T, Seidenari S, Simon D, Ständer S, Stingl G, Szalai S, Szepietowski JC, Taïeb A, Werfel T, Wollenberg A, Darsow U, European Dermatology Forum (EDF); European Academy of Dermatology and Venereology (EADV); European Federation of Allergy (EFA); European Task Force on Atopic Dermatitis (ETFAD); European Society of Pediatric Dermatology (ESPD); Global Allergy and Asthma European Network (GA2LEN). Guidelines for treatment of atopic eczema (atopic dermatitis) part I. J Eur Acad Dermatol Venereol. 2012;26(8):1045–60.
14. Williams HC. Atopic dermatitis. N Engl J Med. 2005;352(22):2314–24.
15. Cuello-Garcia CA, Brożek JL, Fiocchi A, Pawankar R, Yepes-Nuñez JJ, Terracciano L, Gandhi S, Agarwal A, Zhang Y, Schünemann HJ. Probiotics for the prevention of allergy: a systematic review and meta-analysis of randomized controlled trials. J Allergy Clin Immunol. 2015;136(4):952–61.
16. Zuccotti G, Meneghin F, Aceti A, Barone G, Callegari ML, Di Mauro A, Fantini MP, Gori D, Indrio F, Maggio L, Morelli L, Corvaglia L, Italian Society of Neonatology. Probiotics for prevention of atopic diseases in infants: systematic review and meta-analysis. Allergy. 2015;70(11):1356–71.

Chapter 36
Psoriasis

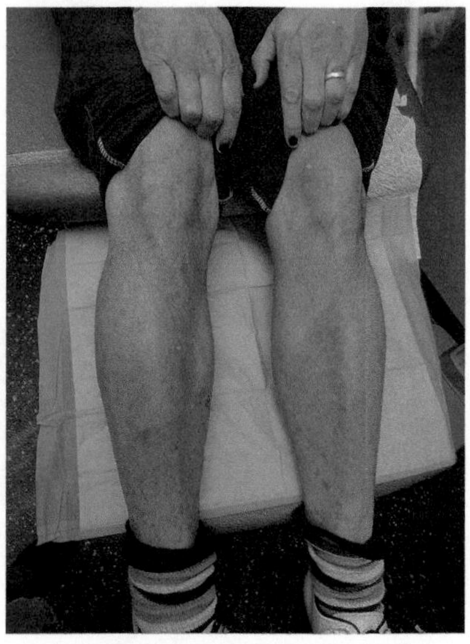

Fig. 36.1 Red hyperkeratotic plaques over knees and pretibia

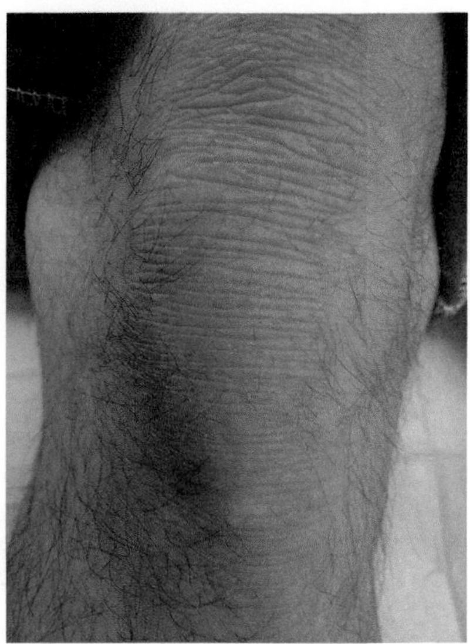

Fig. 36.2 Accentuated skin markings overlying erythematous, well-marginated plaque

D. Reich et al., *Top 50 Dermatology Case Studies for Primary Care*,
DOI 10.1007/978-3-319-18627-6_36

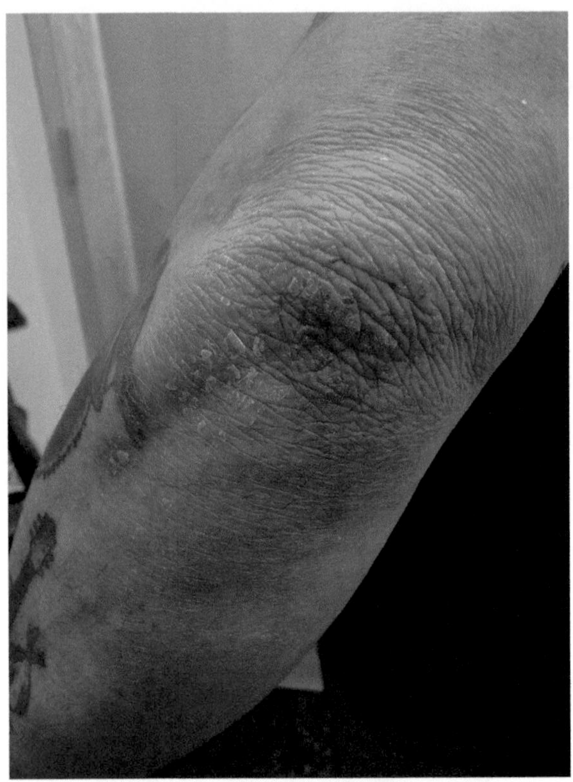

Fig. 36.3 Extensor surfaces predominate in this inheritable condition

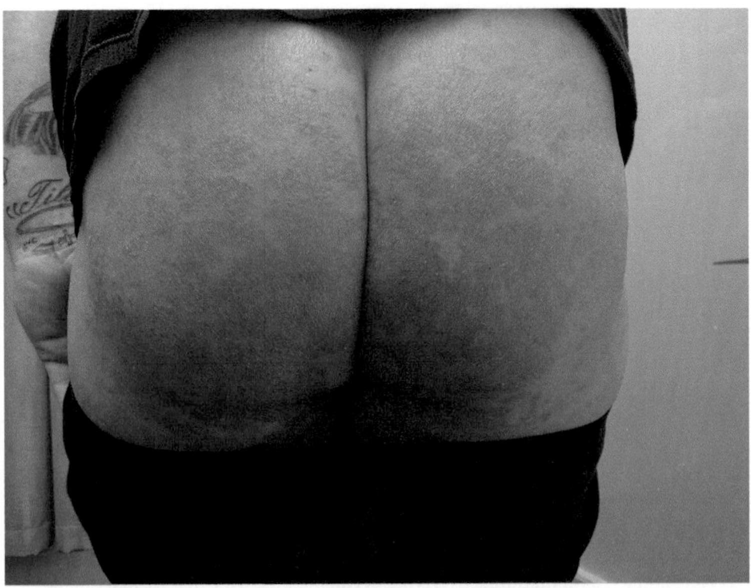

Fig. 36.4 Buttocks with polycyclic scaly erythematous plaques

Primary Care Visit Report

A 47-year-old male with past medical history of asthma and psoriasis presented with a psoriatic flare. The patient had been without health insurance until recently and this visit was his first time seeing a doctor in years. He had been able to control his flares by soaking in water and Epsom salts, and occasionally using a cream.

Vitals were normal. On exam, there were large erythematous scaly plaques on extensor surfaces of the bilateral forearms, bilateral lower legs, and bilateral dorsal hands, as well as on his buttocks and bilateral medial thighs.

Given the patient's extensive history of psoriasis and the extent of the areas affected, he was referred to dermatology to explore further treatment options.

Discussion from Dermatology Clinic

Differential Dx

- Psoriasis
- Atopic dermatitis
- Nummular eczema
- Lichen planus
- Lichen simplex chronicus
- Tinea corporis
- Pityriasis rosea
- Subacute cutaneous lupus erythematosus

Favored Dx

The lesion distribution and erythematous, thickened, plaque-like appearance are indicative of psoriasis.

Overview

Psoriasis is a chronic, relapsing, immune-mediated disease estimated to affect 0.5–4.6 % of the population [1, 2]. It affects men and women equally, and is about twice as likely to occur in Caucasians [1, 2]. Onset of psoriatic symptoms is most likely between the ages of 15 and 30 [3]. One large study reported a median age of 28 years [1]. Global epidemiology of psoriasis is varied, with highest incidence in Western Europe, North America, southern Latin America, Australasia, and Asia Pacific [4]. Higher incidence is also associated with higher geographic latitudes (i.e., closer to the North or South Pole) [1, 2].

The exact cause of psoriasis is not known [3]. There is a strong genetic basis for the disease, and its expression is thought to result from contribution by multiple genes. Monozygotic twin studies show a concordance rate of 35–73 %, suggesting there are environmental factors contributing to the pathogenesis of psoriasis [3, 5]. HLA genes on chromosome 6 have been implicated, but the disease is thought to be caused by an interaction of several genes and environmental factors [1–3, 5]. UV exposure may be one environmental factor, supported by the efficacy of UV therapy in treating psoriasis [3].

Onset of psoriasis occurs after predisposed individuals experience a triggering event, such as trauma, infection, allergic drug reaction, or emotional stress [3, 5]. T cell mediated immune responses are activated and proinflammatory cytokines are released. Natural killer cells, TNF-α, and interleukins IL-12, 17, 22, and 23 are frequently involved [3, 5, 6]. These mediators lead to a range of changes on the skin, and nails, and dilation of capillaries causing erythema.

Presentation

There are several phenotypic variants of psoriasis. They include plaque, inverse, guttate, erythrodermic, and pustular psoriasis. The most common is plaque psoriasis, also called psoriasis vulgaris, and accounts for over 80–90 % of cases [1, 3, 7]. It is characterized by erythematous plaques with well-defined borders, occurring on the extensor surfaces of arms and legs, the lower back, scalp, and neck. Plaques may feature a silvery-white scale. The lesions usually occur symmetrically, and range from coin-sized to large plaques [3]. They are often asymptomatic but can be accompanied by pruritus. Nail changes, pitting and onycholysis (separation of the nail from the nail bed) are eventually seen in about half of patients with chronic psoriasis [1, 3]. Psoriatic arthritis occurs in up to 25 % of patients with psoriasis [3]. This usually manifests as joint swelling, particularly at the distal interphalangeal joints, inflammation of an entire finger or toe (dactylitis), and inflammation of the vertebra (spondylitis). It can precede psoriasis in 20 % of patients [1].

Inverse psoriasis occurs in intertriginous areas where skin touches or rubs together, such as the axilla, inguinal folds, and retroauricular folds. This variant accounts for 2–6 % of psoriatic patients, and is more likely to present in obese people [7]. Lesions usually do not feature the scaling typical of psoriasis, and may be confused for tinea infections.

Guttate psoriasis is usually self-limiting (resolution within 6–12 weeks) and occurs following streptococcal throat infection [1, 3, 7]. It is characterized by an eruption of small erythematous papules, most often on the trunk and extremities. Guttate psoriasis is more common in young adults, and is associated with an increased risk of developing plaque psoriasis [7].

Erythrodermic psoriasis is a variant whose most prominent feature is erythema. It can affect all parts of the body and have up to 100 % cutaneous surface area involvement. It can develop slowly in patients with plaque psoriasis, with lesions coalescing over time, or suddenly and unexpectedly [3]. Patients with this variant are at risk of developing hypothermia and hyperthermia in cold and warm climates respectively, due to body temperature loss through extensive vasodilation.

Pustular psoriasis is a rare and severe variant that can be life-threatening [7]. There are several variants of pustular psoriasis: generalized, localized, annular, and impetigo herpetiformis [3]. Generalized pustular psoriasis usually includes systemic symptoms, e.g., fever, and is characterized by the development of sterile pustules on psoriatic plaques. These can coalesce and form large areas of pus. The large pustules compromise the skin's barrier function, and can have severe consequences due to fluid loss, and susceptibility to infection [1]. Palmoplantar pustulosis is a common variant of pustular psoriasis, with debilitating pustules forming on the palms and soles of feet. It is more common in older women and smokers [7]. Annular pustular psoriasis describes pustules that form rings, and may occur in generalized pustular psoriasis. Impetigo herpetiformis is a pustular psoriasis that occurs during the final trimester of pregnancy, usually in women without any prior or family history of psoriasis [3, 7].

Workup

Diagnosis is generally made based on the classic clinical features of psoriasis. Erythematous, scaling plaques with well-demarcated borders are strongly suggestive of psoriasis. Characteristic areas of psoriasis such as the scalp, nails, and intergluteal cleft may be examined for further correlation [1].

If the diagnosis is unclear, biopsy may be done. Histopathology typically reveals thickened or acanthotic epidermis with prominent rete pegs, parakeratosis with keratinocyte nuclei found within the stratum corneum, loss of the granular cell layer, increased presence of T cells in the dermis and epidermis, increased mitotic activity in basal cells (consistent with hyperproliferation), and dilated dermal capillaries [5]. A bacterial culture of the throat may be performed on patients with guttate psoriasis.

Treatment

Treatment options for psoriasis include topical and systemic medications, and phototherapy. Treatment approach should take into account the type, severity and surface area involvement of lesions. This is typically measured using the Psoriasis Area Severity Index (PASI), which generates a score based on location of lesions, body surface area of involvement, erythema, desquamation, and induration. Treatment should also consider the patient's perspective of severity, their desired speed to resolution, and satisfaction with any prior treatment methods, as a substantial proportion of patients report dissatisfaction with treatment effectiveness [3]. Additionally, since psoriasis is usually chronic and recurrent, treatments should address both symptomatic relief and long-term management.

Topical corticosteroids are the most commonly prescribed topical treatment for psoriasis and are considered first line therapy [1, 3, 8]. They can be effective in managing mild to moderate plaque psoriasis. Lesion location and thickness determine the choice of topical steroid - the thicker the lesion, the stronger the steroid. Superpotent corticosteroids (Class I) are indicated for thick plaques on the extremities, trunk, and scalp, but should not be used on the face or intertriginous areas, which would warrant a milder steroid (i.e., Class V or VI). Effective potent corticosteroids include clobetasol propionate and betamethasone dipropionate (both Class I) twice daily. Ointments tend to be more effective than creams [3]. These are generally recommended for a period of up to 2 weeks to avoid long-term side effects of skin atrophy, telangiectasia, and effects on the hypothalamic–adrenal–pituitary axis.

Vitamin D analogues such as calcipotriene 0.005 %, calcitriol, and tacalcitol are also effective, slightly more so as a twice daily combination therapy with corticosteroids [8–10]. These can be irritating and are thus contraindicated for pruritic, erythrodermic, and pustular psoriasis [3]; however, they can be very useful for patients who do not tolerate corticosteroids. For scalp psoriasis, corticosteroids alone, e.g., clobetasol propionate, are most effective [9]. Special formulations such as shampoos, solutions, oils, and foams are often preferable for the scalp.

The topical retinoid tazarotene 0.05 or 0.1 % is effective in reducing scaling and plaque thickness when applied nightly, but it can cause irritation [1, 3]. It is more effective when used in combination with corticosteroids [3]. Tacrolimus 0.1 %, a calcineurin inhibitor, is most effective against inverse and facial psoriasis [3, 11]. However, there has been limited and controversial evidence suggesting an association with neoplasms, which gave the drug an FDA black-box warning [3, 12]. Other topical treatments include salicylic acid and coal tar. Coal tar is an option that has been available for 2000 years; however, its efficacy is limited, it is carcinogenic, and its use is declining due to unwanted characteristics like malodor and tendency to stain [3].

Despite the association with bacteria, there are no strong data to support antibiotic treatment of guttate psoriasis [1, 3, 7]. However, antibiotics may be given in cases with a positive strep culture in order to treat the underlying strep pharyngitis.

Cases of psoriasis that are severe, recalcitrant, and/or resistant to topical therapy should be referred to dermatology. Variants other than plaque psoriasis should also be referred. Further effective treatment options that may be investigated include UVB phototherapy, PUVA photochemotherapy, methotrexate, and anti-TNF biologics etanercept, adalimumab, and ustekinumab [1, 3, 13]. Biologics may be the most effective treatment against nail psoriasis [14]. Systemic corticosteroids are generally avoided as they are the most frequent cause of erythrodermic and pustular psoriasis in patients who already have psoriatic predisposition.

Follow-Up

Psoriasis is a multifactorial, polygenic disease whose pathogenesis is not yet entirely understood. Psoriasis presentation and response to treatment may vary greatly from patient to patient. As such, initial therapy may involve trial-and-error of topicals of different strengths, classes, and combinations. Psoriasis can have a significant effect on quality of life, thus treatment follow-up should aim to provide patient satisfaction while taking into account short- and long-term safety, and cost [2–4].

Patients treated with topical corticosteroids should be reevaluated after 2 weeks, as they are not safe for continuous long-term use. If patients are responsive to steroid treatment, they may switch to a weekend-only schedule (applying steroid twice daily on Saturdays and Sundays) to maintain clearance. As stated earlier, resistance to therapy, and complications should be referred to dermatology.

Questions for the Dermatologist

– *Are there home remedies that can help control psoriasis, such as Epsom salt water soaks?*

Yes, there are over-the-counter remedies that can be somewhat helpful. Baths with colloidal oatmeal packs or Epsom salts may help provide relief by softening plaques and reducing inflammation. The baths should be with lukewarm water to avoid further irritation. Moisturizers might be sufficient treatment for mild psoriatic presentations. Moderate and severe cases would warrant additional pharmacologic therapy.

– *Are there dietary choices that can help control, or that cause flares of, psoriasis?*

There are data indicating improvement of psoriasis with omega-3 and omega-6 fatty acids [15, 16]. There may also be an association between a low glycemic index diet and improvement of psoriasis symptoms. Weight loss is positively correlated with psoriatic improvement as well, so overweight patients with psoriasis may be advised to try to lose weight. Many people ask about gluten free diet; however, there is little evidence to support any correlation with psoriatic symptoms. However, if someone wants to try going gluten-free, there is no harm in doing so.

– *With what dose of steroid cream is it appropriate to start treatment for someone experiencing a flare-up?*

The location and severity of psoriatic plaques determine the appropriate dosage. Plaques on the face, intertriginous areas, or genitals should be treated with a mild corticosteroid (i.e., Class V or VI). A steroid of moderate potency may be used if there is severe psoriasis in those areas. Thick plaques on the trunk and extremities may be treated with potent corticosteroids (Class I–III).

– *Is there a role for oral steroids in treating a flare-up with extensive surface area of involvement, as in this case?*

No, systemic corticosteroids are contraindicated in psoriasis. They can cause psoriatic flares, and are the most common cause of palmoplantar pustular psoriasis.

– *What risks are there to untreated psoriasis?*

From a purely dermatological perspective, there are very few risks. Psoriasis does not lead to an increased incidence of malignancy. However, it can lead to social isolation and depression, and have a significant psychosocial impact. It can also lead to irreversible joint destruction from long-standing inflammation. There is a higher incidence of cardiac events in patients with psoriasis due to increased presence of inflammatory mediators. The incidence of coronary artery disease, for example, is higher in patients suffering from psoriasis. Unchecked inflammation in the dermis leads to complexes being deposited in the lamina media of the heart, which gives rise to more atherosclerotic plaques. Systemic effects make a case for systemic control with biologic medications or methotrexate, for example.

References

1. Lebwohl M. Psoriasis. Lancet. 2003;361(9364):1197–204.
2. Rachakonda TD, Schupp CW, Armstrong AW. Psoriasis prevalence among adults in the United States. J Am Acad Dermatol. 2014;70(3):512–6.
3. Gudjonsson JE, Elder JT. Chapter 18. Psoriasis. In: Goldsmith LA, Katz SI, Gilchrest BA, Paller AS, Leffell DJ, Wolff K, editors. Fitzpatrick's dermatology in general medicine. 8th ed. New York: McGraw-Hill; 2012. [cited 2015 Feb 11]. Available from: http://accessmedicine.mhmedical.com.ezproxy.cul.columbia.edu/content.aspx?bookid=392&Sectionid=41138713.
4. Goff KL, Karimkhani C, Boyers LN, Weinstock MA, Lott JP, Hay RJ, Coffeng LE, Norton SA, Naldi L, Dunnick C, Armstrong AW, Dellavalle RP. The global burden of psoriatic skin disease. Br J Dermatol. 2015. doi:10.1111/bjd.13715.
5. Hugh JM, Newman MD, Weinberg JM. Chapter 2. The pathophysiology of psoriasis. In: Weinberg JM, Lebwohl M, editors. Advances in psoriasis: a multisystemic guide. New York: Springer; 2014. p. 9–19.
6. Krueger GG, Langley RG, Leonardi C, Yeilding N, Guzzo C, Wang Y, Dooley LT, Lebwohl M, CNTO 1275 Psoriasis Study Group. A human interleukin-12/23 monoclonal antibody for the treatment of psoriasis. N Engl J Med. 2007;356(6):580–92.
7. Grozdev I, Korman NJ. Chapter 3. Psoriasis: clinical review and update. In: Weinberg JM, Lebwohl M, editors. Advances in psoriasis: a multisystemic guide. New York: Springer; 2014. p. 21–6.
8. Tajirian AL, Kircik L. Chapter 6. Topical therapy I: corticosteroids and vitamin D analogues. In: Weinberg JM, Lebwohl M, editors. Advances in psoriasis: a multisystemic guide. New York: Springer; 2014. p. 63–72.
9. Mason A, Mason J, Cork M, Hancock H, Dooley G. Topical treatments for chronic plaque psoriasis: an abridged Cochrane systematic review. J Am Acad Dermatol. 2013;69(5):799–807.
10. Soleymani T, Hung T, Soung J. The role of vitamin D in psoriasis: a review. Int J Dermatol. 2015. doi:10.1111/ijd.12790.
11. Martin Ezquerra G, Sánchez Regaña M, Herrera Acosta E, Umbert Millet P. Topical tacrolimus for the treatment of psoriasis on the face, genitalia, intertriginous areas and corporal plaques. J Drugs Dermatol. 2006;5(4):334–6.
12. Reitamo S, Rustin M, Harper J, Kalimo K, Rubins A, Cambazard F, Brenninkmeijer EE, Smith C, Berth-Jones J, Ruzicka T, Sharpe G, Taieb A, 0.1% Tacrolimus Ointment Long-term Follow-up Study Group. 4-Year follow-up study of atopic dermatitis therapy with 0.1% tacrolimus ointment in children and adult patients. Br J Dermatol. 2008;159(4):942–51.
13. Takahashi H, Tsuji H, Ishida-Yamamoto A, Iizuka H. Comparison of clinical effects of psoriasis treatment regimens among calcipotriol alone, narrowband ultraviolet B phototherapy alone, combination of calcipotriol and narrowband ultraviolet B phototherapy once a week, and com-

bination of calcipotriol and narrowband ultraviolet B phototherapy more than twice a week. J Dermatol. 2013;40(6):424–7.

14. de Vries AC, Bogaards NA, Hooft L, Velema M, Pasch M, Lebwohl M, Spuls PI. Interventions for nail psoriasis. Cochrane Database Syst Rev. 2013;1, CD007633.
15. Mayser P, Mrowietz U, Arenberger P, Bartak P, Buchvald J, Christophers E, Jablonska S, Salmhofer W, Schill WB, Krämer HJ, Schlotzer E, Mayer K, Seeger W, Grimminger F. Omega-3 fatty acid-based lipid infusion in patients with chronic plaque psoriasis: results of a double-blind, randomized, placebo-controlled, multicenter trial. J Am Acad Dermatol. 1998;38(4):539–47.
16. Millsop JW, Bhatia BK, Debbaneh M, Koo J, Liao W. Diet and psoriasis, part III: Role of nutritional supplements. J Am Acad Dermatol. 2014;71(3):561–9.

Chapter 37
Vitiligo

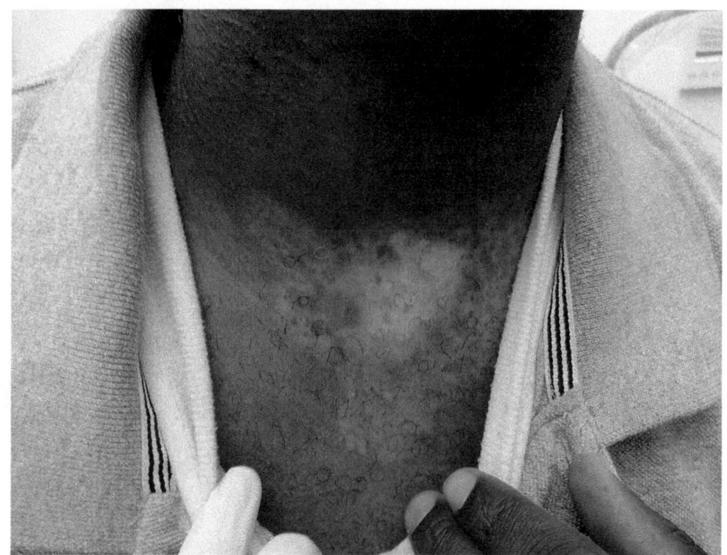

Fig. 37.1 Note repigmentation occurs first around the hair follicle

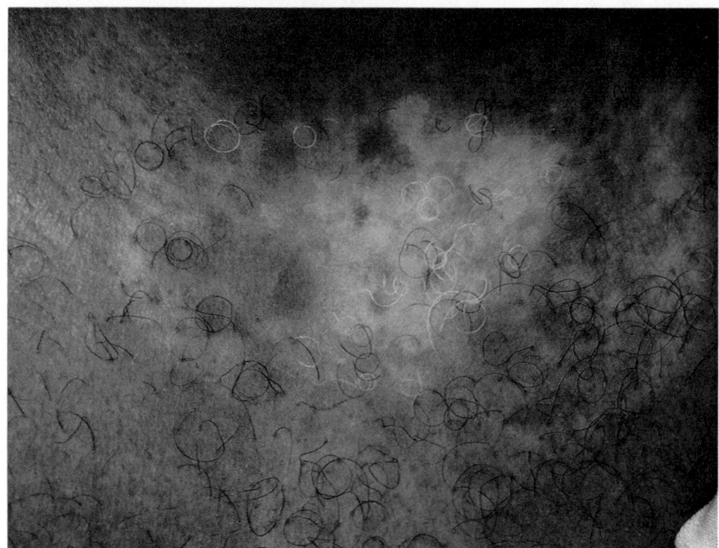

Fig. 37.2 Achromic, asymptomatic well demarcated patch on the chest

D. Reich et al., *Top 50 Dermatology Case Studies for Primary Care*,
DOI 10.1007/978-3-319-18627-6_37

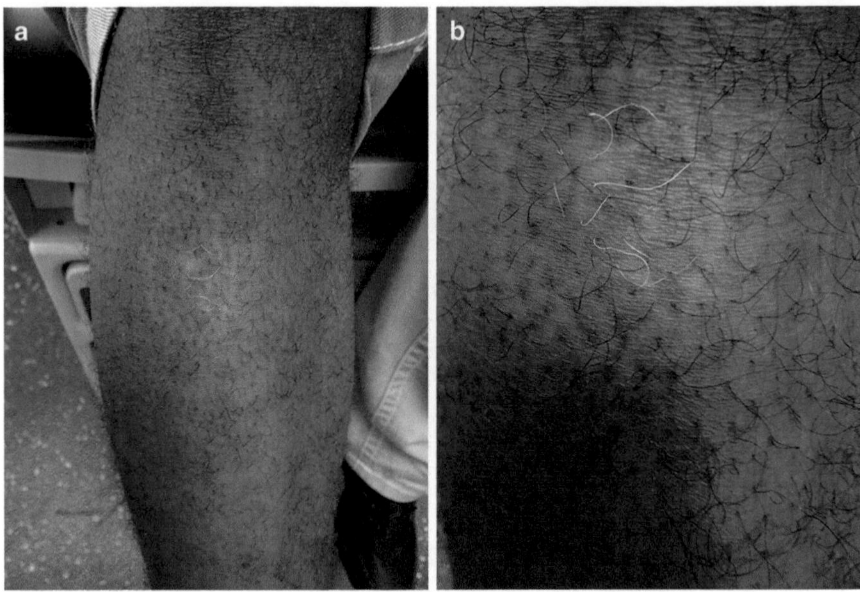

Fig. 37.3 (**a** and **b**) Lesions present on extensor surface of lower leg

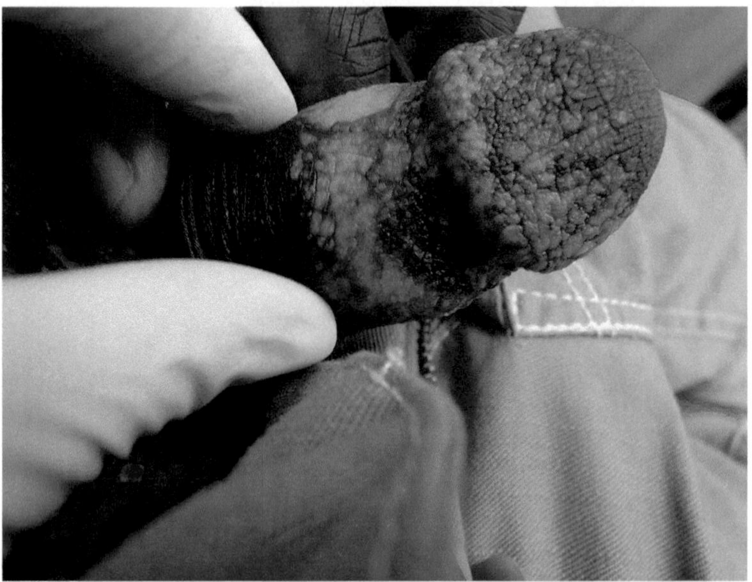

Fig. 37.4 Lesions affecting the genitals can cause significant psychological distress

Primary Care Visit Report

A 33-year-old male with past medical history of schizoaffective disorder, taking olanzapine, presented with a new hypopigmented rash on his penis. About 1 month prior, the patient had unprotected sex with a new partner. Then 2 weeks after that, he noted a red rash on his penis which was slightly uncomfortable, eventually became a scab, and then when healed was hypopigmented. It was not itchy. He had tried putting cocoa butter on it, which did not help. Prior to this incident, at around age 7, he developed a hypopigmented area on his inferior neck. At around age 12, he developed another hypopigmented area on his right shin following an abrasion.

Vitals were normal. On exam, the glans and distal shaft of his penis had well-defined scattered hypopigmented patches. His inferior neck had a 5 cm × 5 cm hypopigmented patch with white hair growing within the patch. His anterior right shin had a 5 cm × 5 cm mildly hypopigmented patch with white hair growing within the patch.

The differential diagnosis considered was vitiligo vs. hypopigmented scarring (given the history of the area scabbing before healing), and the patient was referred to dermatology for further evaluation.

Discussion from Dermatology Clinic

Differential Dx

- Vitiligo
- Post-inflammatory hypopigmentation
- Tinea versicolor
- Pityriasis alba
- Idiopathic guttate hypomelanosis
- Albinism
- Chemical leukoderma
- Hypopigmented mycosis fungoides

Favored Dx

The history of onset and characteristics of the patches are consistent with vitiligo. Furthermore, vitiligo is sometimes associated with a history of local trauma. This patient's vitiligo would be considered an example of generalized or non-segmental vitiligo, as it affects his neck, leg and genital area.

Overview

Vitiligo is an acquired, idiopathic, chronic disorder of depigmentation. It is the most common cause of depigmentation worldwide and affects 0.5–1 % of the population [1, 2]. Vitiligo affects genders and races equally, and it can occur at any age. Epidemiological studies suggest the mean age of onset is 24 years, however there are mixed reports on age predominance [1, 2]. It is likely the majority of vitiligo cases present before the age of 20 years [1, 3, 4]. The exact cause of vitiligo is unknown; however, it is thought to involve multiple genetic and environmental factors. The current understanding of pathogenesis is that autoimmune-mediated processes lead to destruction of the skin's pigment cells, the melanocytes.

Vitiligo has two distinct subtypes: generalized or non-segmental, and segmental vitiligo. Generalized vitiligo, which can involve widespread loss of pigment in patches that are often symmetrical, accounts for 85–90 % of vitiligo cases. It is associated with other autoimmune conditions, such as diabetes, rheumatoid arthritis, psoriasis, hypothyroidism and hyperthyroidism, and Addison's disease, in 20–30 % of cases [1–4]. Generalized vitiligo shows polygenic inheritance patterns. There is a 23 % concordance rate in monozygotic twins [2]. Segmental vitiligo, which involves loss of pigment in smaller patches on one side of the body in a limited area, is thought to be a genetically distinct entity. Factors predisposing specific areas of the body to developing vitiligo include sun exposure, physical trauma, inflammation, and vitamin deficiency. Hormonal changes associated with pregnancy have also been implicated in the formation of patches [2].

Presentation

Vitiligo is characterized by chalk-white macules of varying sizes, resulting from autoimmune destruction of melanocytes. Depigmentation of the macules tends to be uniform, with sharp borders. In addition to the epidermis, depigmentation affects hair follicles, and patches of vitiligo may feature white hair (leukotrichia). A key characteristic of vitiligo is the absence of textural changes in the affected skin. Vitiligo is usually asymptomatic but about 20 % of patients experience pruritus prior to the onset of a new macule [4].

Generalized/non-segmental vitiligo often presents bilaterally and symmetrically. Macules can be scattered or exhibit an acrofacial distribution pattern that affects the face and hands or feet. There are often halo nevi, moles that are surrounded by an area of depigmentation, surrounding the vitiliginous patches [3]. Common sites of presentation are the face, neck, scalp, and extensor surfaces [1]. Areas surrounding the mouth, eyes, and ears are frequently involved. Up to 100 % of skin can be affected in universal vitiligo. Segmental vitiligo typically presents unilaterally, in a dermatomal distribution. Its extent of involvement tends to be limited. Segmental vitiligo is more likely to affect children [2]. Patients with vitiligo may experience stigmatization and significant psychosocial distress [4].

Workup

Vitiligo is diagnosed on clinical presentation. Many of the differential diagnoses can be ruled out by identifying depigmentation (complete loss of pigment with chalk white appearance) versus hypopigmentation (reduced pigment compared to surrounding tissue). This can be achieved by Wood's lamp examination, which would cause skin to fluoresce bright white or blue-white. Wood's lamp examination may be especially useful in diagnosing fair-skinned individuals with vitiligo. Family history, extensive involvement, or evidence of autoimmune disorders warrants appropriate blood tests (antinuclear antibody, TSH, etc.), and may benefit from referral to a specialist.

Treatment

Vitiligo treatment should take into account personal and family history, extent of the disease, and psychosocial effect on the patient. In some cases it is possible to achieve repigmentation; however, there is no way to prevent new macules from developing. Treatment inhibits the immune response associated with vitiligo in order to restore function to existing melanocytes, and to stimulate migration of melanocytes from adjacent skin [2].

The available treatment modalities for vitiligo are topical therapy, phototherapy, oral medication, and surgical interventions. Combination regimens are more effective than monotherapy [4]. First line treatment is topical medications, including corticosteroids, vitamin D analogues (e.g., calcipotriene), and calcineurin inhibitors (e.g., tacrolimus).

Topical steroids are appropriate for treating small, localized lesions. Class III or IV mid-potency steroids are recommended. Alternatively, clobetasol propionate 0.05 % (Class I) may be used on a discontinuous schedule, e.g., daily for 2 weeks per month for 2 months, in order to avoid side effects. Topical tacrolimus or pimecrolimus are preferred for lesions on the face and neck [3]. They may be used twice daily for 6 months. They have a direct effect on melanocytes and are more effective in combination with UV phototherapy [1, 2, 4]. Vitamin D analogues have mixed reports on efficacy. They are more effective as combination therapy with PUVA (ultraviolet photochemotherapy) [4].

Oral therapies with some demonstrated efficacy are *Ginkgo biloba* and oral minipulses of betamethasone. *Ginkgo biloba* is an anti-inflammatory supplement that may be taken as a 40 or 60 mg tablet twice daily. One study demonstrated an effect of repigmentation when taken as a monotherapy, however the evidence is limited [4–6]. *Ginkgo biloba* would not be considered first line therapy but may provide an alternative option for patients desiring a natural approach to treatment. Oral minipulses of betamethasone are taken at a dose of 0.1 mg/kg twice weekly on two consecutive days for 3 months, then tapered to 1 mg monthly for the following 3 months. This regimen is more effective when combined with narrow-band ultraviolet light therapy [7].

Vitiligo that does not respond to topical or oral therapy may be referred to dermatology for phototherapy or photochemotherapy. Narrow-band UVB tends to be more effective than PUVA. It requires twice weekly treatments of 5–10 min, and may achieve over 75 % repigmentation after 1 year of treatment [3, 4]. Surgical interventions, such as tissue grafts, are an option for patients with segmental, limited, or stable vitiligo. Melanocyte transplant is a new and emerging surgical intervention. Both tissue grafts and melanocyte transplants are not common practice in the USA; however, they are predicted to become more available in the future [8]. Patients may be referred to dermatology to discuss these interventions.

Follow-Up

Patients should be advised that topical medications may require several months before they cause any repigmentation. Patients should be monitored for adverse effects of topical corticosteroids such as atrophy, telangiectasia, folliculitis, and steroid acne.

Vitiliginous skin lacks melanin, which protects skin from ultraviolet radiation. Thus individuals with vitiligo should be advised of an increased risk of sunburns on areas of the skin with vitiligo and to apply sunblock to those areas when they are exposed to the sun.

The course of vitiligo is unpredictable. Patients may experience stable lesions, or the lesions may rapidly spread. If they experience a rapid increase in vitiligo distribution, patients may return to the office for a referral to dermatology. Extensive vitiligo is best managed by dermatology, where more extensive treatments with PUVA or narrow-band UVB may be administered.

Questions for the Dermatologist

– *Is it common for vitiligo to develop slowly, over decades, as occurred with this patient?*

It is. Patches can be aggressively rapid, with a new one forming every month, or they can develop slowly over years. It is not uncommon to have a static patch, for example around the mouth, and then not develop another one for years.

– *Is there anything that can be done to stop the progression?*

No, there is nothing that can prevent the progression. Light therapy is the best tool we have for vitiligo treatment. It is good, but not great. A new drug called Afamelanotide, an agonistic analogue of α-melanocyte stimulating hormone, is under development and may provide greater success at repigmentation.

– *Could unprotected sex have anything to do with developing vitiligo on the penis? Could the reported abrasion have anything to do with developing vitiligo on the shin?*

Trauma has been implicated as a predisposing factor to developing new patches. Unprotected sex is most likely unrelated. It is possible the previous abrasion to the knee is related.

– *How often does vitiligo treatment achieve repigmentation?*

Vitiligo treatment can be very helpful, but it is not necessarily a home run. Treatment success depends on the body surface area involved. A single patch is easier to treat. If there is extensive involvement, with most of the body affected, it will be more difficult to achieve extensive repigmentation. Ultimately most treatment is successful at gaining some repigmentation. It may not be 100 % repigmentation, but some pigment will return. The typical treatment story ends in gaining some of the pigment back on some the vitiliginous patches. For example we recently treated a patient with 70 % body surface area involvement, and the patient was able to regrow 50–60 % of pigment on some of the plaques. There was repigmentation on the hands and face, highly visible areas, which is important for many patients.

– *Does vitiligo ever spontaneously regress? For example, if a patient chooses not to treat their vitiligo because it is on a part of their body where it is not bothersome to them, are there any long term negative implications to that choice?*

Vitiligo does not usually spontaneously regress. It may be the case that depigmentation occurs in waves. The extent of involvement could increase and then plateau. The course of vitiligo is difficult to predict and varies between individuals. There is no danger is leaving vitiligo untreated and it will not influence the course of the disease, as treatment generally aims to improve the appearance of depigmented patches.

– *If a patient develops vitiligo and in the ensuing workup is subsequently found to have an autoimmune disease (like diabetes or autoimmune thyroiditis), if the autoimmune disease is treated and brought under control, does the vitiligo then regress?*

No, treating the associated autoimmune disease would not affect vitiligo. Autoimmune diseases like diabetes and vitiligo track together, however there are different underlying etiologies. They indicate a propensity for autoimmune disease generally. Treatment of one disorder will not make the other one go away.

References

1. Ezzedine K, Eleftheriadou V, Whitton M, van Geel N. Vitiligo. Lancet. 2015;386(9988):74–84. pii: S0140-6736(14)60763-7.
2. Birlea SA, Spritz RA, Norris DA. Chapter 74. Vitiligo. In: Goldsmith LA, Katz SI, Gilchrest BA, Paller AS, Leffell DJ, Wolff K, editors. Fitzpatrick's dermatology in general medicine. 8th ed. New York: McGraw-Hill; 2012. Available from: http://accessmedicine.mhmedical.com.ezproxy.cul.columbia.edu/content.aspx?bookid=392&Sectionid=41138776. Accessed 26 Feb 2015.
3. Taïeb A, Picardo M. Vitiligo. N Engl J Med. 2009;360(2):160.
4. Whitton ME, Pinart M, Batchelor J, Leonardi-Bee J, González U, Jiyad Z, Eleftheriadou V, Ezzedine K. Interventions for vitiligo. Cochrane Database Syst Rev. 2015;2, CD003263.
5. Szczurko O, Shear N, Taddio A, Boon H. Ginkgo biloba for the treatment of vitiligo vulgaris: an open label pilot clinical trial. BMC Complement Altern Med. 2011;11:21.
6. Whitton ME, Ashcroft DM, González U. Therapeutic interventions for vitiligo. J Am Acad Dermatol. 2008;59(4):713–7.
7. Rath N, Kar HK, Sabhnani S. An open labeled, comparative clinical study on efficacy and tolerability of oral minipulse of steroid (OMP) alone, OMP with PUVA and broad/narrow band UVB phototherapy in progressive vitiligo. Indian J Dermatol Venereol Leprol. 2008;74(4):357–60.
8. American Academy of Dermatology. New surgical techniques hold promise for treating vitiligo | aad.org [Internet]. 2015 [cited 26 February 2015]. Available from: https://www.aad.org/stories-and-news/news-releases/new-surgical-techniques-hold-promise-for-treating-vitiligo

Chapter 38
Drug Reaction

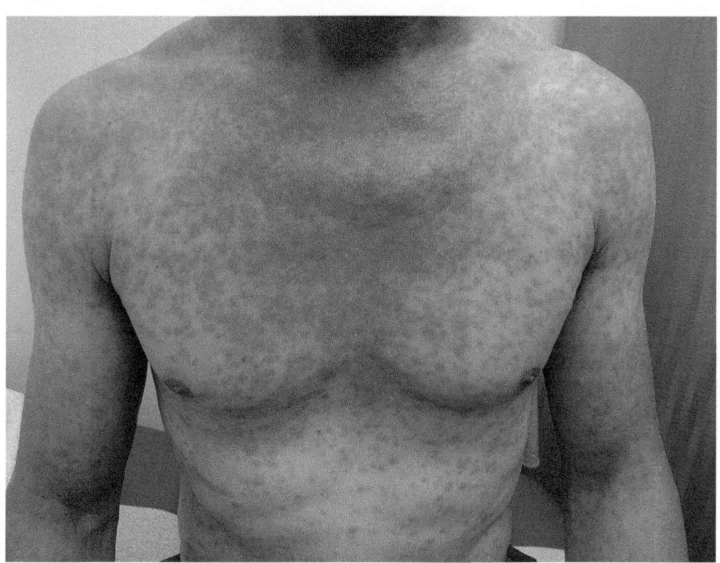

Fig. 38.1 The true "maculopapular" rash involving trunk diffusely

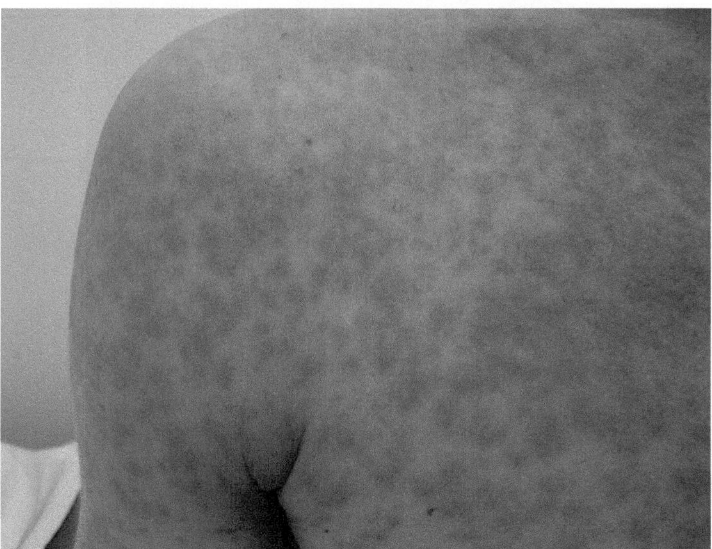

Fig. 38.2 Slight edema and bright red color are characteristic of this condition

D. Reich et al., *Top 50 Dermatology Case Studies for Primary Care*,
DOI 10.1007/978-3-319-18627-6_38

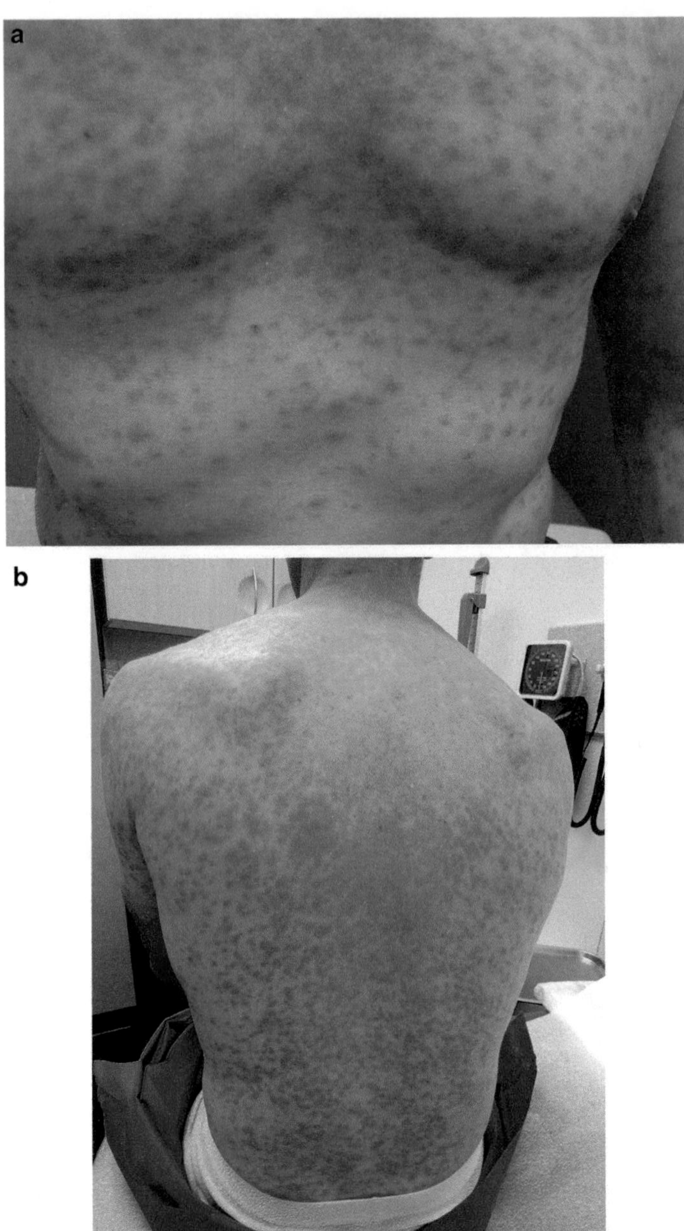

Fig. 38.3 (**a** and **b**) Truncal plaque areas of sparing

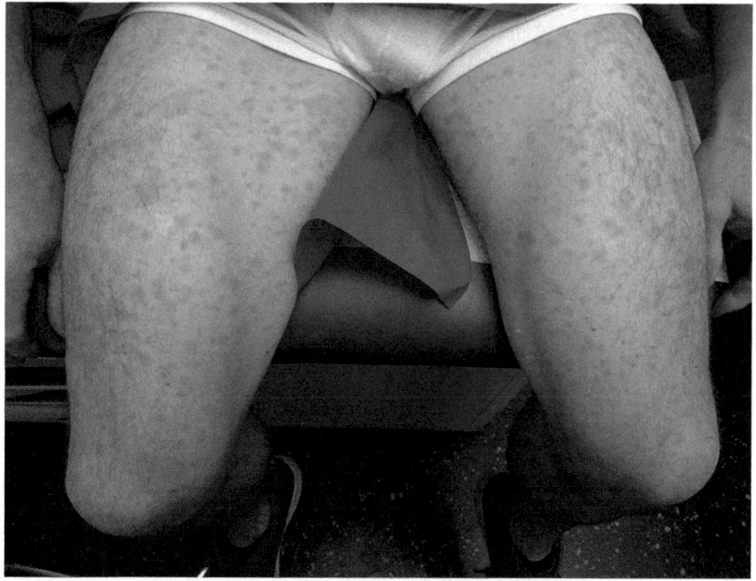

Fig. 38.4 This rash tends to start on the trunk and then spread to extremities

Primary Care Visit Report

A 44-year-old male with no past medical history presented with a rash on his face, chest, back, arms, and legs. One day prior, he had noticed the rash upon waking. It had started on his face and progressively spread down his trunk, and then to his arms and legs. It was not itchy. The day prior was the final day of a 7-day course of amoxicillin (prescribed by a different doctor), which the patient had taken for a tick bite. The patient had no known drug allergies.

Vitals were normal. On exam, there was a diffuse, erythematous morbilliform rash on bilateral arms, bilateral legs, chest, abdomen and back. The rash spared the palms and soles. His face was erythematous but did not have the rash.

The patient was treated for a drug reaction, assuming it was caused by amoxicillin even though the patient had no prior reaction to that medication. Since he had finished the course of amoxicillin already, we did not have to discontinue it or switch to a different antibiotic. We started the patient on a 15-day prednisone taper starting with 80 mg for 3 days, then 60 mg for 3 days, then 40 mg for 3 days, then 20 mg for 3 days, then 10 mg for 3 days. We advised the patient that going forward he should consider himself allergic to penicillins.

Discussion from Dermatology Clinic

Differential Dx

- Drug eruption
- Erythema multiforme
- Viral exanthem
- Urticaria
- Collagen vascular disease

Favored Dx

Drug-induced eruption is favored given the extent of cutaneous involvement, and onset of rash while taking an antibiotic commonly associated with adverse reactions.

Overview

Acute cutaneous drug reaction is an umbrella term, inclusive of any abnormal skin findings that manifest as a result of an adverse response to a systemic or topical drug. Drug eruptions can occur as a result of immunologic or non-immunologic responses, which include allergies, overdose, dose accumulation, or drug interactions. Consequently, drug eruptions do not necessarily indicate an allergy to a particular medication. Drug-induced eruption describes a sudden-onset rash that coincides with starting a new drug, or occurs in patients who take multiple medications.

Hives and rashes are among the most common adverse reactions to drugs. Cutaneous drug reactions occur in up to 8 % of the population, and 12 % of children treated with antibiotics [1]. According to the American College of Allergy, Asthma, and Immunology, up to 10 % of the population is allergic to β-lactam (penicillin family) antibiotics [2].

Any oral medication can cause an adverse reaction; however, they most frequently occur following treatment with antibiotics, anticonvulsants, nonsteroidal anti-inflammatories, allopurinol, dapsone, nevirapine, and abacavir. Some of these medications can lead to severe cutaneous drug eruptions, like toxic epidermal necrolysis or Stevens–Johnson syndrome, that cause significant morbidity or death [1, 3].

Presentation

The most common presentation of drug eruptions, occurring in 95 % of cases, is a morbilliform erythematous rash [1, 4]. The eruption presents as pruritic erythematous macules and papules that blanch on application of pressure. There is variable involvement, but it tends to begin on the trunk and spread to extremities. Rashes tend to appear within 7–14 days after initiating medication; however, it is not uncommon for the rashes to appear up to 3 weeks later. Lesions desquamate and become scaly as they resolve. In more severe reactions, patches can coalesce and form erythroderma (erythema and scaling that can affect almost the entire cutaneous surface). Any systemic involvement such as fever may be indicative of a more serious drug-induced hypersensitivity reaction.

Workup

Drug-induced eruptions are usually diagnosed based on patient history and clinical findings. A skin biopsy may be performed; however, it has limitations. In cases of drug eruption, a biopsy would not be able to identify the offending medication. The presence of eosinophils on biopsy was once considered a classic sign of drug reactions; however, that belief is now controversial. Furthermore, the presence of eosinophils cannot reliably distinguish between drug eruptions, viral exanthem, and acute graft-versus-host disease. When accompanied by systemic symptoms such as fever, lymphadenopathy, or organ involvement, a biopsy with high concentration of eosinophils could point to a rare, severe syndrome called drug reaction with eosinophilia and systemic symptoms (DRESS) [5].

If eruptions are very severe, or there is indication of systemic involvement such as fever, lymphadenopathy, or organ involvement, further tests should be ordered, including complete blood count and serum chemistry. Prick, intradermal, specific IgE, and lymphocyte transformation tests (LTT) can help determine true allergies to medications, and are performed by an allergist or immunologist.

Non-allergic drug eruptions may occur in up to 70 % of adults and 100 % of children with acute Epstein-Barr virus infection who are treated with amoxicillin [6]. Patients presenting with a recent history of fatigue, sore throat, and swollen lymph nodes in the neck should be tested for EBV.

Treatment

The first step in treating cutaneous drug reactions is identifying and eliminating the responsible drug. If possible, a structurally different substitute should be given [7]. Symptom resolution can take up to 2 weeks following discontinuation of the offending medication. Pruritus can be treated with antihistamines such as hydroxyzine. A systemic corticosteroid may accelerate resolution of the rash but its benefits are controversial. A 2-week prednisone taper with a starting dose of 1 mg/kg daily would be appropriate for the patient in this case.

Follow-Up

Patients should be instructed to return to the office if the rash does not start resolving after prednisone is initiated, or if fever develops. Patients should be advised that adverse reactions to penicillin may not reflect a true drug allergy. It is possible for people to have drug reactions to a medication they have previously taken without complications. It is also possible for drug sensitivity to decrease over time, and for patients to resume taking the offending drug in the future without incident. There is inherent risk in taking a drug that has previously caused a reaction, especially one that involves the airway. The safest approach would be to avoid that class of medication altogether.

Questions for the Dermatologist

– *Could a drug reaction turn into anaphylaxis?*

No, usually not. Patients who have anaphylactic reactions to penicillin have a very specific kind of response, moderated by acute T cell hypersensitivity. A patient with a drug eruption following ingestion of the drug has a delayed T cell response with a rash.

– *Is it common for a drug reaction to start at the end of taking the drug? What is the typical timeframe from ingestion to rash?*

A common misconception is that a drug eruption should be immediate. It can happen up to a month after a drug is taken. Even after stopping a medication, developing a rash the following week elicits suspicion of a drug reaction. Beyond a month, the incidence of drug eruptions drops. There is no typical timeframe; a rash could occur anytime from the following day to a month later. The rash most commonly occurs within a week; however, that should not be used as a guideline to rule out drug eruptions that occur in a different timeframe.

– *Is it true that, with skin rashes, a longer steroid taper is necessary or the rash will recur (vs. a 5-day course with no taper)?*

Correct. Five day courses of prednisone can do beautifully in clearing a rash and then it pops back up. Our practice usually does a 2-week taper, with initial dosing of 1 mg/kg/day.

– *Is a drug eruption considered an allergy or an adverse reaction? Should the patient now say he is allergic to penicillins?*

Drug eruptions can be caused either by an allergy or an adverse reaction – it depends on the case and the patient history. For example, you can have a drug toxic affect causing rash. Think benzoyl peroxide and irritated cheeks. Or nitroglycerin and flushing. Or amoxicillin in someone who has mononucleosis. Those are true drug reactions that affect everyone. You can also have allergic drug reactions like penicillin and a full body rash which only affect those patients who form antibodies to the beta lactam ring of penicillin. This case is likely an allergy to penicillin given the patient's history, but without allergy testing we can't know for sure. It would be appropriate, however, for the patient to say he is allergic to penicillin until proven otherwise. If he is truly allergic to penicillin, if he ever took it again, the reaction should be reproducible – meaning he should get the same rash again.

– *Is there a way to test if amoxicillin caused the reaction? Is there any utility in doing this?*

An allergist could test for penicillin allergy, if it is important for the patient to get penicillin in the future, or if he will be somewhere where penicillin is the only class of antibiotics available. The worst-case scenario for this patient would be getting another rash. Otherwise we would recommend he avoid that class of medications in the future. Anaphylaxis is harder to test for, and any potential for suspected airway involvement should rule this class of medication out altogether.

References

1. Shear NH, Knowles SR. Chapter 41. Cutaneous reactions to drugs. In: Goldsmith LA, Katz SI, Gilchrest BA, Paller AS, Leffell DJ, Wolff K, editors. Fitzpatrick's dermatology in general medicine. 8th ed. New York: McGraw-Hill; 2012.
2. American College of Allergy, Asthma & Immunology. Drug Allergies [Internet]. 2014 [cited 2014 Dec 6]. Available from: http://www.acaai.org/allergist/allergies/Types/drug-allergy/Pages/penicillin-allergy.aspx
3. Knowles SR, Shear NH. Recognition and management of severe cutaneous drug reactions. Dermatol Clin. 2007;25(2):245–53. viii.
4. Gerson D, Sriganeshan V, Alexis JB. Cutaneous drug eruptions: a 5-year experience. J Am Acad Dermatol. 2008;59(6):995–9.
5. Ganeva M, Gancheva T, Lazarova R, Troeva J, Baldaranov I, Vassilev I, Hristakieva E, Tzaneva V. Carbamazepine-induced drug eruption with eosinophilia and systemic symptoms (DRESS) syndrome: report of four cases and brief review. Int J Dermatol. 2008;47(8):853–60.
6. Renn CN, Straff W, Dorfmüller A, Al-Masaoudi T, Merk HF, Sachs B. Amoxicillin-induced exanthema in young adults with infectious mononucleosis: demonstration of drug-specific lymphocyte reactivity. Br J Dermatol. 2002;147(6):1166–70.
7. Riedl MA, Casillas AM. Adverse drug reactions: types and treatment options. Am Fam Physician. 2003;68(9):1781–91.

Chapter 39
Scarring

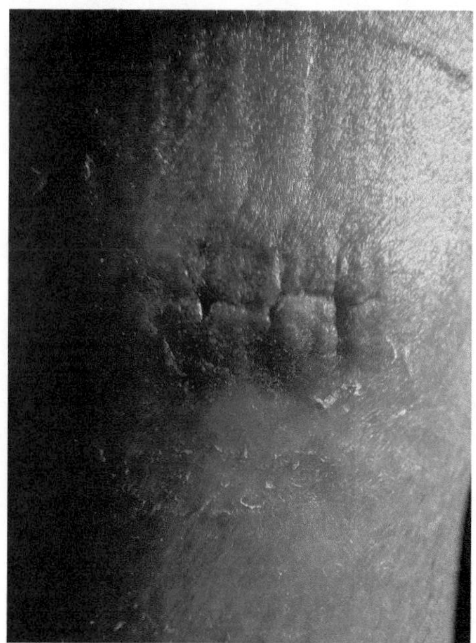

Fig. 39.1 Post suture removal with good approximation of edges in this arm wound

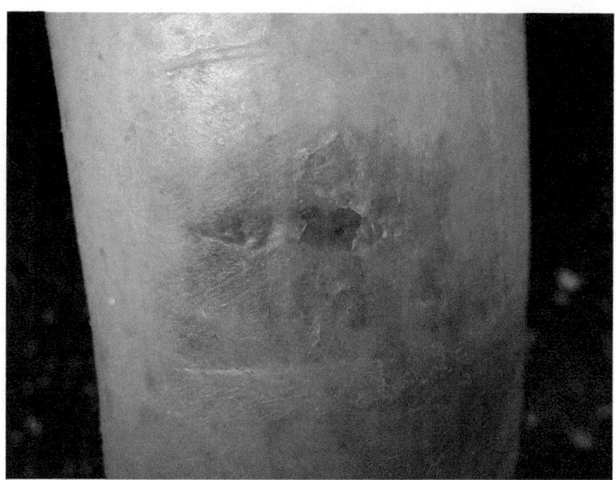

Fig. 39.2 Mild wound gaping noted centrally, poor approximation of edges, and higher risk of cosmetically less desirable scarring in this leg wound

D. Reich et al., *Top 50 Dermatology Case Studies for Primary Care*,
DOI 10.1007/978-3-319-18627-6_39

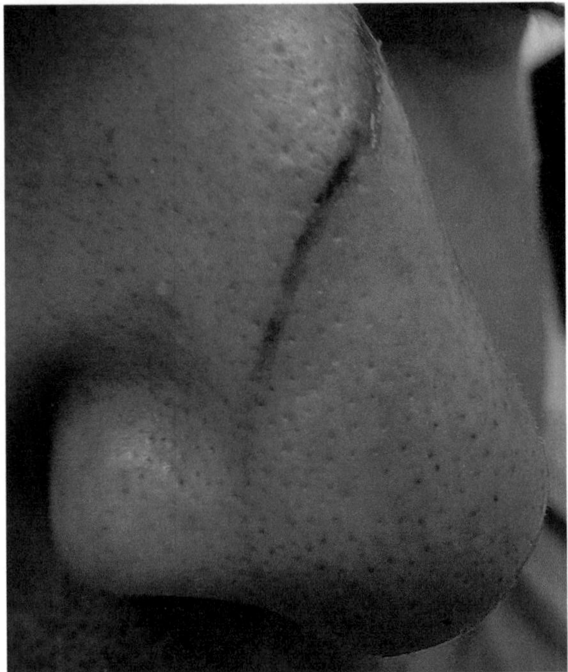

Fig. 39.3 Linear abrasion, partial thickness

Primary Care Visit Report

The first patient, a 56-year-old female with newly diagnosed invasive squamous cell carcinoma on her lower leg, presented for removal of stitches from a recently biopsied lesion on her left upper arm. The sutures had been placed 14 days prior to this visit.

Vitals were normal. On exam, her left upper arm had a 2 cm × 2 cm erythematous raised lesion with three sutures, knots buried, and some erythematous papular irritation surrounding the lesion from the bandage. Her left lower leg featured a well-healing lesion from prior SCC removal.

The stitches were removed from the left arm lesion.

The second patient was a 28-year-old male with no past medical history who presented with a laceration on his nose. About an hour prior, a fluorescent light box had fallen from the ceiling and cut his nose.

Vitals were normal. On exam, there was a 3 cm linear laceration extending from the left side of his nose superiorly to the right side of his nose inferiorly (crossing the bridge of his nose) with minimal bleeding.

A plastic surgeon was consulted, and advised that, even though this laceration appeared to be superficial, stitching would help reduce scarring. The patient was referred to this plastic surgeon for suturing.

In both cases, the patients were concerned with scarring from these skin lesions and wanted to know how to minimize or prevent scarring. They were advised to ensure the lesions were covered with sunblock and to avoid direct sun exposure.

Discussion from Dermatology Clinic

Differential Dx

- Scar
- Hypertrophic scar
- Keloid

Favored Dx

Both patients have actively healing partial thickness wounds that may result in scarring.

Overview

Scars are formed by fibrous tissue, which replaces normal tissue after an insult or injury to the skin. Following damage to tissue, wounds undergo a dynamic healing process that is characterized by four stages: hemostasis, inflammation, proliferation or granulation, and maturation or remodeling [1]. This healing process can last between months and years [2]. Depending on the depth and nature of the wound, the healing process can result in formation of a scar.

Hemostasis is the first stage of tissue healing. After the continuity of skin is disrupted, platelet activation and the coagulation cascade act to stop hemorrhage. The inflammatory phase is marked by initiation of the inflammatory cascade, with neutrophils, macrophages, and other mediators infiltrating the wound site, and contributing to removal of damaged tissue. Tissue loss triggers vascularization and formation of new tissue, termed granulation tissue, and over the course of up to 2 years, fibroblasts and collagen are produced and deposited, and the skin is remodeled [3]. Rather than occurring sequentially, these events are dynamic and represent an interplay between several healing mediators.

A number of different characteristics of wounds affect the prognosis of healing and scar formation. Wounds can be classified according to the depth of injury, with superficial wounds limited to the epidermis, partial thickness wounds involving some of the dermis, and full-thickness wounds extending fully through the dermis, and into subcutaneous tissue in some cases. Superficial wounds, caused by friction, mild burns, or abrasions, often resolve without scarring, as the healing process typically only requires re-epithelialization of the epidermis of otherwise continuous, intact skin [4]. Partial thickness wounds typically heal in a similar fashion to superficial wounds; however, their size and shape would influence the healing outcome. Wounds that cover a large surface area, or involve jagged edges, are more likely to result in a scar. Full thickness wounds often require suturing and resolve with a scar.

Surgical incisions are the most common cause of scarring, with an estimated incidence of 100 million new scars per year following elective procedures in the developed world [2]. Acne scars are estimated to affect up to 14 % of people suffering from acne [5]. Other common causes of scarring are discoid lupus erythematosus, scarring alopecia, and varicella. Exaggerated healing responses can lead to hypertrophic and keloid scarring. Between 5 and 15 % of wounds are thought to result in keloid scars [6]. Keloid scars are more common in people under the age of 30, are 15 times more likely to occur in African Americans and 5 times more like to occur in Asians than Caucasians [5, 7]. Scars can cause anxiety and depression, and more than half of people with scars report dissatisfaction with their scars' appearance [2].

Presentation

Scar presentation varies by subtype. Surgical scars are typically linear, and may be hyperpigmented, pink, or ivory in color. Atrophic scars, commonly caused by varicella, smallpox, and acne, are white or ivory depressions in the skin. Acne scars have distinct presentations, referred to as ice-pick, rolling, and boxcar scarring [8]. Icepick scars are under 2 mm in diameter and extend to the deep dermis. Rolling scars are wide depressions that give the skin an undulating appearance. Boxcar scars can be shallow or deep, and they are similar to varicella scars—round and oval depressions with sharp edges [8].

Hypertrophic scars are raised and red or pink in color, and they do not extend beyond the borders of the initial wound. Keloid scars extend beyond the border of the wound edge. They are also raised, nodular, and typically red-colored in their early stage; however, they may darken over time. Keloids are more likely to present on the earlobes, chest, and shoulders.

Workup

Scars are diagnosed on history and clinical examination. Scar surface area, thickness, color, and texture are important parameters to assess and record, as they affect prognosis and treatment approach [2]. Furthermore, they are parameters that can be reevaluated at later visits to monitor healing progression.

Treatment

Treatment of healing wounds should aim to minimize scarring. The specific approach depends on the type of wound being treated. Any surgical incisions and suturing should ideally occur along Langer's lines (which correspond to the orientation of collagen in the dermis) to minimize tension on the wound. The edges of the laceration or wound should be matched up as neatly as possible. Superficial lacerations, and wounds that require internal sutures, can have their apposing edges bound by a chemical adhesive, such as Dermabond. A chemical bonding agent has several advantages in that it does not require anesthesia, it is not typically painful, and it may be more agreeable to children who are uncooperative with sutures [1]. Chemical bonding agents have similar cosmetic outcomes to suturing [7, 9]. They are not appropriate for use in areas of high skin tension, like the hands, feet, and joints. While wounds are healing, adhesive dressings should be avoided as they can remove newly formed superficial tissue when they are changed. Over-the-counter hydrogel dressings have demonstrated efficacy in promoting normal wound healing [10]. An optimal wound healing environment is the first step to scar prevention.

There are several nonsurgical and surgical approaches to prevent and minimize scarring after wounds have healed. These include moisturizers, gel sheeting, sunscreen, intralesional steroid injections, surgical excision, laser therapy, and cryotherapy [6]. Keeping the immature scar in a well-hydrated environment can help prevent or minimize permanent scar formation. This can be achieved with non-irritating over-the-counter moisturizes and emollients like Aveeno, Cerave, Aquafor, or Cetaphil. Sunscreen is recommended as it can reduce post-inflammatory hyperpigmentation. Silicone gel sheets are another option for a conservative approach to treatment, and they are available over-the-counter. There is little evidence of their prophylactic benefit; however, they may reduce the size of hypertrophic scars [3, 6]. Silicone gel sheets should not be used on open wounds. While Vitamin E ointment is often mentioned in the context of scar prevention, there is little evidence that it improves cosmetic outcomes. Additionally it has been found to cause significant contact dermatitis [11].

Intralesional corticosteroid injections are considered first-line treatment for abnormal scars, as they have been found to prevent hypertrophy and reduce the size of keloids [3, 7]. Triamcinolone acetonide suspension (Kenalog) is a commonly used agent, which the author's practice injects at a concentration of 10 mg/cc. This concentration should be reduced to 2.5–5 mg/cc for facial scars. These are typically repeated monthly for 5–6 months, or until the scars have reached satisfactory response. While they are greatly effective at reducing scar formation, intralesional corticosteroids are associated with a number of adverse effects, including atrophy, hypopigmentation, and telangiectasia [3, 7].

Patients interested in surgical excision may be referred to a dermatologist or plastic surgeon. Surgical excision is not usually recommended for keloids, as there are extremely high recurrence rates [7]. However, there is some evidence to suggest surgical excision combined with intralesional corticosteroid injections may minimize the risk of recurrence [7]. Acne scar treatment warrants a referral to a dermatologist, as the best treatment options are chemical peels, dermabrasion, filler injections, or laser resurfacing [5, 8].

Follow-Up

Patients opting for conservative approaches do not require follow-up, unless they are dissatisfied with outcomes and would like to consider alternative options. Those treated with intralesional corticosteroids should be monitored for adverse side effects, including atrophy, hypopigmentation, and telangiectasia. They will likely need to return for several treatments in order to see substantial improvement in their scars. Further minimization of scars may be achieved by applying sunblock to the area, as UV exposure can result in significant hyperpigmentation [2].

Questions for the Dermatologist

– *What can be done to prevent scarring?*

Perhaps the most important factors would be to keep the healing wound away from any source of infection, to keep it hydrated by applying emollients or moisturizers, and to avoid exposing the wound to sunlight.

– *Should the area be massaged or left alone?*

While the wound is healing, it should be left alone. After the wound has fully closed and healed, it would be okay to massage the area in order to break down any banding or firmness of the scar tissue. There are no evidence-based recommendations for this practice; however, it could theoretically be beneficial [12].

– *What is the role of sun exposure and sunblock in scarring? Why does sun exposure lead to more severe scarring?*

UV light is a macrophage inhibitor. It acts to suppress the immune system, which is why it can be a successful treatment for psoriasis and eczema. When scars are forming, macrophages play a large role in laying down new bands of collagen and removing damaged tissue. If macrophages are inhibited, the area ends up being crowded by inflammatory mediators that prevent optimal healing.

– *Does stitching help reduce scarring?*

Stitching does help reduce scarring; however it is not always necessary. If the wound is superficial and the edges match up neatly, the wound will likely heal nicely without stitches.

References

1. Rivera AE, Spencer JM. Clinical aspects of full-thickness wound healing. Clin Dermatol. 2007;25(1):39–48.
2. Junker JP, Philip J, Kiwanuka E, Hackl F, Caterson EJ, Eriksson E. Assessing quality of healing in skin: review of available methods and devices. Wound Repair Regen. 2014;22 Suppl 1:2–10.
3. Reish RG, Eriksson E. Scar treatments: preclinical and clinical studies. J Am Coll Surg. 2008;206(4):719–30.
4. Irion G, editor. Chapter 2, Normal wound healing. Comprehensive wound management [internet]. 2nd ed. Thorofare (NJ): SLACK Incorporated; 2009. [cited 23 March 2015]. Available from: ProQuest ebrary.
5. Rivera AE. Acne scarring: a review and current treatment modalities. J Am Acad Dermatol. 2008;59(4):659–76.
6. O'Brien L, Jones DJ. Silicone gel sheeting for preventing and treating hypertrophic and keloid scars. Cochrane Database Syst Rev. 2013;9, CD003826.
7. Juckett G, Hartman-Adams H. Management of keloids and hypertrophic scars. Am Fam Physician. 2009;80(3):253–60.
8. Jacob CI, Dover JS, Kaminer MS. Acne scarring: a classification system and review of treatment options. J Am Acad Dermatol. 2001;45(1):109–17.
9. Bruns TB, Worthington JM. Using tissue adhesive for wound repair: a practical guide to Dermabond. Am Fam Physician. 2000;61(5):1383–8.
10. Wasiak J, Cleland H, Campbell F, Spinks A. Dressings for superficial and partial thickness burns (Review). Cochrane Database Syst Rev. 2013;3, CD002106.
11. Baumann LS, Spencer J. The effects of topical Vitamin E on the cosmetic appearance of scars. Dermatol Surg. 1999;25(4):311–5.
12. Shin TM, Bordeaux JS. The role of massage in scar management: a literature review. Dermatol Surg. 2012;38(3):414–23.

Chapter 40
Bedbug Bites

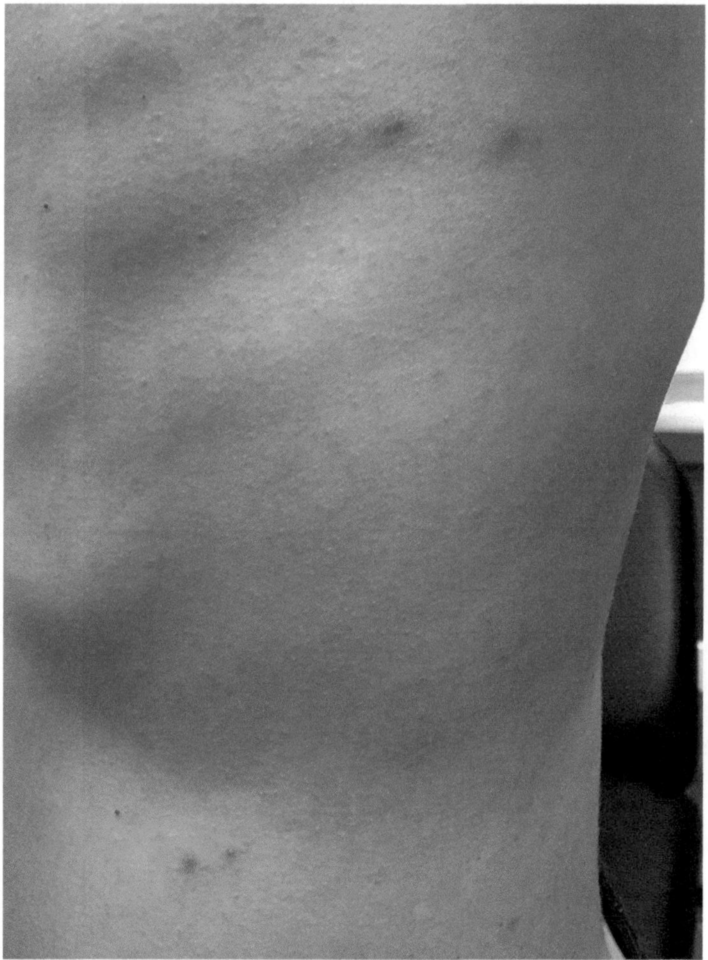

Fig. 40.1 Grouped erythematous, edematous papules with surrounding wheal

D. Reich et al., *Top 50 Dermatology Case Studies for Primary Care*,
DOI 10.1007/978-3-319-18627-6_40

Primary Care Visit Report

A 24-year-old male with no prior medical history presented with a rash on his trunk after a weekend away with friends at an upstate New York rental property. The patient slept in pajama bottoms only, without any clothes covering his torso or arms. The patient woke up with discrete papular lesions on his trunk. The lesions were very itchy, and they developed surrounding welts over a few hours after waking. No blood was noted on the sheets. His partner in bed did not have any lesions.

Vitals were normal. On examination, on his left lateral trunk, there were four 3–4 mm erythematous papules with surrounding erythema.

Given that the lesions were very itchy, they presented in pairs, and the patient had slept in a different bed in a rental property, the possibility of bed bugs was considered to be high. The lesions were treated as bed bugs. The patient was advised to take an over-the-counter anti-histamine to help relieve the pruritus, and was prescribed Desonide 0.05 % (Class VI) steroid cream to reduce inflammation and associated pruritus.

The patient was advised to take precautions with his clothing and any belongings he brought to the rental property so as not to introduce bed bugs into his own home. He was advised to wash anything he had with him in hot water and to inspect his suitcase for bed bugs and bug fecal matter.

Discussion from Dermatology Clinic

Differential Dx

- Bedbug bites
- Scabies
- Flea bites
- Urticaria
- Body lice (pediculosis corporis)

Favored Dx

Bedbug bites can be difficult to differentiate from other insect bites. In this case, finding new bites in the morning on areas of the body that were exposed, coupled with sleeping in a new location that may be particularly vulnerable to bedbugs due to higher numbers of travelling visitors, are factors that support a diagnosis of bedbug bites.

Overview

The common bedbug, *Cimex lectularius*, is a blood-feeding insect of the order Hemiptera. *C. lectularius* is flat, wingless, brown, and typically 2–5 mm in size [1]. They are nocturnal feeders and spend the daytime hiding often in the cracks of headboards, crevices of bed frames, and mattress seams. They emerge from their hiding places when they sense the body warmth and expired carbon dioxide of their victims [2]. Bedbugs feed every 3–5 days, but they can go up to 1 year without feeding [1–3].

Bedbug infestations are becoming increasingly prevalent in the USA and worldwide, perhaps owed to increased travel and insecticide resistance [1, 3–5]. They were once associated with disadvantaged socioeconomic status; however, bed bugs can affect individuals of all socioeconomic strata. Infestations can be found in hotels, homes, offices, nursing homes, trains, buses, or ships. Bedbugs may spread through clothing, luggage, used furniture, and mattresses. They are not thought to be vectors for human viruses or disease [1, 2].

Presentation

Bedbug bites typically appear as erythematous papular lesions with a central hemorrhagic punctum. Bites are usually located on uncovered parts of the body, and may appear in groups of 3–4 lesions along a line or curve. These are often referred to as the "breakfast, lunch, and dinner" arrangement. Bites are usually painless, but may be severely pruritic. Individuals who are more sensitive to bedbug bites may experience morbilliform (widespread erythematous macules or papules that blanch with pressure) or urticarial eruptions, and in severe cases, anaphylactoid reactions and bullae [3, 5]. Some people may not experience any skin reaction to bedbug bites, and one study identified 30 % of those living in infested households did not experience a reaction [1].

Workup

Bedbugs bites are usually diagnosed based on clinical presentation and history. Clues suggestive of bedbug bites are new lesions in the morning, similar symptoms in people sharing a bed, change of symptoms upon changing sleeping location, onset of symptoms during or after recent travel, detecting bedbug fecal matter (dark spots) around the bed or mattress seams, and blood on the sheets [1]. Other arthropod bites may be excluded from the differential based on presence of burrows (scabies), or pets in the household (fleas). Once clinical diagnosis is made, it is recommended patients evaluate their homes for infestation. If diagnosis is unclear, a biopsy may be done, or the patient may be referred to a specialist.

Treatment

Bedbug treatment targets symptomatic relief. Topical corticosteroids are usually an adequate treatment for controlling pruritus. A mid-potency steroid (Class III or IV), such as triamcinolone 0.1 % or fluocinonide 0.05 % twice daily for 1–2 weeks, is appropriate for the trunk and extremities. A milder (Class V or VI) steroid (e.g., Desonide 0.05 %) is appropriate for the face. Oral antihistamines, such as diphenhydramine 25–50 mg or hydroxyzine 10–25 mg twice daily, may be added if patients' sleep is disrupted due to itching. If the lesions are complicated by secondary infection, a topical or systemic antibiotic may be needed. This should be treated empirically, or based on culture results if available. Discussion of treatment should include recommendations to eradicate the insects, through professional pest exterminators if possible.

Follow-Up

While treatment can control symptoms of bedbug bites, new lesions will present unless the infestation is controlled. Patients may be shown pictures of bedbugs and their fecal traces so they are able to search for, and identify the pest. If they find evidence of an infestation, patients should wash their clothes and linens in hot water. Extermination through professional services will also be necessary to eradicate the bugs.

Questions for the Dermatologist

– *Is there a tell-tale sign that insect bites are from bedbugs vs. other bugs?*

Unfortunately, there is no definitive sign. Bedbug bites are generally more urticarial and slightly larger than other bug bites; however, I would be careful to call a lesion a bedbug bite based only on those two factors. The presentation of a bite is based on the individual immune system's response to a particular antigen, which varies greatly. One person may have a mosquito sensitivity and experience huge, pruritic mosquito bites but have little reaction to bedbug bites. Although the pattern of three bites is associated with bedbug bites, it is a more common finding in flea bites. History gives more helpful clues in diagnosing bedbug bites. New bites in the morning, blood on the sheets, increased itch at night—those would be better clues than the look of the bite.

– *Is it common that one person could get bitten by bedbugs and someone else sharing the same bed or residence would be bite-free? Or would this rule out bed bugs?*

It is common, and in fact usually the case, that not everyone in the house is getting bites, because not everyone is sensitive to bedbug bites. There are two different schools of thought on what attracts bedbugs to their victims. One is that bedbugs follow carbon dioxide to find fresh blood, which would not explain why some people do not get bites since we all exhale CO_2. Another suggestion is that the epidermal lipid milieu—ceramides, free fatty acids, cholesterols, etc.—of some hosts is more hospitable to bed bugs.

– *Is there a role for treating the itch with steroid cream? If so, what class is best?*

Steroid creams are the recommended treatment of bedbug bites, and both the inflammation from the bite and the associated itch are targeted. The class depends on the anatomical location of the bite, and the severity of the reaction.

– *Is there a role for treating the bites with an antihistamine like benadryl, or with topicals like calamine lotion?*

Oral antihistamines can help patients whose sleep is disrupted by the itch or discomfort associated with bites. Calamine lotion probably will not do much in terms of calming inflammation, improving the appearance of the bite, or relieving pruritus. However, if an individual finds it soothing, there is no problem in using it.

– *Do bed bugs ever just go away on their own or do they always need to be eradicated?*

I am not aware of a reason bedbugs would go away without being actively eradicated. They tend to be more active in winter months, perhaps because of people clustering closer to home, and being present as a food source more often. However, I am not aware of them going away on their own, regardless of the season. I would always recommend eradication.

References

1. Bernardeschi C, Le Cleach L, Delaunay P, Chosidow O. Bed bug infestation. BMJ. 2013;346:f138.
2. Schwartz RA, Steen CJ. Chapter 210. Arthropod bites and stings. In: Goldsmith LA, Katz SI, Gilchrest BA, Paller AS, Leffell DJ, Wolff K, editors. Fitzpatrick's dermatology in general medicine. 8th ed. New York: McGraw-Hill; 2012. Available from: http://accessmedicine.mhmedical.com.ezproxy.cul.columbia.edu/content.aspx?bookid=392&Sectionid=41138941. Accessed 3 Mar 2015.
3. Melnick L, Samimi S, Elder D, Xu X, Vittorio CC, Rosenbach M, Wanat KA. Targetoid lesions in the emergency department. Bed bug bites (Cimex lectularius) with targetoid lesions on initial presentation. JAMA Dermatol. 2013;149(6):751–6.
4. Baumblatt JA, Dunn JR, Schaffner W, Moncayo AC, Stull-Lane A, Jones TF. An outbreak of bed bug infestation in an office building. J Environ Health. 2014;76(8):16–8.
5. Goddard J, Edwards KT. Effects of bed bug saliva on human skin. JAMA Dermatol. 2013;149(3):372–3.

Chapter 41
Scabies

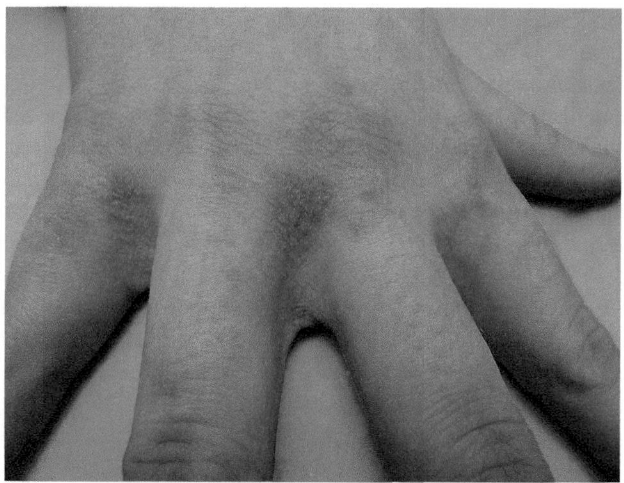

Fig. 41.1 Web spaces with a mix of papules and excoriations

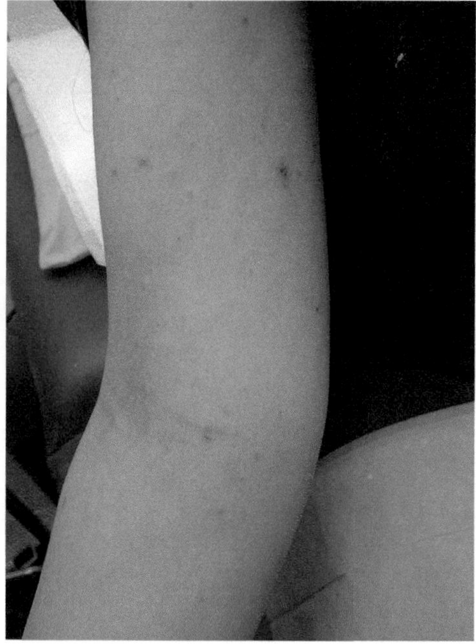

Fig. 41.2 Nonspecific excoriations and abrasions with occasional papules arms

D. Reich et al., *Top 50 Dermatology Case Studies for Primary Care*,
DOI 10.1007/978-3-319-18627-6_41

Primary Care Visit Report

A 24-year-old female with no past medical history presented with an itchy red rash on her arms and hands that had started 2 weeks prior. The rash started in the webbing between her left thumb and pointer finger, then she noticed it in other finger webbings, and eventually on her upper and lower arms. The rash was itchiest during the day. The patient worked in a kitchen and wore gloves that covered only her hands (not arms) while at work. Sometimes at night her legs itched, but there was no rash on them. The patient had tried cutting gluten out of her diet, which seemed to improve the rash, and also tried moisturizing lotion. She had not tried any steroid creams.

Vitals were normal. On exam, in the webbing between the third and fourth fingers, and fourth and fifth fingers of her right hand there was a 1 cm × 1 cm erythematous scaly rash. Similarly, in the webbing between the thumb and second finger of her left hand, there was a 1 cm × 1 cm erythematous scaly rash. There were multiple scattered erythematous papules on the bilateral upper arms, and a patch of erythematous scale on her right back and hip area.

Due to the improvement with decreased gluten, the possible irritant from wearing gloves at work, and the rash's spread to the upper arms and right hip, this case was treated as atopic dermatitis and the patient was prescribed hydrocortisone valerate 0.2 % cream—an intermediate potency (Class V) topical steroid—twice daily for 10 days. However, the patient was uninsured, and the steroid cream was too expensive for her, so over-the-counter hydrocortisone cream was recommended first. If there was no improvement noted, the patient was instructed to try the higher strength steroid next. It was also suggested that she try taking shorter warm (not hot) showers and using an over the counter barrier cream, like Eucerin or Aveeno.

Discussion from Dermatology Clinic

Differential Dx

- Scabies
- Atopic dermatitis
- Dyshidrotic eczema
- Insect bite
- Contact dermatitis

Favored Dx

Dermatology ruled out atopic dermatitis and reclassified the diagnosis as scabies due to the distribution of lesions, excoriations, and associated pruritus.

Overview

Scabies is a highly contagious ectoparasitic infestation by *Sarcoptes scabiei* mites. Scabies mites are arthropods that do not fly or jump. Scabies are spread by prolonged skin-to-skin contact. Rarely they can also be spread through shared clothing, towels, and linens [1]. Scabies affects people of all ages, races, and socioeconomic levels worldwide, with an estimated incidence of 300 million cases per year [1–4]. Scabies is considered a neglected skin disease by the World Health Organization due to its endemic nature in developing countries, its high economic burden, its association with poverty and its relative neglect by the scientific and healthcare communities [5]. Risk factors making people especially susceptible to mite infestation are immunocompromised status, homelessness, poverty, poor nutritional status, dementia, and living in conditions with overcrowding and poor hygiene [3]. It has also been associated with hospital and nursing home outbreaks [2, 3].

Scabies mites spend their entire life cycle in the epidermis [1, 2]. Adult female mites burrow into the stratum corneum layer of the skin, and lay eggs that typically hatch after 10 days. After a 4–6 week incubation period, hosts experience a hypersensitivity reaction to the mites, their saliva, and excretions [2]. Between 10 and 50 mites are thought to typically infect a host at any time [2–4]. Thousands of mites may be present in immunocompromised hosts, representative of a more severe form of the disease called crusted or Norwegian scabies. This variant is more difficult to treat and can lead to bacterial sepsis [1].

Presentation

Scabies typically presents with burrows at the site of infestation. Mites burrow within the epidermis and leave behind a fine, serpiginous line that can be up to 1 cm long. Sometimes a black dot is visible at the end of the burrow, representing the mite. These may be accompanied by a small number of papules, and are typically seen in the interdigital webbing, flexor surfaces of the wrist, the extensor aspects of the elbows, axilla, umbilical area, groin, and areolae. Scabies in children may additionally present on the palms and soles of feet. Patients tend to experience severe pruritus that becomes worse at night. They may present with excoriations from scratching, and an eczema-like dry, scaly, erythematous rash in the affected areas.

Patients with crusted scabies present with diffuse erythema, scaling and widespread thick crusts over the skin. Areas that are typically spared in common scabies infestations, such as the head and neck, may be involved in crusted scabies. Patients with crusted scabies may not experience pruritus due to a reduced ability to mount an immune response.

Workup

Diagnosis of scabies is usually made based on severe pruritus and excoriations in classic areas, such as the interdigital webbing, groin, elbow extensors, and wrist flexors. History of household members experiencing similar symptoms is another indication. The presence of burrows is not required to make an accurate diagnosis of scabies.

Lesion scraping may be performed to confirm the diagnosis. Mineral oil is applied to a burrow or lesion, which is then scraped laterally with a number 15 blade. The scrapings are placed on a glass slide and viewed under a microscope. Microscopy may reveal eggs, mites, or fecal matter. If there is no mineral oil available, antibacterial gel such as Purell may be substituted instead.

Treatment

The goal of scabies treatment is to eliminate mites using a scabicide, to prevent reinfestation by fomites (objects or substances that carry the scabies mites) by washing bedding and clothes, and to minimize risk of reinfestation by treating all family members at the same time.

Permethrin 5 % cream is the most effective topical treatment for scabies [1, 6]. It has selectively neurotoxic effects on arthropods and well studied efficacy on eradicating scabies, with a 97–98 % clearance rate [1–3, 6]. Permethrin cream is applied two times with a 1-week interval between applications. The medication is applied at night to the whole body from the neck down, kept on for 8–14 h, and washed off in the morning. It should not be used in children under 6 months of age. Permethrin is associated with a faster improvement in symptoms, which can occur within 3 days of treatment [2, 6, 7]. Crotamiton and lindane are alternative topical medications; however, they are not first-line as crotamiton is less effective than permethrin, and lindane has been associated with neurotoxicity [1–3].

Ivermectin is an oral antiparasitic that may be used off-label in cases that are resistant to permethrin. Ivermectin has a 70 % cure rate when given one time, and a 95 % cure rate when given two times at a dosage of 200 μg/kg spaced by 2 weeks [1–3, 6]. It should be taken with food to increase the drug's bioavailability [3]. Combination treatment of ivermectin and permethrin is recommended for people with crusted scabies [2]. Crusted scabies may require 3–7 doses of ivermectin [3]. Ivermectin is not FDA-approved for scabies treatment, has not been studied in pregnant or nursing women, and is not recommended for children weighing less than 15 kg.

Patients may be given adjunctive antihistamines to treat pruritus, such as hydroxyzine 10–25 mg.

Follow-Up

Patients should be evaluated after 1 week of treatment. Scabies lesions may persist even after mites have been eradicated but they should improve after 1 week. Patients should be informed pruritus may persist for up to 4 weeks (referred to as postscabetic itch) [2].

Clothes, linens, and towels should be washed in hot water in order to prevent recurrence. There is no need for fumigation or treating pets [2]. At the time of publication, there were no controlled studies on the effect of prophylactic treatment on family members or those in close contact with people with scabies; however, this practice is standard of care in our office [4]. It is possible for scabies to be asymptomatic initially, and for carriers to transmit the mites before they develop symptoms. Therefore, it is recommended to treat all members of the household in order to prevent recurrence.

Questions for the Dermatologist

– *What are some ways to distinguish scabies from atopic dermatitis?*

Eczema would be accompanied by a rash in a typical area, such as the antecubital or popliteal fossa. Scabies appear in the interdigital webbing, axilla, nipples, groin, periumbilical area, and top of the intergluteal cleft. Scabies is sometimes referred to as the itch with no rash, meaning there may be diffuse itching but no visible rash. There may be excoriations from scratching. Atopic dermatitis features a rash indicative of inflamed, irritated skin.

– *Is a rash in the interdigital webbing more likely to be caused by scabies until proven otherwise?*

Not necessarily. It is important to consider the context of presentation. If there is diffuse itching accompanying the interdigital excoriations with a small number of papules, the diagnosis is most likely scabies. Hand eczema and "winter itch" can mimic scabies in the interdigital space. In that context, we might expect to see some eczematous plaques without complaints of diffuse itching.

– *Do scabies respond to steroid cream?*

They do not. Topical steroids may relieve the associated itching, but a dedicated anti-mite therapy is needed to treat scabies.

– *Is a rash on the upper arms consistent with presentation of scabies?*

Scabies are fiercely pruritic. They can cause diffuse itching and scratching can lead to red, irritated excoriations anywhere on the body. The presence of excoriations on classic areas of presentation such as interdigital webbing helps to make a diagnosis.

– *What contact precautions should the patient take with roommates or partners?*

It is good practice to treat everyone in the household in order to eliminate any mites in the house. This does not include people who spend a few hours in the household, but anyone who sleeps in the house overnight. There is no need for isolation, or fumigation of the house; however, it would be a good idea to wash the linens, towels, and clothes used by household members.

References

1. Currie BJ, McCarthy JS. Permethrin and ivermectin for scabies. N Engl J Med. 2010;362(8):717–25.
2. Burkhart CN, Burkhart CG. Chapter 208. Scabies, other mites, and pediculosis. In: Goldsmith LA, Katz SI, Gilchrest BA, Paller AS, Leffell DJ, Wolff K, editors. Fitzpatrick's dermatology in general medicine. 8th ed. New York: McGraw-Hill; 2012. Available from: http://accessmedicine.mhmedical.com.ezproxy.cul.columbia.edu/content.aspx?bookid=392&Sectionid=41138939. Accessed 22 Feb 2015.
3. Shimose L, Munoz-Price LS. Diagnosis, prevention, and treatment of scabies. Curr Infect Dis Rep. 2013;15(5):426–31.
4. FitzGerald D, Grainger RJ, Reid A. Intervention for preventing the spread of infestation in close contact of people with scabies. Cochrane Database Syst Rev. 2014;2, CD009943.
5. Karimkhani C, Boyers LN, Prescott L, Welch V, Delamere FM, Nasser M, Zaveri A, Hay RJ, Vos T, Murray CJ, Margolis DJ, Hilton J, MacLehose H, Williams HC, Dellavalle RP. Global burden of skin disease as reflected in Cochrane Database of Systematic Reviews. JAMA Dermatol. 2014;150(9):945–51.
6. Ranjkesh MR, Naghili B, Goldust M, Rezaee E. The efficacy of permethrin 5% vs. oral ivermectin for the treatment of scabies. Ann Parasitol. 2013;59(4):189–94.
7. Sharma R, Singal A. Topical permethrin and oral ivermectin in the management of scabies: a prospective, randomized, double blind, controlled study. Indian J Dermatol Venereol Leprol. 2011;77:581–6.

Chapter 42
Shingles

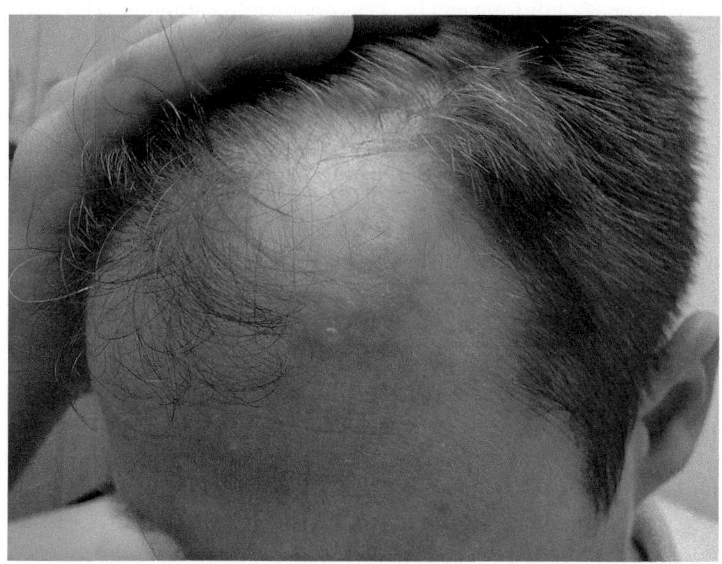

Fig. 42.1 This eruption corresponds to the V1 branch of the trigeminal nerve

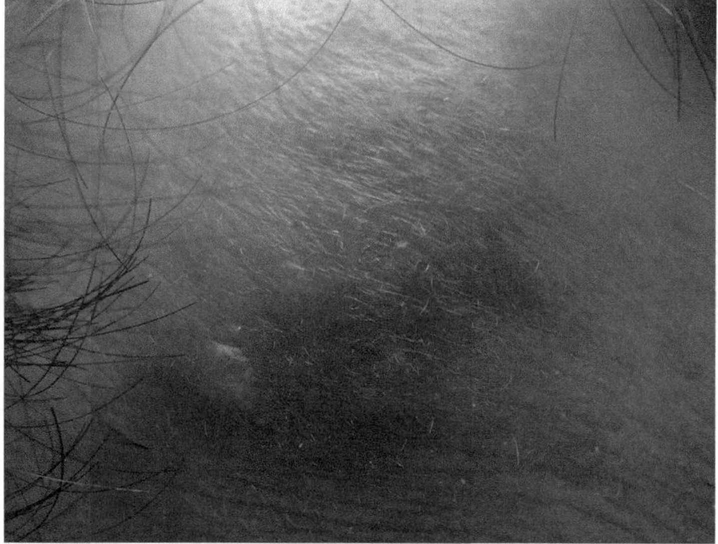

Fig. 42.2 The classic clustered vesicles on an erythematous base

D. Reich et al., *Top 50 Dermatology Case Studies for Primary Care*,
DOI 10.1007/978-3-319-18627-6_42

Primary Care Visit Report

A 29-year-old male with no past medical history presented with bumps on his forehead, behind his left ear, and near his left eye. One week prior, the patient was accidentally hit on his left forehead by a car door while getting in. The next day, he woke up with a bump on his left frontal forehead area where he had been hit. The following day, he noticed a bump behind his left ear. Two days after that, his left medial eye area started to become red and then developed bumps. While his forehead was itchy, none of the other bumps or associated areas were painful. He was afebrile and felt well. He reported having chickenpox as a child. He had tried moisturizer and ice on the lesions; however, neither helped.

Vitals were normal. On exam, on his left superolateral frontal scalp, there was a 3.2 cm × 2 cm area of macular erythema with one fluid-filled vesicle inferiorly. This was non-tender to palpation. Lateral to the left superior aspect of his nose and medial to his left eye, there was a 1 cm × 0.5 cm erythematous macule containing 2 small (1 mm) papules centrally. The left infraorbital area featured edema and erythema. Tender, enlarged lymph nodes were noted at the left occipital and left posterior auricular areas.

This was treated as trigeminal (ophthalmic division) shingles. Given the history of blunt trauma immediately preceding the development of the rash, a bacterial culture was taken to rule out infection. Viral and bacterial cultures were taken from fluid from the forehead lesion, and a CBC, varicella zoster IgM and varicella zoster IgG antibody tests were sent. The patient was started on valacyclovir 1000 mg three times daily for 7 days, and an over-the-counter hydrocortisone cream for the eyelid edema. The viral culture eventually grew out varicella zoster. The patient's blood tested positive for zoster IgG antibody, but negative for zoster IgM antibody. The bacterial culture grew out normal skin flora only, and the CBC was normal. The patient did well on valacyclovir and hydrocortisone cream. The patient was referred to ophthalmology because of possible eye involvement, but due to cost concerns, lack of vision involvement, and rash improvement with valacyclovir he opted not to go.

Discussion from Dermatology Clinic

Differential Dx

- Herpes zoster (shingles)
- Contact dermatitis
- Insect bites
- Herpes, simplex

Favored Dx

Although it is unusual for shingles to present without pain, the erythematous papular and vesicular lesions appear in a unilateral distribution and have a presentation typical of shingles.

Overview

Herpes zoster, or shingles, is caused by the same virus that causes chickenpox. It is a herpesvirus known as varicella zoster virus (VZV), chickenpox virus, or human herpesvirus type 3 (HHV-3). Initial infection causes chickenpox, a once ubiquitous childhood infection in the United States, whose incidence has decreased by as much as 90 % since the introduction of varicella vaccines in 1995 [1]. After the initial acute chickenpox illness, the latent virus persists in the sensory dorsal root ganglia and autonomic ganglia. Once reactivated, VZV causes herpes zoster, an erythematous, vesicular unilateral rash that is accompanied by dermatomal pain.

The lifetime risk of herpes zoster is up to 30 % [2]. The decreased incidence of varicella in children has not affected the prevalence of herpes zoster, perhaps because there is reduced repeat exposure to the virus in individuals who already had chickenpox and therefore reduced immune boosting. Herpes zoster can occur at any age, but most commonly occurs in ages 50–59 and generally affects older adults [1–3]. Age is a strong risk factor due to inherently reduced immunity in older individuals, as well as being female and white [1–3]. Although commonly thought to affect immunocompromised populations, and certainly immunocompromised status is a risk factor, one large study found only 8 % of patients with herpes zoster were immunocompromised [3]. The immunocompromised populations most affected are people with HIV, organ transplant recipients, and people on immunosuppressants for autoimmune disorders. Reactivation of VZV can also be triggered by emotional stress and physical trauma to the affected dermatome. Physical trauma can increase risk of herpes zoster by up to eight times [4].

Presentation

Unlike varicella rashes which are more scattered and diffuse due to spread by viremia, herpes zoster lesions are unilateral and tend to be isolated to a single dermatome. The thoracic region and face, especially the ophthalmic branch of the trigeminal nerve, are the most commonly affected sites. The vesicles may be preceded by 1–3 days of prodromal symptoms of burning, tingling, or aching in the affected dermatome. More rarely, patients may also experience headaches, fever, and malaise. The lesions typically appear in groups, as either distinct or confluent vesicles over an erythematous background. In most cases they are restricted to a single dermatome, or two adjacent dermatomes;however, they may sometimes spread to distal sites. Vesicles form over several days, and may ulcerate and then crust. Patients typically complain of pain in the affected area, which can last up to a month in acute cases. Symptoms tend to increase in severity with age.

Trigeminal herpes zoster is associated with ophthalmological symptoms when the ophthalmic (and especially nasociliary) branch is involved, including conjunctivitis, keratitis, chronic ulceration, and glaucoma [1]. The condition of the eye should be carefully examined when patients present with a herpetiform rash on the nose.

Workup

If diagnosis cannot be made based on history and presence of painful unilateral rash, the Tzanck smear test is a fast way to diagnose herpes zoster. This involves scraping a new vesicle, spreading material onto a glass slide and fixing in methanol, staining with Giemsa or Papanicolaou, and viewing under a microscope. Multinucleated giant cells would appear. These also appear in chickenpox and herpes; however, patient history would distinguish between these conditions.

Viral culture swab, immunofluorescence, and PCR amplification are other standard tests of choice. Bacterial cultures should be performed if there is suspicion of an overlaying infection.

Treatment

The main goals of treatment are to limit the extent and duration of involvement and pain, and to prevent post-herpetic neuralgia (PHN). Valacyclovir is first line treatment for immunocompetent patients with herpes zoster, preferred over acyclovir because of increased bioavailability, reduced viral resistance, and more convenient dosing [1, 5]. Appropriate valacyclovir dose is 1000 mg three times daily for 7 days. Valacyclovir, acyclovir, and famciclovir all demonstrate efficacy in reducing the duration of lesions, and sometimes temporarily reduce pain [1, 5–7]. Antiviral treatment should be initiated within 72 h of symptom onset [1, 6]. Even if more time has elapsed, antivirals are still recommended, especially for older patients, or patients with ocular involvement. Patients with ocular involvement should be referred to an ophthalmologist.

Patients with herpes zoster may experience significant pain. Lidocaine 5 % and capsaicin 8 % patches may provide relief. Over-the-counter or prescription analgesics may also be given. Gabapentin and tricyclic antidepressants have been shown to provide pain relief in older patients with PHN [1].

Follow-Up

Patients should be monitored for symptom resolution. Vesicles tend to resolve within 2 weeks. Discoloration may persist for longer, and herpes zoster lesions often scar, especially in more severe cases and older patients. Prompt treatment, keeping affected areas clean to avoid infection, and avoiding touching or scratching the lesions may help to lower the scarring risk. Patients may inquire about the herpes zoster vaccination. It is recommended for people over 60 years old; however, it is of no benefit to patients with acute herpes zoster [6, 8]. Patients who have experienced an episode of herpes zoster may be vaccinated to help prevent future occurrences. There is no specific time period that someone must wait after having the shingles rash before getting the vaccine, but they must at least wait until after the herpes rash has resolved. The vaccine is effective in reducing the risk of developing herpes zoster, as well as reducing the severity of symptoms (especially post-herpetic neuralgia) in those who do develop the condition.

The most common complication of herpes zoster is PHN, defined as pain lasting longer than 90 days after diagnosis. PHN occurs in 13 % of cases and the incidence increases with age [3]. Other complications include eye disease and motor neuropathies. Any new or persisting complications warrant a follow-up visit.

Questions for the Dermatologist

– *What special considerations do I need to make for ophthalmological involvement?*

Any involvement of the V1 or V2 branches of the trigeminal nerve should be referred to ophthalmology to rule out corneal abrasions.

– *Could the trauma to the patient's forehead have triggered a shingles outbreak, or was that a red herring?*

Trauma can trigger a shingles outbreak. Even heavy chemical peels and treatment with CO_2 lasers can cause herpetic outbreaks, which is why those patients are often given prophylactic valacyclovir prior to deeper procedures.

– *What is the argument for treating with antivirals vs. letting the disease run its natural course? Is this different for different age groups?*

Prior recommendations were to definitively treat uncomplicated zoster with valacyclovir only if the patient was over the age of 50. The current standard of care is to treat adults of any age with 1 g of valacyclovir three times a day for 7 days within 72 h of clinical presentation. The standard of care also includes referrals to specialists when cosmetically sensitive areas like the face are involved, or there is ophthalmic involvement. Antivirals are critical in these cases, and when treating older patients. Antiviral treatment decreases the incidence of postherpetic neuralgia, and this is particularly true for older age groups. While the efficacy of valacyclovir in patients less than 50 years old has not been well studied, it is still recommended as there is low risk of adverse events, and there are potential benefits, such as decreasing nerve pain and resolving skin lesions more rapidly.

– *Why is the shingles vaccine only recommended for people 60 years and up, even though young people are also affected? Is the incidence higher or are complications greater?*

Both the incidence is higher and the complications are greater. The majority of people experiencing shingles are over 60 years old. Incidence of post-herpetic neuralgia also increases with age. There is greater risk of varicella-related pneumonitis and cerebritis.

– *The Varicella IgM test was done 6 days after symptoms started and it was negative. When would we expect IgM to be positive?*

Once IgM is positive, it stays elevated for 2–4 weeks. In this case, since the IgM test was done just 6 days after the prodromal symptoms started and only 2 days after the shingles rash started, it is likely it was too early to detect any IgM antibodies. If confirmation of varicella zoster is necessary via IgM antibodies (i.e., if viral culture was not available or was inconclusive), the test can be repeated 2–3 weeks later. However, clinical symptoms alone are used to diagnose herpes zoster, and a positive viral culture of the vesicular fluid confirms the diagnosis (A positive IgG just tells us that the patient has had chickenpox or the zoster vaccine in the past.).

References

1. Schmader KE, Oxman MN. Chapter 194. Varicella and herpes zoster. In: Goldsmith LA, Katz SI, Gilchrest BA, Paller AS, Leffell DJ, Wolff K, editors. Fitzpatrick's dermatology in general medicine. 8th ed. New York: McGraw-Hill; 2012. p. 2382–401.
2. Thomas SL, Hall AJ. What does epidemiology tell us about risk factors for herpes zoster? Lancet Infect Dis. 2004;4(1):26–33.
3. Yawn B, Saddier P, Wollan P, St Sauver J, Kurland M, Sy L. A population-based study of the incidence and complication rates of herpes zoster before zoster vaccine introduction. Mayo Clinic Proceedings [serial on the Internet]. (2007, Nov), [cited January 25, 2015]; 82(11):1341–1349. Available from: MEDLINE with Full Text.
4. Thomas SL, Wheeler JG, Hall AJ. Case-control study of the effect of mechanical trauma on the risk of herpes zoster. BMJ. 2004;328(7437):439.
5. Shaikh S, Ta CN. Evaluation and management of herpes zoster ophthalmicus. Am Fam Physician. 2002;66(9):1723–30.
6. Harpaz R, Ortega-Sanchez IR, Seward JF, Advisory Committee on Immunization Practices (ACIP) Centers for Disease Control and Prevention (CDC). Prevention of herpes zoster: rec-

ommendations of the Advisory Committee on Immunization Practices (ACIP). MMWR Recomm Rep. 2008;57(RR-5):1–30.
7. Chen N, Li Q, Yang J, Zhou M, Zhou D, He L. Antiviral treatment for preventing postherpetic neuralgia. Cochrane Database Syst Rev. 2014;2, CD006866.
8. Gagliardi AM, Gomes Silva BN, Torloni MR, Soares BG. Vaccines for preventing herpes zoster in older adults. Cochrane Database Syst Rev. 2012;10, CD008858.

Chapter 43
Lyme Disease

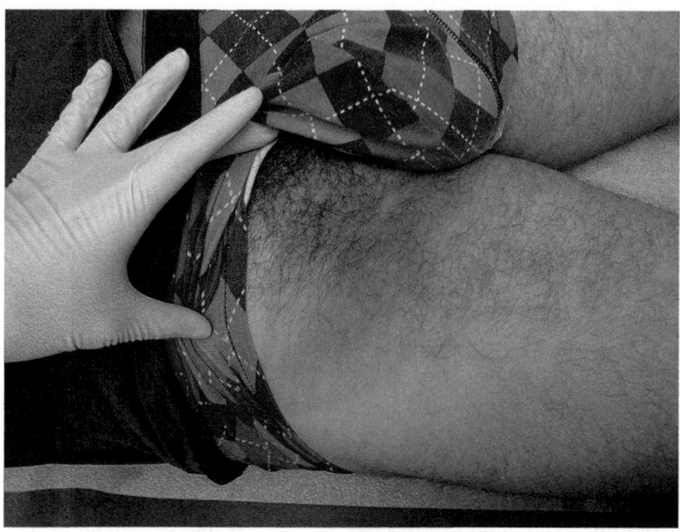

Fig. 43.1 Do not get hung up looking for a perfect target; sometimes this two toned patch is all you will get

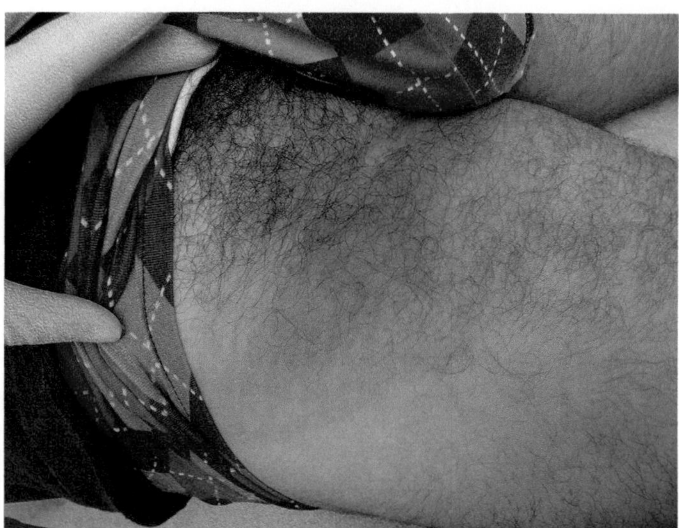

Fig. 43.2 Two-toned inguinal ovoid patch without scale

D. Reich et al., *Top 50 Dermatology Case Studies for Primary Care*,
DOI 10.1007/978-3-319-18627-6_43

Primary Care Visit Report

A 38-year-old male with no past medical history presented with a rash in his right inguinal area that had been growing in size. About 10 days prior to his visit, the patient had some mouth sores, a fever, neck stiffness, and a severe headache. The fever and mouth sores resolved; however, the patient's neck remained stiff and he continued to have intermittent headaches. Then about 6 days prior to his visit, the rash in his right inguinal area developed. It started with one sore spot, which the patient thought might have been an infected hair follicle. He tried putting a warm compress on the rash; however, the rash continued to get bigger. The patient had no known exposure to Lyme disease.

Vitals were normal. On examination, in his right inguinal area there was an 18 cm × 10 cm mildly erythematous blanchable macular lesion. Within that lesion was a 10 cm × 3 cm macule with darker erythema, which was also blanchable. Within the smaller macule, there was a central 2 mm × 2 mm tender, peeling area (3/10 pain). There was no induration, and no abscess noted. The skin texture was irregular.

The rash was treated as cellulitis and the patient was given Bactrim DS twice daily for 10 days. The appearance of the rash was suspicious for Lyme; however, attempts to draw blood in order to test for Lyme titers were unsuccessful, and the patient was advised to return when he was better hydrated. The borders of the rash were marked with permanent marker and the patient was instructed to return if the rash extended beyond its marked borders.

The patient returned 2 days later because the rash continued to spread beyond its original borders. The patient reported no fever or headache, and said the rash was very itchy.

Vitals remained normal. On examination, his right inguinal area had a 22 cm × 13 cm erythematous macular rash with a 17 cm × 8 cm central darker erythematous area. The center of the rash was tender on deep palpation.

The rash was still suspicious for Lyme, so the patient was given a 21-day course of doxycycline 100 mg three times daily, while continuing the Bactrim. Blood was drawn for Lyme titers, complete blood count, liver function tests, and erythrocyte sedimentation rate.

The patient returned 1 day later (now status post three doses of doxycycline and seven doses of Bactrim) because the rash continued to extend beyond its prior borders and the patient was feeling "loopy." The rash continued to be highly pruritic. The patient also reported fatigue, increased sleep, and waking up groggy, but noted the onset of his fatigue had been gradual over the preceding 2 months.

Vitals remained normal. On examination, the rash in his right inguinal area had extended beyond its previous borders, and was warm and edematous. Three right inguinal lymph nodes were enlarged and tender. Two left inguinal lymph nodes were enlarged and tender. There was no other lymphadenopathy.

The labs were reviewed. The initial Lyme screening was positive but remaining Lyme tests were still pending. His CBC and LFTs were normal. The ESR was elevated.

The patient was referred to the Emergency Room to address ongoing concern about cellulitis and the potential need for IV antibiotics.

The patient went to the ER later that day after he developed a severe headache, neck pain, and back pain in addition to the rash. In the ER, they gave him a 900 mg dose of clindamycin for possible cellulitis. They stopped the Bactrim and sent him home on clindamycin 300 mg twice daily for 7 days for cellulitis, and instructed him to continue the doxycycline (for Lyme). They also gave him a referral to follow up with an Infectious Disease specialist.

The following day, all Lyme titers were received, with Lyme IgM positive and Lyme IgG negative. The rash was improving, and the headache and neck pain were starting to resolve. The clindamycin was discontinued, and the doxycycline 100 mg twice a day was continued for Lyme disease treatment. The patient had a follow-up appointment with an infectious disease doctor scheduled.

One week later, the infectious disease specialist saw the patient and thought perhaps the patient had Lyme and coxsackie, as Lyme disease could not explain the presence of mouth sores. He advised that 10–14 days of doxycycline were adequate to treat Lyme and that the patient did not need to finish the 21-day course. The patient continued to improve, the rash gradually became lighter in color, and the neck pain and headache were resolving.

Discussion from Dermatology Clinic

Differential Dx

- Lyme disease
- Babesiosis
- Human granulocytic anaplasmosis (HGA)
- Erysipelas
- Cellulitis
- Arthropod bite
- Southern tick-associated rash illness (STARI, caused by *Amblyomma americanum* tick)

Favored Dx

The characteristic erythema migrans rash and confirmed titers indicate Lyme disease in this patient.

Overview

Lyme disease is an infectious disease caused by *Borrelia* spirochete bacteria, lending the disease the alternate name Lyme borreliosis. It was first diagnosed in Lyme, Connecticut in 1977 following a cluster of unusual cases of recurrent arthritis [1].

In the USA, Lyme disease is caused primarily by *Borrelia burgdorferi*, bacteria which are transmitted by *Ixodes* ticks of the species *Ixodes scapularis* and *Ixodes pacificus* [2]. In Europe and Asia, the disease is also caused by *B. afzelii*, *B. garinii*, and other related species [3]. *I. scapularis* ticks also carry *Anaplasma phagocytophilum* and *Babesia microti*, making them vectors for human granulocytic anaplasmosis and babesiosis, infections that sometimes occur with Lyme disease. Ticks must be attached for at least 36 h in order to transmit Lyme disease, with peak infection in the 48–72 h range [2, 4]. The overall risk of developing Lyme disease following a bite with an infected tick is 1–3 %, although this may be higher in endemic areas [4].

Lyme disease is the most common vector-borne and tick-borne disease in the USA [2, 3]. There were over 27,000 cases reported in the USA in 2013 with an overall incidence of 8.6 per 100,000, and a much higher incidence in endemic areas [5]. Lyme is most common in the Northeastern States and upper Midwest, with 95 % of cases diagnosed in Connecticut, Delaware, Maine, Maryland, Massachusetts, Minnesota, New Hampshire, New Jersey, New York, Pennsylvania, Rhode Island, Vermont, Virginia, and Wisconsin [5]. Lyme disease is more common in summer months, and people who are active outdoors in woods and tall grasses are at increased risk of infection.

Presentation

Erythema migrans is the most common clinical manifestation of Lyme disease [2–4, 6]. Up to 80 % of patients develop the characteristic rash, usually within 1–2 weeks of the tick bite, with a range of 3–32 days [3, 7]. Other symptoms include nonspecific flu-like symptoms, such as headache, arthralgia, malaise, and fever. Two to 3 % of patients are estimated to present with facial palsy, trigeminal neuropathy, or Lyme arthritis [7].

Erythema migrans begins as a small erythematous papule or macule at the site of the bite, which develops erythema that expands centrifugally over a period of several days to become a large plaque. Rarely, the bite site may demonstrate bullous, vesicular, hemorrhagic, or necrotic changes [8]. The rash is often described as having a "bull's eye" appearance, as the erythema may have central clearing as it expands. Up to 2/3 of cases do not have the bull's eye appearance and are instead either uniformly erythematous, or more erythematous centrally [3]. Erythema migrans may present anywhere on the body, with the most common sites of presentation being the axilla, groin, waist, and back in adults, and the head and neck in children [3].

Workup

In cases where erythema migrans is present, clinical findings are sufficient to diagnose Lyme disease, and serological testing is not necessary; however, it may be used to confirm the diagnosis. For nonspecific symptoms, blood tests are required in order to confirm the diagnosis [2]. An enzyme immunoassay, such as ELISA (enzyme-linked immunosorbent assay) is typically used; however, it may not detect IgM antibodies to *B. burgdorferi* within the first 1–2 weeks, or IgG antibodies within the first 4–6 weeks of infection [4]. As ELISA may provide false-positive results due to other medical conditions, a two-tiered system is recommended, with a Western blot test serving as the next step in confirming the diagnosis.

Treatment

Lyme disease is treated with a 14-day course of oral antibiotics (range 10–21 days). Doxycycline is recommended for adults and children over 8 years of age who have early Lyme disease associated with erythema migrans and without neurological or cardiac involvement. The recommended doxycycline dose for adults is 100 mg twice daily, while children over 8 years old may be dosed at 4 mg/kg/day divided in two doses that are not to exceed 100 mg each. Women who are pregnant or breast-feeding and children under 8 years old may take amoxicillin (500 mg TID for adults; 50 mg/kg/day divided in three doses of max 500 mg for children) or cefuroxime axetil (500 mg BID for adults; 30 mg/kg/day divided in two doses of max 500 mg for children) [2]. Each of these antibiotics has demonstrated cure rates of up to 90 % [3]. Patients who are intolerant to all three of the above antibiotics may be treated with a macrolide such as azithromycin or clarithromycin; however, macrolides are not as effective at curing Lyme disease.

Untreated Lyme disease may lead to neurological complications, including meningitis and radiculopathies, and more rarely cardiac involvement, in the form of atrioventricular heart block and myopericarditis [2]. Patients with neurological symptoms require 14 days of intravenous antibiotics. Intravenous ceftriaxone is recommended at 2 g once daily for adults, and 50–75 mg/kg/day (max 2 g) for children. Patients with cardiac symptoms may be treated with oral or intravenous antibiotics, and should be referred to a hospital for monitoring [2].

Follow-Up

All patients should be monitored for resolution of clinical symptoms. Erythema migrans tends to resolve within a few weeks of initiating treatment, while nonspecific symptoms such as myalgia, arthralgia, fatigue, and neck stiffness may last for several months [4]. Neurological complications such as Bell's palsy, as well as cardiac and arthritic complications may also take longer to resolve. Within 1 year after initiating treatment, up to 90 % of patients are symptom-free.

When symptoms persist for more than 6 months they are classified as post-treatment Lyme disease syndrome (PTLDS). The etiology of PTLDS is unknown. Use of the term "chronic Lyme disease" is discouraged as it lacks a clear definition and its existence is controversial [3, 6]. Evidence suggests that extending antibiotic therapy in order to treat PTLDS is of little or no benefit [3, 6, 9–12].

The best way to prevent recurrence of Lyme disease infection is by preventing tick bites. This can be achieved by wearing tall socks, pants, and long sleeves while spending time outdoors in endemic areas. In addition, insect repellent with at least 20 % DEET can help prevent bites [3]. Checking the body for ticks after spending time outdoors can minimize the risk of infection following a tick bite. If a tick is found and is thought to have been attached for more than 36 h, is confirmed to be the *I. scapularis* type, and this occurs in a geographical area with >20 % local rate of infection of ticks with *B. Burgdorferi*, then a single 200 mg prophylactic dose of doxycycline (or 4 mg/kg in children over 8 years old) may be taken within 72 h of the tick removal. That patient should subsequently be monitored for development of any symptoms suggestive of Lyme disease [13].

Questions for the Dermatologist

– *How common is it to get Lyme disease without any known or obvious exposure?*

In my clinical experience, I would estimate over half of the patients recognize some kind of tick bite prior to the onset of symptoms.

– *Is there a way to distinguish cellulitis from the erythema migrans rash?*

During the examination, if you palpate infected tissue, a patient with cellulitis would be quite uncomfortable. Cellulitis presents as flush red throughout. It is indurated, or hard, with signs of tissue inflammation. Cellulitis weeps fluid. Erythema migrans on the other hand is asymptomatic. The lesion looks like a target, with usually two different tones. EM is typically smooth, with no surface changes, except for rare instances when the bite site features bullae or vesicles.

References

1. Oliveira CR, Shapiro ED. Update on persistent symptoms associated with Lyme disease. Curr Opin Pediatr. 2015;27(1):100–4.
2. Wormser GP, Dattwyler RJ, Shapiro ED, Halperin JJ, Steere AC, Klempner MS, Krause PJ, Bakken JS, Strle F, Stanek G, Bockenstedt L, Fish D, Dumler JS, Nadelman RB. The clinical

assessment, treatment, and prevention of Lyme disease, human granulocytic anaplasmosis, and babesiosis: clinical practice guidelines by the Infectious Diseases Society of America. Clin Infect Dis. 2006;43(9):1089–134.

3. Shapiro ED. Lyme disease. N Engl J Med. 2014;371(7):684.
4. Borchers AT, Keen CL, Huntley AC, Gershwin ME. Lyme disease: a rigorous review of diagnostic criteria and treatment. J Autoimmun. 2015;57:82–115.
5. Centers for Disease Control and Prevention. Reported cases of Lyme disease by state or locality, 2004–2013. [Online] 2015. Available from: http://www.cdc.gov/lyme/stats/chartstables/reportedcases_statelocality.html. Accessed 27 Mar 2015.
6. Feder Jr HM, Johnson BJ, O'Connell S, Shapiro ED, Steere AC, Wormser GP, Ad Hoc International Lyme Disease Group, Agger WA, Artsob H, Auwaerter P, Dumler JS, Bakken JS, Bockenstedt LK, Green J, Dattwyler RJ, Munoz J, Nadelman RB, Schwartz I, Draper T, McSweegan E, Halperin JJ, Klempner MS, Krause PJ, Mead P, Morshed M, Porwancher R, Radolf JD, Smith Jr RP, Sood S, Weinstein A, Wong SJ, Zemel L. A critical appraisal of "chronic Lyme disease". N Engl J Med. 2007;357(14):1422–30.
7. Steere AC, Sikand VK. The presenting manifestations of Lyme disease and the outcomes of treatment. N Engl J Med. 2003;348(24):2472–4.
8. Tiger JB, Guill III MA, Chapman MS. Bullous Lyme disease. J Am Acad Dermatol. 2014;71(4):e133–4.
9. Marques A. Chapter 16: Chronic Lyme Disease. In: Halperin JJ, editor. Lyme disease: an evidence-based approach. Wallingford, England: CABI Publishing; 2011.
10. Klempner MS, Hu LT, Evans J, Schmid CH, Johnson GM, Trevino RP, Norton D, Levy L, Wall D, McCall J, Kosinski M, Weinstein A. Two controlled trials of antibiotic treatment in patients with persistent symptoms and a history of Lyme disease. N Engl J Med. 2001;345(2):85–92.
11. Krupp LB, Hyman LG, Grimson R, Coyle PK, Melville P, Ahnn S, Dattwyler R, Chandler B. Study and treatment of post Lyme disease (STOP-LD): a randomized double masked clinical trial. Neurology. 2003;60(12):1923–30.
12. Fallon BA, Keilp JG, Corbera KM, Petkova E, Britton CB, Dwyer E, Slavov I, Cheng J, Dobkin J, Nelson DR, Sackeim HA. A randomized, placebo-controlled trial of repeated IV antibiotic therapy for Lyme encephalopathy. Neurology. 2008;70(13):992–1003.
13. Nadelman RB, Nowakowski J, Fish D, Falco RC, Freeman K, McKenna D, et al. Prophylaxis with single-dose doxycycline for the prevention of Lyme disease after an Ixodes scapularis tick bite. N Engl J Med. 2001;345(2):79–84.

Chapter 44
Urticaria

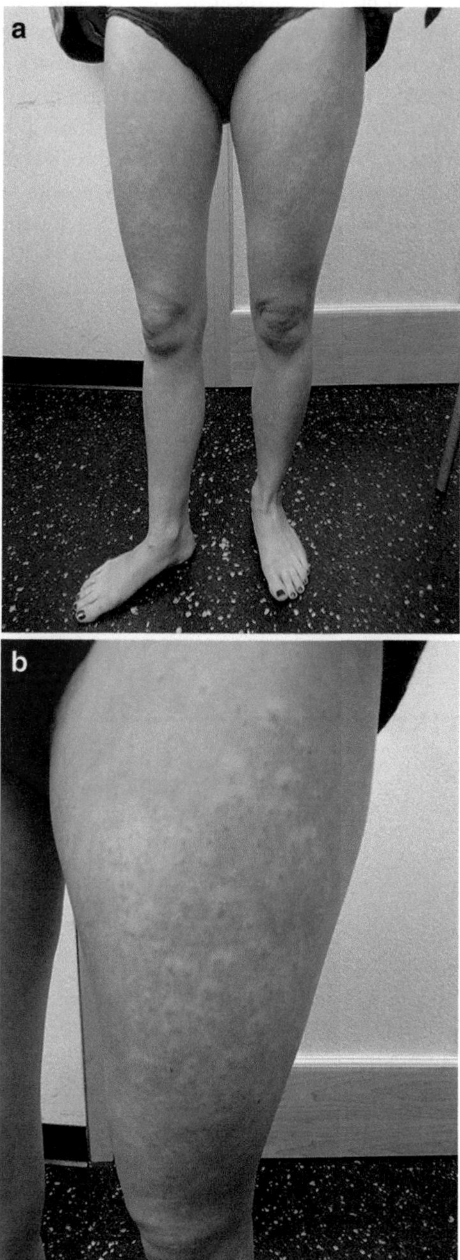

Fig. 44.1 (**a** and **b**) Edematous wheals with perilesional pallor on the bilateral lower extremities

D. Reich et al., *Top 50 Dermatology Case Studies for Primary Care*,
DOI 10.1007/978-3-319-18627-6_44

Primary Care Visit Report

A 29-year-old female with no past medical history presented with a diffuse, itchy, erythematous papular rash. The rash was most severe on her anterior and posterior lower extremities bilaterally, and less prominent on her lower abdomen and lower forearms. The rash started 2 days prior to her visit and got progressively worse over that time. She felt well otherwise. She reported no new lotions, detergents, or clothes. She got a flu shot 2 days prior (which she had received in the past without incident and she denied an egg allergy), otherwise there were no new medications. The rash started later in the afternoon after she got her flu shot. The rash on her hands worsened with contact with hot water. She had taken 50 mg of benadryl the day before and the day of the visit, and the rash continued to progress and to become more itchy.

Vitals were normal. On exam, there was a diffuse, papular, erythematous blanchable rash on her anterior and posterior thighs, lower legs, and ankles bilaterally. Hypopigmentation surrounded the erythematous papules. The rash was less severe but similar in appearance on her lower abdomen and bilateral forearms and hands. There was one 3 cm × 3 cm erythematous wheal on the patient's right medial ankle area.

The patient was treated for hives or a possible allergic reaction (to an unknown allergen). She was put on a 15-day prednisone taper (80 mg for 3 days, 60 mg for 3 days, 40 mg for 3 days, 20 mg for 3 days, 10 mg for 3 days).

Discussion from Dermatology Clinic

Differential Dx

- Urticaria
- Viral exanthem
- Contact dermatitis
- Erythema multiforme
- Urticarial vasculitis

Favored Dx

Urticaria is favored.

Overview

Urticaria, commonly known as hives, is a raised, pruritic edematous rash. It occurs when a stimulus activates mast cells, causing a massive release of histamine and inflammatory mediators that results in leaky capillaries and, consequently, the appearance of wheals.

Urticaria is common, affecting one in five people at some point in their lifetime [1–3]. It can affect people of any age and gender, but commonly occurs in children and middle-aged women [2]. Urticaria is classified as acute (resolving within 6 weeks) or chronic (recurrent, lasting longer than 6 weeks). Chronic urticaria is much less common, with a 0.5 % incidence [3], and twice as likely to occur in women than men [2]. Chronic urticaria is subtyped as autoimmune and idiopathic. Chronic urticaria is associated with underlying health conditions, including thyroid problems and lupus. A common type of chronic urticaria is dermatographism, which is characterized by the appearance of raised welts after the skin is scratched, rubbed, or slapped.

Urticaria can be triggered by a number of allergic or nonallergic factors, and can be further categorized according to the causative agent. These triggers include foods, medications, insect bites, plants, pollen, animal dander, pressure, emotional stress, sweat (cholinergic urticaria), some viral, bacterial, and fungal infections, and exposure to heat, cold, water, or sunlight. Fewer than half the cases of acute urticaria have an obvious cause.

Presentation

Urticaria presents as raised, pruritic wheals (areas of localized edema) which are surrounded by erythema. The lesions are pale or evanescent in the center, and blanchable. They may be accompanied by stinging or burning sensations, as well as varying degrees of pruritus. Hives are variable in size, from a few millimeters to 30 cm, and can appear on any part of the body. They can present within minutes of exposure to a stimulus, or have a delayed onset within a few hours. Lesions invariably migrate within a 24-h period, with old lesions fading and new ones appearing. They can last between several days and up to 6 weeks in acute urticaria.

Workup

History is essential in establishing diagnosis, so physicians should thoroughly question patients to determine any time of onset, exposure to allergens, history of allergies, initiation of new medications, recent viral symptoms, gastrointestinal problems, stress, type of occupation, and family history. Physical examination should pay attention to the number, size, and distribution of wheals [4].

Skin biopsies and lab testing are not usually required for ordinary urticaria; however, a biopsy should be performed if lesions persist for longer than 24 h, or if urticarial vasculitis is suspected. Chronic urticaria warrants CBC, ESR, CRP, and thyroid function blood tests [4]. Chronic urticaria has been associated with *H. pylori* infection, in which case GI investigations may also be indicated in some cases. Patients may be referred to an allergist if systemic allergy is suspected. Cryoproteins should be evaluated in patients with urticaria from exposure to a cold stimulus.

Treatment

When the causative agent is known, the first point of treatment for urticaria is eliminating or avoiding the trigger, or treating the underlying etiology. In many cases the cause is unknown, so therapy focuses on symptomatic relief.

Nondrowsy second generation H_1 antihistamines, e.g., cetirizine or loratadine 10 mg once or twice daily, are recommended first-line treatment for urticaria [4, 5]. Second generation H_1 antihistamines can be administered safely at up to four times the recommended dose when symptoms persist after 2 weeks of initial treatment [4, 6]. Sedating antihistamines, such as 25 mg of hydroxyzine at night, may be used for acute control of pruritus that interrupts sleep.

Patients who do not experience adequate symptomatic relief with antihistamines may benefit from a short course of oral corticosteroid treatment [3, 5]. If conventional therapy fails, patients should be referred to dermatology, where cyclosporine or leukotriene inhibitors may be trialed.

Follow-Up

Acute urticaria is self limiting but may require up to 6 weeks for full clearance. Patients should be monitored for improvement after 2 weeks of treatment, and should be instructed to return to the office if symptoms worsen or change. If urticaria persists or recurs after 6 weeks, daily treatment with antihistamines may become necessary.

Questions for the Dermatologist

– *Is there a way to distinguish between viral rashes and urticaria?*

Distinguishing between viral exanthem and urticaria can be tricky. Urticaria is histamine-mediated versus viral rashes, which are T cell-mediated. Urticarial lesions are always migratory, from one body site to another, within hours. Viral rashes may be preceded by symptoms such as a runny nose and sore throat 1–2 weeks before rash onset. When the diagnosis is unclear, it is best to start with the T cell treatment approach. Starting with a prednisone treatment versus antihistamine is an acceptable choice. Alternatively, the patient can be treated with both prednisone and antihistamines when rash etiology is unclear. Antihistamines would mitigate any itch, and prednisone is a good treatment for viral rashes. If the correct diagnosis is urticaria, the rash will rebound if the patient is only treated with prednisone and no antihistamines. A biopsy would give a more definitive answer if there are not enough clues from patient history and physical exam.

- *Is a 5-day course of 60 mg daily prednisone or a 6-day Medrol Dosepak likely to result in a rebound reaction of the hives after the treatment course is over? Is a longer course necessary with rashes (vs. asthma for example)?*

The authors would not routinely use a Medrol Dosepak because of the risk of rebound rash. Instead of a 5-day course of prednisone, a prednisone taper would be used starting at a dose of 1 mg/kg, taken as a single dose in the morning. The standard tapering time is 2 weeks. Treatment can be extended to 3 weeks if full clearance has not been achieved; however, the extra week is not usually necessary.

- *Could this have been a reaction to a flu shot?*

It is frequently difficult to ascertain the exact cause of urticaria but history can give some clues. It could have been the flu shot that caused hives, which would put the diagnosis in the drug reaction category; however, flu shots are not generally regarded as causing drug-induced urticaria. Drug-induced urticaria typically presents within minutes to hours of exposure to a drug. The offending drugs are most frequently penicillins, sulfonamides and NSAIDs, none of which are in this patient's history. Another diagnosis to consider would be urticarial viral exanthem. It looks the same as idiopathic urticaria; however, it is associated with a viral illness. Onset of the rash would typically be preceded by symptoms of a viral infection, such as runny nose, fever, or headache. It is more common to see viral exanthem in children, however, and the patient did not present with any systemic involvement. Acute idiopathic urticaria is the best diagnosis for this patient based on her history.

- *If this were a viral exanthem, would the treatment be any different?*

For a viral exanthem, drug reaction, or contact dermatitis, an immunosuppressant like prednisone should be used. If a diagnosis of hives is certain, the patient can be treated with solely antihistamines. When the diagnosis is uncertain, as it is in this case, both diagnoses can be covered by treating with antihistamines and topical or oral steroids.

References

1. American College of Allergy, Asthma & Immunology. Hives (Urticaria) [Internet]. 2015 [cited 2015 Jan 13]. Available from: http://acaai.org/allergies/types/skin-allergies/hives-urticaria
2. NHS Choices. Urticaria (hives) [Internet]. 2015 [cited 2015 Jan 13]. Available from: http://www.nhs.uk/conditions/Nettle-rash/Pages/Introduction.aspx

3. Kaplan AP. Chapter 38. Urticaria and angioedema. In: Goldsmith LA, Katz SI, Gilchrest BA, Paller AS, Leffell DJ, Wolff K, editors. Fitzpatrick's dermatology in general medicine. 8th ed. New York: McGraw-Hill; 2012. p. 414–30.
4. Zuberbier T, Aberer W, Asero R, Bindslev-Jensen C, Brzoza Z, Canonica GW, Church MK, Ensina LF, Giménez-Arnau A, Godse K, Gonçalo M, Grattan C, Hebert J, Hide M, Kaplan A, Kapp A, Abdul Latiff AH, Mathelier-Fusade P, Metz M, Nast A, Saini SS, Sánchez-Borges M, Schmid-Grendelmeier P, Simons FE, Staubach P, Sussman G, Toubi E, Vena GA, Wedi B, Zhu XJ, Maurer M. The EAACI/GA(2) LEN/EDF/WAO Guideline for the definition, classification, diagnosis, and management of urticaria: the 2013 revision and update. Allergy. 2014;69(7):868–87.
5. Bernstein JA, Lang DM, Khan DA, Craig T, Dreyfus D, Hsieh F, Sheikh J, Weldon D, Zuraw B, Bernstein DI, Blessing-Moore J, Cox L, Nicklas RA, Oppenheimer J, Portnoy JM, Randolph CR, Schuller DE, Spector SL, Tilles SA, Wallace D. The diagnosis and management of acute and chronic urticare: 2014 update. J Allergy Clin Immunol. 2014;133(5):1270–7.
6. Mitchell S, Balp MM, Samuel M, McBride D, Maurer M. Systematic review of treatments for chronic spontaneous urticaria with inadequate response to licensed first-line treatments. Int J Dermatol. 2014. doi:10.1111/ijd.12727.

Chapter 45
Irritant Dermatitis

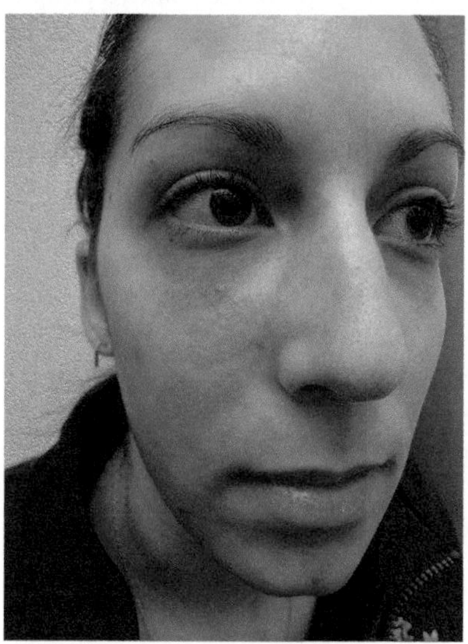

Fig. 45.1 Poorly defined eczematous plaques on the right face

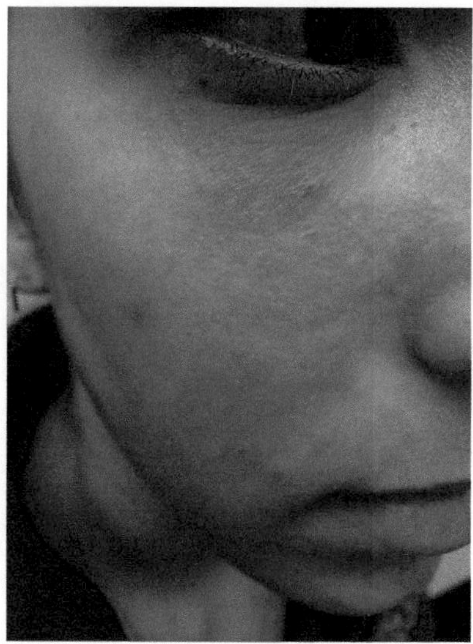

Fig. 45.2 Splotchy erythematous plaques with fine scale

D. Reich et al., *Top 50 Dermatology Case Studies for Primary Care*,
DOI 10.1007/978-3-319-18627-6_45

Primary Care Visit Report

A 24-year-old female with no past medical history presented with a rash on her right cheek and chin which started 3 days prior, when she put her roommate's Epiduo (combination retinoid and benzoyl peroxide) on two pimples on her chin. The next day, she had a large itchy red rash on her chin, right cheek, and right eyelid. She had some clobetasol 0.05 % cream which she applied to the rash, and it improved the itching but not the redness. She also took 25 mg of diphenhydramine on the day the rash appeared and the following day, and applied mupirocin to the rash as well. Despite all of this, the patient said the redness was spreading so she came in for an evaluation. She reported having a similar reaction in the past to a topical ointment (she was unsure which one) and to benzoyl peroxide.

Vitals were normal. On exam, there were erythematous, non-blanchable macular patches on her chin and right cheek, extending superiorly to the right infra-orbital area. The right supra-orbital area featured edema but no erythema. The left supra-orbital area featured slight edema.

This was treated as irritant contact dermatitis. Given that the patient had already used topical steroids without resolution, an oral steroid (6 day methylprednisolone taper pack) was added. The patient was advised to continue using clobetasol twice daily on her face for 1 week, as well as to continue the diphenhydramine daily in case there was an allergic component.

Discussion from Dermatology Clinic

Differential Dx

- Irritant dermatitis
- Allergic contact dermatitis
- Atopic dermatitis
- Psoriasis
- Drug eruption
- Id reaction (autoeczematization)
- Fungal infection

Favored Dx

Irritant and allergic contact dermatitis can be difficult to distinguish. A thorough medical history and identification of potential allergens and irritants is necessary to arrive at a correct diagnosis. One clue is the strong temporal association between exposure to the irritant and onset of dermatitis. In this case, irritant contact dermatitis is favored as the patient reacted to a common irritant (benzoyl peroxide), and the onset of the rash occurred soon after exposure.

Overview

Irritant dermatitis (ID) is a type of dermatitis that occurs following direct injury to the outermost layer of the epidermis, the stratum corneum, caused by a chemical or physical irritant. The response involves local inflammation and is not mediated by the immune system. In contrast, allergic contact dermatitis occurs after exposure to an allergen, and it is characterized by a delayed T cell hypersensitivity response.

Individuals with diminished skin barrier function, such as those with atopic dermatitis, are predisposed to ID [1]. One study found the median affected age to be 38 years, although it can occur at any age, and skin sensitivity to irritants tends to decrease over the lifespan [1–3]. More women are affected than men [1, 4].

ID is often associated with occupational exposure to irritants, and it is the most commonly diagnosed type of occupational contact dermatitis (OCD). Certain occupations place individuals at higher risk for developing ID, including health care workers, food workers, hairdressers, housekeepers and cleaners, and those involved in wet work (classified as contact with water >2 h daily, or hand washing >20 times daily) [1, 4, 5]. Individuals are more prone to ID when there is lower air humidity, so some seasonal variation may be seen [1, 2].

Presentation

Irritant dermatitis is characterized by erythema, pruritus, burning sensation, and dry skin. Severe cases may include edema, vesicle formation and bullae. Patients with chronic exposure to irritants may develop hyperkeratosis (thickening of stratum corneum), diffuse epidermal thickening (acanthosis), and fissured skin. ID most frequently presents on the hands and face; however, irritant diaper dermatitis and irritant dermatitis of the lips from excessive licking are often seen in young children [2, 3]. Irritant dermatitis can occur immediately after contact, or within a few hours.

Workup

Diagnosis is made on clinical examination and patient history. Patch testing can exclude allergic contact dermatitis. A KOH test should be done if there is any suspicion of a fungal infection.

Treatment

The first step in treatment is to identify the underlying cause of irritant dermatitis, and avoid exposure to the irritant. Common irritants are cosmetics, detergents, acids, and friction. Topical corticosteroids are first line treatment for contact dermatitis, but they are only effective if the irritant is removed[A]. Weaker steroids (Class V to VII) such as desonide cream are recommended for the face, or any areas of the body with thinner skin. High potency steroids (Class I or II) are appropriate for the hands. Topical steroids can be used twice daily until inflammation subsides, and patients should be instructed to discontinue their use after 2 weeks to avoid skin atrophy. If there is extensive involvement or severity, patients can be given a systemic corticosteroid [1, 3]. Our practice typically prescribes a 15-day prednisone taper, starting at 1 mg/kg/day for severe cases.

Follow-Up

Patients should be instructed to avoid irritants in the future. Daily use of moisturizers or emollients, which form a protective barrier against water loss from the skin and come in the form of creams, ointments and lotions, may help prevent future irritation by maintaining the skin barrier. There are a variety of emollients and moisturizers available over the counter, and finding one that patients like may involve trial-and-error. Some of the manufacturers include Cutemol, Aquaphor, Aveeno, CeraVe, Curél, and Cetaphil. They may be used in conjunction with topical steroids during treatment course; however, patients should be advised to apply the steroid first. In ID related to the workplace, patients can try protective gear, such as gloves for affected hands. They may also benefit from making every effort to keep their hands well hydrated with emollients after washing.

Questions for the Dermatologist

– *Which steroids are okay to use on the face, and for how long?*

Steroid potency classes V through VII are appropriate to use on the face. They can be used twice daily in the acute phase until dermatitis resolves, for up to 2 weeks. In this case, the clobetasol 0.05 % that the patient had been using on her own (and was instructed to continue to use) is a Class I (superpotent) steroid cream and is usually too strong to use on the face.

– *When is it appropriate to add oral steroids to a rash treatment plan? Is the decision related to failure of topicals, or extent of surface area involved?*

The decision is based on severity and body surface area involvement. It would be reasonable to add oral steroids if the patient has not responded to a few days of treatment with topicals. Other symptoms like itchiness would be another indication for oral steroids. The decision should be made after a risks and benefits discussion with the patient.

– *If you are prescribing oral steroids, why do you prescribe a 15-day prednisone taper instead of, for example, a 5-day course of 60 mg prednisone or the 6-day methylprednisolone taper (Medrol dose pack)?*

Rebound reactions are common with irritant and allergic skin rashes. It is standard practice in our office to prescribe a longer taper (i.e., 2 weeks) with initial dosing of 1 mg/kg/day, in order to avoid achieving temporary clearance followed by a rebound rash.

– *Are topical steroids discontinued after oral steroids are added?*

The patient would typically continue to use the topical corticosteroid along with the oral preparation.

– *Is it common to see irritant dermatitis on sites other than where the irritant was applied?*

Patients can have id reactions (autoeczematization caused by an immune response) to irritants on areas distal to the site of primary application. In this case, it seems more likely that benzoyl peroxide triggered inflammation in certain areas, and then the benzoyl peroxide migrated (perhaps as the patient touched her face) and caused a reaction distally.

– *Does diphenhydramine help with irritant dermatitis?*

It can only help with symptoms such as itchiness. It will not work to improve the rash itself.

References

1. Tan CH, Rasool S, Johnston GA. Contact dermatitis: allergic and irritant. Clin Dermatol. 2014;32(1):116–24.
2. Morris-Jones R, Robertson SJ, Ross JS, White IR, McFadden JP, Rycroft RJ. Dermatitis caused by physical irritants. Br J Dermatol. 2002;147(2):270–5. Review.
3. Usatine RP, Riojas M. Diagnosis and management of contact dermatitis. Am Fam Physician. 2010;82(3):249–55.
4. Dickel H, Kuss O, Schmidt A, Kretz J, Diepgen TL. Importance of irritant contact dermatitis in occupational skin disease. Am J Clin Dermatol. 2002;3(4):283–9.
5. Schwensen JF, Menné T, Johansen JD. The combined diagnosis of allergic and irritant contact dermatitis in a retrospective cohort of 1000 consecutive patients with occupational contact dermatitis. Contact Dermatitis. 2014;71(6):356–63.

Chapter 46
Allergic Contact Dermatitis

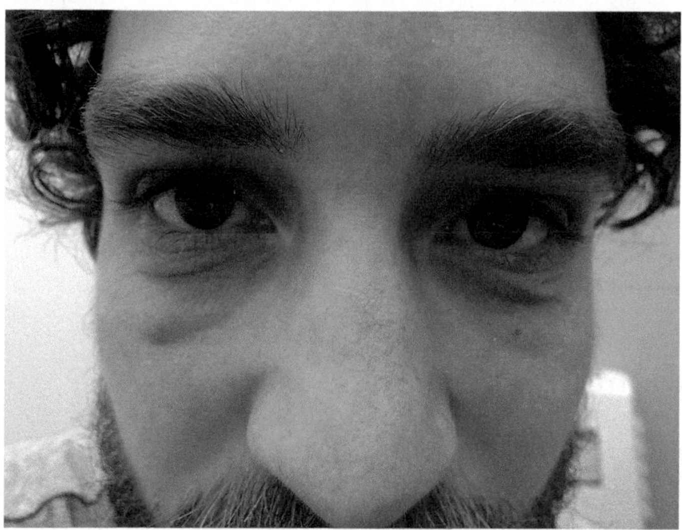

Fig. 46.1 Periocular distribution is one of the more common presentations for this condition

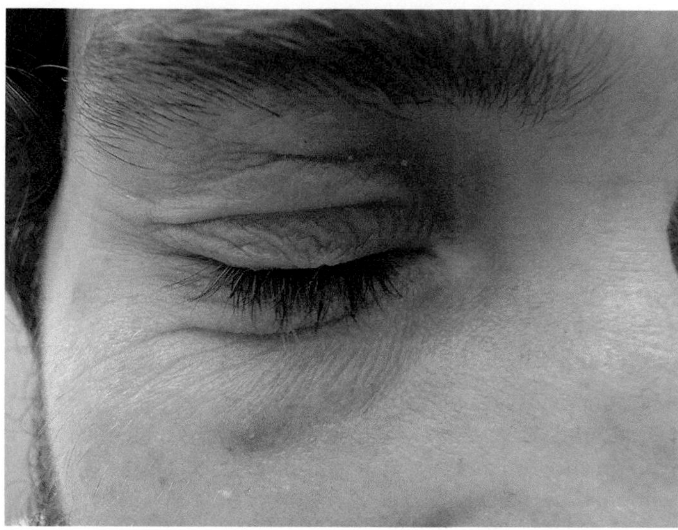

Fig. 46.2 Accentuated skin markings, edema, and redness along with notable itch are hallmarks for this dermatitis

D. Reich et al., *Top 50 Dermatology Case Studies for Primary Care*,
DOI 10.1007/978-3-319-18627-6_46

Primary Care Visit Report

A 33-year-old male with past medical history of thrombophilia, on warfarin, presented with a rash around his eyes starting 1 week prior. He tried using some moisturizer, as well as some over-the-counter eye drops. He also had some erythromycin ophthalmic ointment 0.5 % that he applied to the skin beneath his eyes. None of these things helped.

The patient reported no new skin products and had no known allergens.

Vitals were normal. On exam, on his bilateral infra- and supra-orbital areas there was an erythematous and edematous macular rash. The right inferior infra-orbital area had a 1 mm yellow papule.

The differential considered was contact dermatitis vs. mild blepharitis. To cover for a possible bacterial component of blepharitis as well as to treat a possible contact dermatitis, TobraDex (tobramycin and dexamethasone) 0.3–0.1 % ointment was prescribed twice daily for 7 days.

Discussion from Dermatology Clinic

Differential Dx

- Allergic contact dermatitis
- Irritant dermatitis
- Atopic dermatitis

Favored Dx

Allergic contact dermatitis (ACD) can be difficult to definitively diagnose when there is no identified allergen. However, eyelids are a common area for ACD, and edema is a strong diagnostic clue. In this case, ACD is the favored diagnosis.

Overview

Allergic contact dermatitis is a T cell-mediated type IV (delayed hypersensitivity) reaction that occurs after the skin comes in contact with an allergen. As with other type IV hypersensitivity reactions, the skin must have had prior exposure to the offending substance in order to become sensitized. Subsequent exposure leads to a hypersensitivity reaction that develops over the course of 2–3 days.

ACD accounts for 20 % of new cases of contact dermatitides, with the remaining 80 % being cases of irritant contact dermatitis [1]. A large retrospective study estimated the prevalence of contact allergies in the general population to be 21.2% [2]. The prevalence varies by geographic region, due to differences in exposure, cultural customs, and environmental differences. Workers in certain occupations, especially hairdressers, barbers, metal workers, and health care professionals, are at higher risk for developing contact allergies [3, 4]. Of over 3700 chemicals implicated as causative agents of contact allergy, among the most common are nickel, thimerosal (antiseptic and antifungal agent), fragrance mix, neomycin, and formaldehyde (used as a preservative in many cosmetics) [1, 2, 4, 5]. The estimated prevalence of contact allergy to cosmetics is 6% in the general population [5]. Nickel allergies are more prevalent in women, and have been associated with a history of atopic dermatitis in women [2]. Women with pierced ears tend to present with nickel allergies more often than women without pierced ears [2].

Presentation

Allergic contact dermatitis presents as an eczematous rash that can be severely pruritic. The rash tends to have sharply demarcated borders and is localized to the area exposed to the offending allergen. Any geometric or linear distribution of lesions may reveal a plant allergy, as the shapes are consistent with the area of skin that would come in contact with the plant. It is possible for the rash to develop beyond the site of exposure if the allergen is transferred by hands or clothing. Eyelids are susceptible to this kind of transfer, possibly because the thinner skin of the eyelids is more susceptible to reaction [1]. Eyelid ACD typically presents with edema. More severe cases of ACD may be vesicular or bullous.

Workup

Physical examination and thorough medical history, including history of exposures, often aids in diagnosis. The location and pattern of distribution of lesions can be helpful clues in determining the causal allergen. Allergic rashes on the lower abdomen may be provoked by belt buckles, or the buttons of pants. A rash around the hairline may occur due to allergens in shampoo, or hair dye. Ingredients found in cosmetics may cause rashes on the face.

Patch testing is indicated in order to identify the correct allergen. This may be done in primary care if patch tests (e.g., T.R.U.E. test) are available, otherwise patients can be referred to dermatology. The patches must be worn for 48 h. A biopsy of allergic contact dermatitis would reveal an eczematous process but would not differentiate between eczema and allergic contact dermatitis. More importantly, it would not reveal the offending allergen.

Treatment

The goal of treatment of ACD is to identify the allergen, so that patients may avoid contact with it in the future and prevent recurrence. Patch testing is the method of choice for identifying the allergen. Patients should avoid any immunosuppressive treatments prior to application of patches. Topical and systemic corticosteroids, and sun exposure should be stopped, ideally for 2 weeks, before patch application [1]. In this case, treatment with mild topical corticosteroids on the eyelids would not need to be discontinued prior to patch testing, as local absorption on the eyelids would not affect patch results on the back.

Allergy patches must be worn on the back for 2 days and the site must be kept dry to ensure good test results. The results are read when the patches are removed, 2 days later, and if no allergens are identified, it is recommended they are read again 4 days after patch application, as some allergens are associated with delayed reactions. Metals, antibiotics (neomycin, bacitracin), and paraphenylenediamine (found in hair dye) are common allergens that may require 4–7 days to elicit a response [1]. After the allergen has been identified, it should be strictly avoided.

Topical corticosteroids are the mainstay of symptomatic treatment for ACD [6–8]. Choice of potency class depends on the location of the rash. Mid-potent to potent steroids (Classes II–IV) are appropriate for the trunk and extremities, excluding intertriginous areas which warrant milder steroids, twice daily for up to 2 weeks. Higher-potency steroids may be used on the scalp. The face, neck, intertriginous areas, or any other area with thin, delicate skin, should be treated with a mild (Class V–VII) topical corticosteroid twice daily for 1–2 weeks. Only mild topical corticosteroids are appropriate for the eyelids. The treatment time for eyelids should ideally be limited to 7 days due to the risk of increased intraocular pressure. Treatment with topical tacrolimus 0.1 % ointment may be a safer alternative to corticosteroids for eyelid ACD [9, 10]. It is applied to the eyelids and affected periorbital areas twice daily for 2 weeks.

Although topical corticosteroids are frequently used in treating ACD, they may sometimes be the cause of it [7]. Tacrolimus 0.1 % twice daily for 2 weeks may be used as an alternative, as it has demonstrated comparable efficacy to topical corticosteroids [11]. Severe cases, featuring severe erythema or vesicles, or extensive surface area involvement, may require a course of oral prednisone. This should be tapered over the course of 2 weeks in order to avoid rebound dermatitis. The recommended starting dose is 0.5 mg/kg/day. Severe cases may also be referred directly to dermatology.

Follow-Up

When allergens are correctly identified and subsequently avoided, ACD can often resolve without recurrence. The avoidance of triggering allergens is a key factor in maintaining resolution. Emollients and barrier creams may offer preventative benefits [8, 12]. Any patients with recurrent ACD, severe symptoms, or exacerbation with use of corticosteroids, should be referred to dermatology for further evaluation.

Questions for the Dermatologist

– *Are there special considerations for a rash around the eyes?*

You have to be extra careful with the potency of steroid, because of the risk of increasing intraocular pressure and causing glaucoma. If a patient has a history of glaucoma, a low potency steroid may be used sparingly for a short time, up to 1 week.

– *Which class of steroids is OK to use on the eyelids and infraorbital eye area? And for how long?*

Low potency steroids are okay to use on the eyelids for a short amount of time, up to 1 week. Over-the-counter strength hydrocortisone can be used for a little longer, but no more than 2 weeks. It should be applied sparingly in either case.

– *What is the difference between contact dermatitis, irritant contact dermatitis, and allergic contact dermatitis? Are they all treated similarly?*

Contact dermatitis describes an inflammatory rash that occurs as a result of exposure to a trigger. That trigger could be a chemical or physical irritant (which classifies the rash as irritant dermatitis, or irritant contact dermatitis) or an allergen (allergic dermatitis, or allergic contact dermatitis). Examples of common irritants are detergent soap, bleach, benzoyl peroxide, alcohol, dry air or wind, repeated or prolonged exposure to water, or mechanical friction. Common allergens include poison ivy, nickel, gold, bacitracin, neomycin, and fragrances. Irritant and allergic contact dermatitis are treated similarly, with topical steroids. Body surface area affected, anatomical location, severity of plaques, and size of person are the considerations for determining steroid potency.

References

1. Castanedo-Tardan M, Zug KA. Chapter 13. Allergic contact dermatitis. In: Goldsmith LA, Katz SI, Gilchrest BA, Paller AS, Leffell DJ, Wolff K, editors. Fitzpatrick's dermatology in general medicine [internet]. 8th ed. New York: McGraw-Hill; 2012. Available from: http://accessmedicine.mhmedical.com.ezproxy.cul.columbia.edu/content.aspx?bookid=392&Sectionid=41138708. Accessed 12 Mar 2015.
2. Thyssen JP, Linneberg A, Menné T, Johansen JD. The epidemiology of contact allergy in the general population—prevalence and main findings. Contact Dermatitis. 2007;57(5):287–99.
3. Pesonen M, Jolanki R, Larese Filon F, Wilkinson M, Kręcisz B, Kieć-Świerczyńska M, Bauer A, Mahler V, John SM, Schnuch A, Uter W, ESSCA network. Patch test results of the European

baseline series among patients with occupational contact dermatitis across Europe—analyses of the European Surveillance System on Contact Allergy network, 2002–2010. Contact Dermatitis. 2015;72(3):154–63.

4. Fyhrquist N, Lehto E, Lauerma A. New findings in allergic contact dermatitis. Curr Opin Allergy Clin Immunol. 2014;14(5):430–5.
5. Lundov MD, Moesby L, Zachariae C, Johansen JD. Contamination versus preservation of cosmetics: a review on legislation, usage, infections, and contact allergy. Contact Dermatitis. 2009;60(2):70–8.
6. Cohen DE, Heidary N. Treatment of irritant and allergic contact dermatitis. Dermatol Ther. 2004;17(4):334–40.
7. Schlapbach C, Simon D. Update on skin allergy. Allergy. 2014;69(12):1571–81.
8. Saary J, Qureshi R, Palda V, DeKoven J, Pratt M, Skotnicki-Grant S, Holness L. A systematic review of contact dermatitis treatment and prevention. J Am Acad Dermatol. 2005;53(5):845.
9. Saripalli YV, Gadzia JE, Belsito DV. Tacrolimus ointment 0.1% in the treatment of nickel-induced allergic contact dermatitis. J Am Acad Dermatol. 2003;49(3):477–82.
10. Katsarou A, Armenaka M, Vosynioti V, Lagogianni E, Kalogeromitros D, Katsambas A. Tacrolimus ointment 0.1% in the treatment of allergic contact eyelid dermatitis. J Eur Acad Dermatol Venereol. 2009;23(4):382–7.
11. Katsarou A, Makris M, Papagiannaki K, Lagogianni E, Tagka A, Kalogeromitros D. Tacrolimus 0.1% vs mometasone furoate topical treatment in allergic contact hand eczema a prospective randomized clinical study. Eur J Dermatol. 2012;22(2):192–6.
12. Usatine RP, Riojas M. Diagnosis and management of contact dermatitis. Am Fam Physician. 2010;82(3):249–55.

Chapter 47
Abscess

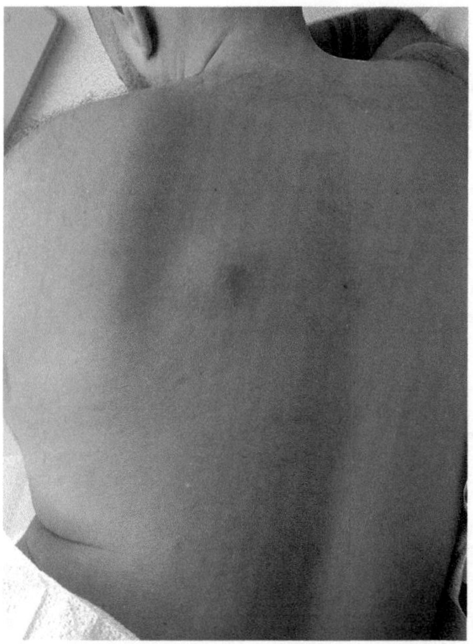

Fig. 47.1 Tender fluctuant ballotable subcutaneous nodule that is tender to touch

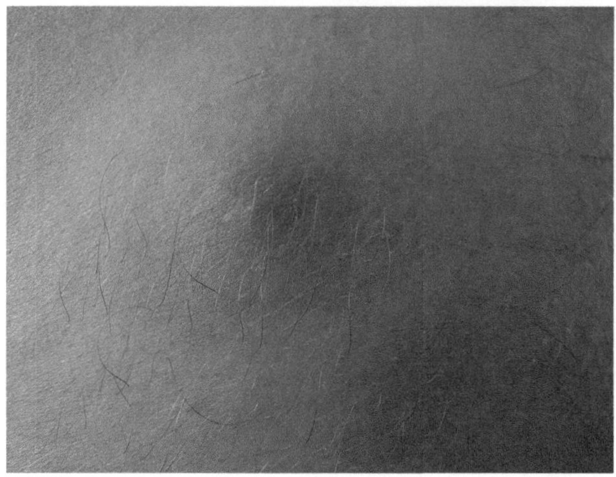

Fig. 47.2 A central pustule is occasionally discernable overlying this lesion

D. Reich et al., *Top 50 Dermatology Case Studies for Primary Care*,
DOI 10.1007/978-3-319-18627-6_47

Primary Care Visit Report

A 29-year-old male with past medical history of depression, anxiety, and ADD (on citalopram and Adderall) presented with a "pimple" on his back. He said it started 3 weeks prior to this visit, while he was in Tanzania volunteering. Recently, the bump became larger and more irritated and he subsequently found it painful to lie on his back. He denied any fever, chills, or systemic symptoms.

Vitals were normal. On exam, on his back, there was a 4 cm × 3.5 cm area of erythema, a 2 cm × 1.5 cm area of induration, and a 1 mm white central papule.

The lesion was treated as an abscess. The abscess was not fluctuant, and therefore it was not ready to be incised and drained. The patient was advised to apply warm compresses twice daily. The area of erythema on the patient's back was marked with a permanent marker, and he was given a prescription for Bactrim DS twice daily with instructions to initiate antibiotics only if the area of erythema spread beyond the marked borders.

Discussion from Dermatology Clinic

Differential Dx

- Abscess
- Ruptured epidermal inclusion cyst
- Foreign body reaction
- Furuncle
- Carbuncle
- Hidradenitis suppurativa

Favored Dx

The dome-shaped, tender nodule with central white pustule and surrounding erythema is consistent with an abscess.

Overview

Skin abscesses are collections of pus in the dermis or subcutaneous tissue that result from an inflammatory response to bacterial infection. Infection can occur following any trauma or break in the skin, or following occlusion of hair follicles. Abscesses that involve hair follicles are called furuncles. Furuncles are an example of deep folliculitis, and carbuncles are groups of furuncles that are interconnected subcutaneously.

Skin abscesses are one of the most common dermatological complaints managed by primary care and emergency physicians [1]. The most frequently implicated pathogens are *S. aureus* and streptococci. Skin and soft tissue infections (SSTIs) account for 3 % of emergency department visits in the United States, and one third of those visits are due to abscesses [2]. The incidence of abscesses overall is increasing, and it is thought to mirror the increased incidence of MRSA infections [2–4]. It is estimated that over 50 % of abscesses are caused by community-associated MRSA [1, 3].

Presentation

Abscesses present as painful, fluctuant, warm, erythematous nodules or masses that vary greatly in size, from 1 to 2 cm to the size of a baseball. They may take anywhere from 1 to 2 days to several weeks to evolve, and can initially present without fluctuance. In some cases a central white pustule may be visualized. Abscesses are common on the lower extremities (often as a complication of cellulitis), trunk, head and neck, and buttock [3]. Some patients may present with fever.

Workup

Abscesses are typically diagnosed on clinical examination. If contents can be expressed, bacterial and fungal cultures with sensitivities should be taken from the exudate; however, results are not necessary in order to initiate antibiotic treatment. Culturing is especially important for recurrent abscesses [5].

Treatment

Incision and drainage (I&D) is the recommended treatment for fluctuant abscesses [5]. Following local anesthetic injection, a small incision is made over the mass, and contents are expressed. The incision should be large enough to allow maximal expression of pus, and made along Langer's tension lines in order to minimize scarring [1]. Although most incisions are left to heal with secondary closure, larger incisions may warrant primary closure with stitches, as it leads to accelerated healing and low recurrence rates [6]. Small abscesses that are not yet fluctuant and cannot be incised and drained, as in this case, can be monitored and treated with hot compresses 1–2 times daily [1].

Oral antibiotic therapy is not necessary for uncomplicated abscesses; however, it is recommended as adjunctive treatment for immunosuppressed patients, if there are systemic symptoms such as fever, tachycardia, or tachypnea, and in cases of recurrent abscesses, or failure to resolve with I&D [1, 5]. The Infectious Diseases Society of America recommends a 10–14 day course of dicloxacillin 500 mg four times daily for methicillin-susceptible *S. aureus* abscesses. A four-times daily dosing regimen may be difficult for patients to follow, so the author's practice often uses cephalexin 500 mg twice daily for 7–10 days as an alternative. MRSA-associated abscesses can be treated with a 5–10 day course of trimethoprim-sulfamethoxazole DS 1–2 tabs twice daily, or clindamycin 300–450 mg four times daily. The two described MRSA regimens have equivalent efficacy [7]. Rapid disease progression with concomitant cellulitis should be referred to a hospital for IV antibiotic therapy.

Follow-Up

Patients treated with I&D should be reevaluated after about 1 week to assess adequate drainage and healing progress. If the mass remains fluctuant, further draining may be required. Patients on oral antibiotic treatment should be seen within 3–4 days to ensure they are responding to treatment. Recurrent abscesses may be reflective of bacterial reservoirs in the nasal mucosa, in which case treatment with intranasal mupirocin 2–3 times daily for 5 days is appropriate. In addition, daily chlorhexidine (e.g., Hibiclens OTC) washes for 5 days may also be beneficial in eliminating bacterial reservoirs. When applicable, it may be appropriate to treat all household members with prophylactic intranasal mupirocin and chlorhexidine wash [1].

Questions for the Dermatologist

- *I was taught that antibiotics do not penetrate an abscess, and the only treatment is incision and drainage. However, sometimes I treated non-fluctuant masses that cannot be incised and drained with oral antibiotics, and they cleared up. Why is that?*

If the mass is not fluctuant, it might not be an abscess, which explains why it would clear up with oral antibiotic treatment. The non-fluctuant mass could be cellulitis, which would respond to antibiotic treatment. Abscesses can spontaneously rupture and drain, but they are sequestered from blood stream and need releasing. They cannot be treated with antibiotics alone.

- *How often should warm compresses be used?*

The evening following I&D, it is a great idea to use a warm compress, and manipulate or massage the abscess to get any residual pus to keep draining. Compresses can be repeated over the next day or two following I&D.

– *Are soaks more effective than warm compresses? Should the soaks contain anything other than water?*

Soaking is not beneficial in the case of abscesses. Warm compresses are preferred, and they should be combined with gentle massage.

– *Is having an abscess an indication to stay out of public pools, spas, etc.?*

Once oral antibiotic therapy is initiated, they are technically no longer considered contagious. However, it would be a good idea to stay out of public pools at minimum until the abscesses stop draining.

References

1. Singer AJ, Talan DA. Management of skin abscesses in the era of methicillin-resistant Staphylococcus aureus. N Engl J Med. 2014;370(11):1039–47.
2. Qualls ML, Mooney MM, Camargo Jr CA, Zucconi T, Hooper DC, Pallin DJ. Emergency department visit rates for abscess versus other skin infections during the emergence of community-associated methicillin-resistant Staphylococcus aureus, 1997–2007. Clin Infect Dis. 2012;55(1):103–5.
3. Gaspari RJ, Blehar D, Polan D, Montoya A, Alsulaibikh A, Liteplo A. The Massachusetts abscess rule: a clinical decision rule using ultrasound to identify methicillin-resistant Staphylococcus aureus in skin abscesses. Acad Emerg Med. 2014;21(5):558–67.
4. Earley MA, Friedel ME, Govindaraj S, Tessema B, Eloy JA. Community-acquired methicillin-resistant Staphylococcus aureus in nasal vestibular abscess. Int Forum Allergy Rhinol. 2011;1(5):379–81.
5. Stevens DL, Bisno AL, Chambers HF, Dellinger EP, Goldstein EJ, Gorbach SL, Hirschmann JV, Kaplan SL, Montoya JG, Wade JC. Practice guidelines for the diagnosis and management of skin and soft tissue infections: 2014 update by the Infectious Diseases Society of America. Clin Infect Dis. 2014;59(2):e10–52.
6. Singer AJ, Thode Jr HC, Chale S, Taira BR, Lee C. Primary closure of cutaneous abscesses: a systematic review. Am J Emerg Med. 2011;29(4):361–6.
7. Miller LG, Daum RS, Creech CB, Young D, Downing MD, Eells SJ, Pettibone S, Hoagland RJ, Chambers HF, DMID 07-0051 Team. Clindamycin versus trimethoprim-sulfamethoxazole for uncomplicated skin infections. N Engl J Med. 2015;372(12):1093–103.

Chapter 48
Hand, Foot, and Mouth Disease

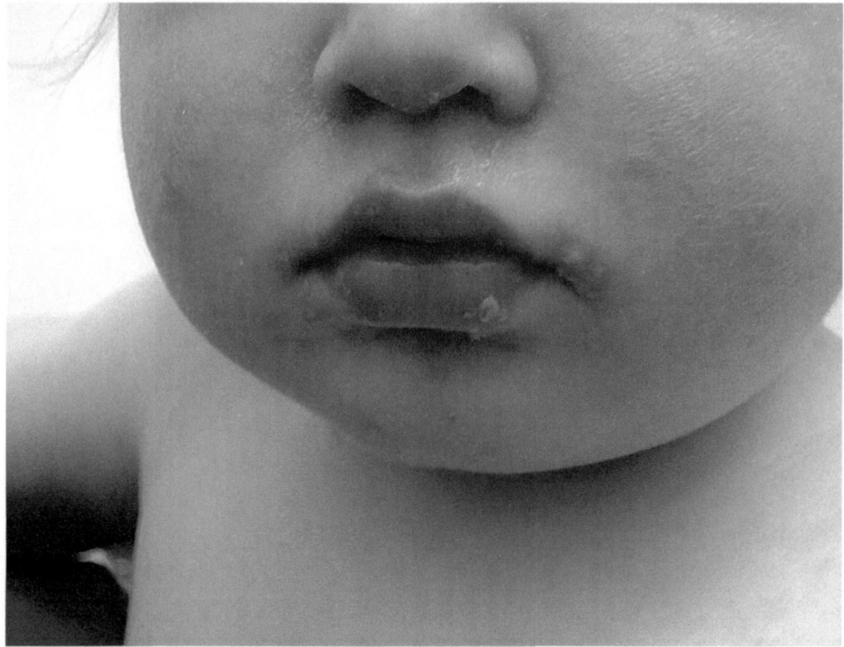

Fig. 48.1 Gray-based ulcers with a rim of erythema on mucosal and perioral surfaces

D. Reich et al., *Top 50 Dermatology Case Studies for Primary Care*,
DOI 10.1007/978-3-319-18627-6_48

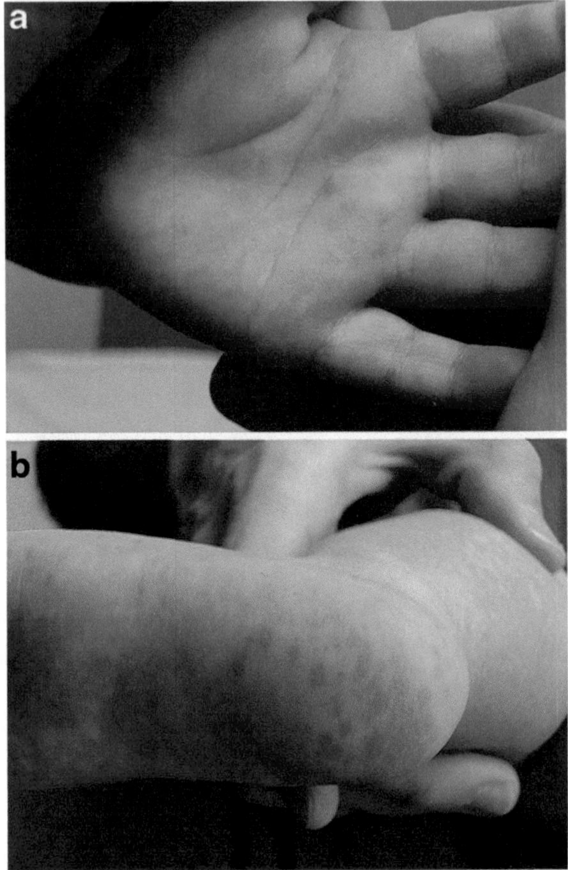

Fig. 48.2 (**a** and **b**) Nonspecific pink papules on the palm, fingers, and soles

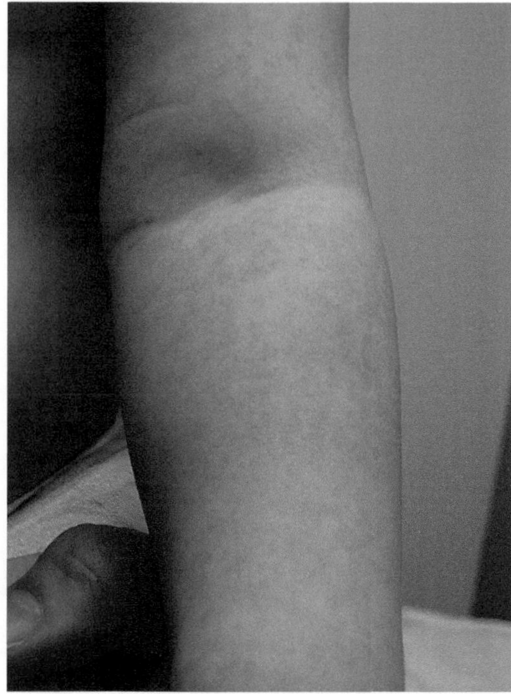

Fig. 48.3 Slightly scaly morbilliform pattern bilateral arms and trunk may also be present in this condition

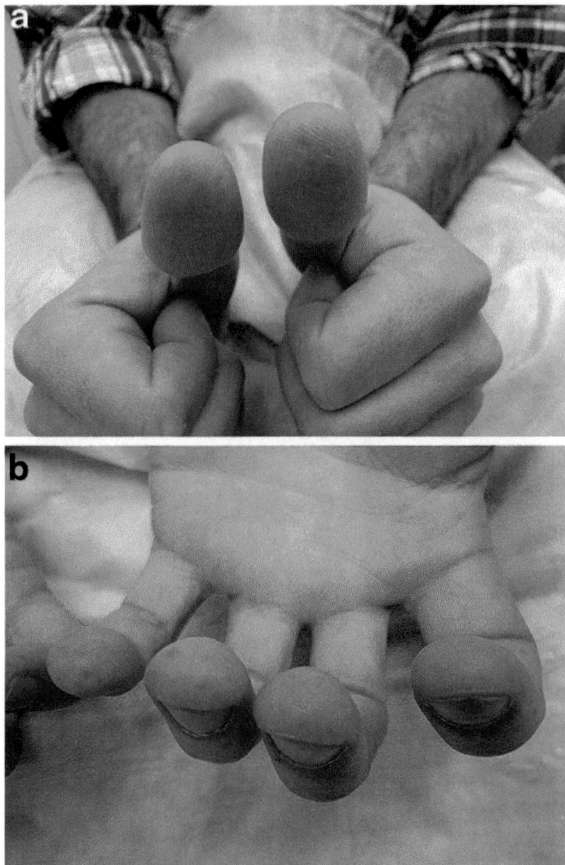

Fig. 48.4 (**a** and **b**) Fingertips with unusual pulp distribution red brown papules

Primary Care Visit Report

Pediatric Case

A 1-year-old male with no past medical history presented with fever and rash. The fever started 4 days prior, with a maximum temperature of 103 degrees Fahrenheit. Three days prior, he developed a rash in his diaper area. Two days prior, he developed a rash on his trunk as well as a white coating, blisters and bumps in his mouth. The parents had been using topical clotrimazole on the diaper area and oral nystatin for possible thrush. He had a decreased appetite and had been cranky.

Vitals were normal except for a temperature of 99.5 degrees Fahrenheit. On exam, there were multiple ulcers around his lips and a papular rash on his face.

There was an erythematous papular rash over his extremities, torso, genital region, palms, and soles, with scattered blisters on his palms and soles as well. A viral culture from the oral lesion was sent to the lab, which was negative for herpes simplex virus (HSV). The lab did not screen the culture for coxsackie.

Adult Case

A 34 year-old male with no past medical history presented with sore throat and "red spots" on his fingers. His wife had presented to the clinic earlier in the day and tested positive for strep throat with the rapid strep test, which is what prompted his visit. The patient's symptoms started 6 days prior with chills, fatigue, and sore throat. Those symptoms lasted about 3 days and then started to resolve. Three days prior, he noticed red spots on his fingers as well as increased sensitivity of his fingertips (not painful, but bothersome if touched).

Vitals were normal. On exam, his tonsils and oropharynx were erythematous, with 1+ tonsillar edema but no exudate and no other mouth lesions. The palmar surfaces of his hands had 2 mm erythematous macules scattered on all fingers. The ventral surfaces of his feet had scattered 2 mm erythematous macules. His rapid strep test was negative, and his throat culture was negative.

Both of these cases were treated as coxsackievirus infections given the lesions on the palms and soles (and in the pediatric case, in the mouth as well) with supportive care, such as NSAIDs or acetaminophen as needed.

Discussion from Dermatology Clinic

Differential Dx

- Hand–foot–mouth disease
- Herpetic stomatitis
- Parvovirus
- Aphthous stomatitis
- Perniosis

Favored Dx

The prodromal syndromes and distribution of the lesions in the mouth, and on the palms and soles, are suggestive of Hand-Foot-Mouth Disease (HFMD).

Herpetic stomatitis was considered in primary care as part of the differential; however, herpetic stomatitis is rarely seen in otherwise healthy babies. Herpetic stomatitis is predominantly seen in severely immunocompromised babies, and it involves a very severe outbreak of oral lesions. Parvovirus was also considered as part of the differential. This typically presents as a distinctive, slapped-cheek facial rash in children, and joint pain in adults. There are usually no oral findings, so parvovirus would not explain the patients' presentation in this case.

Overview

HFMD is a common enteroviral illness that is usually benign and self-limiting. It typically affects infants over 6 months old and children under the age of 5; however, it may sometimes affect adults as well [1]. The disease shows a seasonal variation consistent with other enteroviruses, with most cases presenting during the spring, summer, and fall in temperate climates, and throughout the year in tropical climates. Epidemiology reports indicate a slight male predominance [1, 2]. HFMD is less common in North America; however, it has become increasingly predominant and a cause for concern in Asia-Pacific during the last 15 years [1]. Several large outbreaks have occurred during this time period in Taiwan (where 1.5 million people were affected), China, Singapore, Brunei, Mongolia, and Vietnam [3]. Several smaller outbreaks have occurred in the United States since 2011, with one sample reporting that 25 % of infected patients were adults [3, 4].

HFMD is caused by ssRNA enteroviruses, most commonly coxsackievirus A16, and enterovirus 71. Coxsackievirus A6 is increasingly implicated [3, 5, 6]. HFMD rarely leads to severe complications; however, central nervous involvement, encephalitis, aseptic meningitis, pulmonary edema, myocarditis, and death have been reported, primarily in younger children infected with EV 71 [1, 2]. The illness is transmitted through feces, blister fluid, and secretions of the nose and throat [7]. Transmission typically occurs through the fecal–oral route, and more rarely through particle inhalation. Transmissibility is high in children and within households, while about 11 % of exposed adults become infected [6]. The incubation period lasts 3–5 days.

Presentation

In children, HFMD typically presents with painful oral lesions, and erythematous macules or vesicles on the palms and soles of feet [2, 3]. Other sites of presentation include the dorsal hands and feet, buttocks, and more rarely the genitalia, legs, and face. In adults, the cutaneous findings are similar to those seen in children, typically affecting the mouth, palms, and soles. The lesions initially present as dusky-purple papules and macules, which begin to form vesicles with surrounding erythema, and eventually desquamate and crust. They typically heal without scarring or complications, within 7–10 days of crusting.

Cutaneous findings are usually preceded by 1–2 days of fever, malaise, abdominal pain, and upper respiratory symptoms. As in the above patients, sore throat is a very common preceding symptom, and often leads to decreased eating and drinking.

Workup

HFMD is usually diagnosed based on clinical findings. A viral culture or PCR test (from throat, stool, or vesicular fluid) may be done to identify the exact strain, which is useful to identify strains that are associated with serious complications and increased mortality, i.e., EV 71. Blood may be tested for coxsackie antibodies if confirmation is needed. Fecal analysis may be done; however, it is less sensitive [3]. PCR testing is indicated in patients with central nervous system involvement.

Treatment

Recognizing HFMD is crucial in preventing transmission of the disease to close contacts, and lowering the risk of an epidemic. Treatment for HFMD is typically supportive and aims to provide symptomatic relief. Over-the-counter oral anesthetics such as Orajel and Anbesol may be needed to alleviate discomfort on swallowing. Discomfort on swallowing may lead to dehydration, so patients should be encouraged to stay hydrated. More rare, complicated cases that feature systemic involvement may require hospital management.

Follow-Up

HFMD is typically self-limiting and resolves within 7–10 days [2]. Patients may be evaluated again after a week to monitor symptom resolution. They should be instructed to return to the office urgently if new systemic symptoms present, or existing symptoms worsen.

After symptom resolution, viral shedding may continue for up to 5 weeks, and viral particles may be found in the stool 8 weeks after infection [2, 6]. Complications may occur following infection, such as onychomadesis, which is spontaneous painless separation of the proximal nail plate from the nail bed followed by shedding of the nail as it grows out. Other complications are desquamation of the palms and soles, or eczema coxsackium, which is a coxsackie rash eruption accentuated in areas of eczematous dermatitis in patients with eczema [3, 8]. Contact precautions are recommended for children in diapers, meaning direct body contact with them should be limited as much as is realistically possible due to transmission risks [5]. Further transmission may be prevented by maintaining good hygiene, regularly washing hands (especially after changing diapers), and disinfecting surfaces in child care settings.

Questions for the Dermatologist

- *What other conditions may feature erythematous rash and blistering on the palms and soles?*

The "glove and sock" syndrome of parvovirus can present with painful papules and purpura on the hands and feet. Parvovirus is a common disease of childhood, with estimated seropositivity in at least half of school-aged children. Perniosis (aka chilblains), a hypersensitivity to cold, humid climates, may cause inflammation of blood vessels that gives rise to erythematous, pruritic papules, and nodules on the palms and soles. Perniosis may involve areas that are atypical to HFMD, such as the thighs, lower legs, and face. Additionally, patients with perniosis usually have history of exposure to cold temperatures within a few days of onset of the rash. Less common conditions leading to lesions on the palms and soles are vasculitis, gonococcemia, and multiple emboli, which all primarily affect adults.

- *Is coxsackie generally a clinical diagnosis, or is it worth doing a blood test to screen for coxsackie antibodies?*

The diagnosis is generally clinical, but it would help cement a case to get coxsackie titers. I draw blood in about 50 % of the cases just to get reassurance I am making the correct diagnosis.

- *The oral lesions on the baby were suspicious for herpes. Is there a way to distinguish herpes stomatitis from coxsackie?*

There is no mild presentation of herpes stomatitis. It is very prominent. If there is a patient with one ulcer on the buccal mucosa, the diagnosis is probably not herpetic stomatitis. The condition is seen in babies who are on chemotherapy, or immunosuppressed, or have other severe comorbidities. It is not a normal thing to see in babies, and I would not include it in the differential of an otherwise healthy baby.

- *Would parvovirus infection feature a rash on the body, or just the face? Would there be mouth sores?*

You can get purpuric lesions of the hands and feet with parvo, but it does not typically include mouth sores. A parvo rash can include the proximal extremities and trunk.

References

1. Xing W, Liao Q, Viboud C, Zhang J, Sun J, Wu JT, Chang Z, Liu F, Fang VJ, Zheng Y, Cowling BJ, Varma JK, Farrar JJ, Leung GM, Yu H. Hand, foot, and mouth disease in China, 2008–12: an epidemiological study. Lancet Infect Dis. 2014;14(4):308–18.
2. Belazarian LT, Lorenzo ME, Pearson AL, Sweeney SM, Wiss K. Chapter 192. Exanthematous viral diseases. In: Goldsmith LA, Katz SI, Gilchrest BA, Paller AS, Leffell DJ, Wolff K, editors. Fitzpatrick's dermatology in general medicine. 8th ed. New York: McGraw-Hill; 2012. Available from: http://accessmedicine.mhmedical.com.ezproxy.cul.columbia.edu/content.aspx?bookid=392&Sectionid=41138921. Accessed 3 Mar 2015.
3. Repass GL, Palmer WC, Stancampiano FF. Hand, foot, and mouth disease: identifying and managing an acute viral syndrome. Cleve Clin J Med. 2014;81(9):537–43.
4. Centers for Disease Control and Prevention (CDC). Notes from the field: severe hand, foot, and mouth disease associated with coxsackievirus A6—Alabama, Connecticut, California, and Nevada, November 2011–February 2012. MMWR Morb Mortal Wkly Rep. 2012;61(12):213–4.
5. Flett K, Youngster I, Huang J, McAdam A, Sandora TJ, Rennick M, Smole S, Rogers SL, Nix WA, Oberste MS, Gellis S, Ahmed AA. Hand, foot, and mouth disease caused by coxsackievirus a6. Emerg Infect Dis. 2012;18(10):1702–4.
6. Downing C, Ramirez-Fort MK, Doan HQ, Benoist F, Oberste MS, Khan F, Tyring SK. Coxsackievirus A6 associated hand, foot and mouth disease in adults: clinical presentation and review of the literature. J Clin Virol. 2014;60(4):381–6.
7. Centers for Disease Control. Hand, foot, and mouth disease (HFMD). Transmission [Internet]. 2013 [cited 3 March 2015]. Available from: http://www.cdc.gov/hand-foot-mouth/about/transmission.html
8. Kim EJ, Park HS, Yoon HS, Cho S. Four cases of onychomadesis after hand-foot-mouth disease. Ann Dermatol. 2014;26(6):777–8.

Chapter 49
Nevi

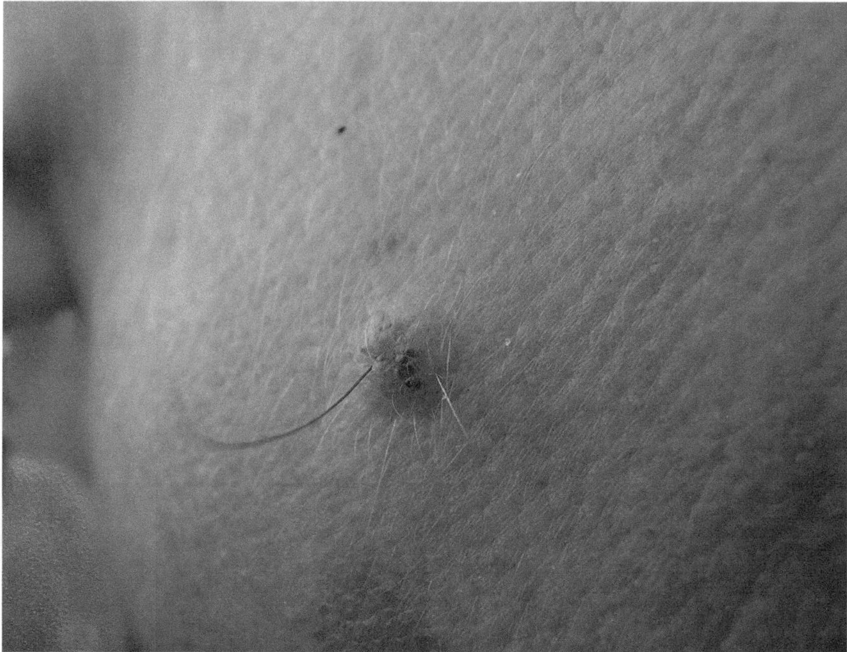

Fig. 49.1 Clear margined pink papule with central pigmentation. Hair growth has zero prognostic significance for the behavior of a mole

D. Reich et al., *Top 50 Dermatology Case Studies for Primary Care*,
DOI 10.1007/978-3-319-18627-6_49

Primary Care Visit Report

A 47-year-old female presented with a mole on her right cheek. Per patient, this mole had been present throughout her life. Until 5 years prior, the mole had been more uniformly dark brown in color. In the past 5 years, the patient noted that the coloring was more varied, with the center remaining darker colored but the periphery becoming lighter. The mole grew a single black hair out of its center, which she regularly plucked.

Vitals were normal. On exam, there was a 0.5 cm brown, raised, round nevus with central dark brown pigmentation and surrounding lighter brown coloring. The borders were regular. There was a single dark-colored hair growing from the center of the nevus as well as several lighter colored hairs.

This patient was referred to dermatology for further evaluation.

Discussion from Dermatology Clinic

Differential Dx

- Congenital nevus
- Dysplastic nevus
- Acquired melanocytic nevus

Favored Dx

Given its presence for the entirety of the patient's life, the growth is most likely a congenital nevus.

Overview

Nevi, or moles, are a class of cutaneous pigmented growths. They are ideally well-circumscribed, can be macular or papular, and are typically round or oval in shape. They can be brown, pink, or flesh colored.

Moles present at birth are called congenital nevi. The American Academy of Dermatology estimates 1 in 100 people are born with one or more such lesions [1]. Men and women of all races are equally likely to have congenital nevi at, or within a few weeks, of birth, and the lesions grow proportionately with the child [2]. Congenital nevi are classified by size (small <1.5 cm; medium 1.5–19.9 cm, giant >20 cm) and they are most likely to occur on the trunk and extremities. They are often indistinguishable from common acquired nevi [3]. Most congenital nevi are benign and asymptomatic through life [2].

Presentation

Congenital nevi can exhibit great variance from patient to patient. They are generally brown in color but can feature shades of black, gray, red, yellow, or blue, and in some cases they may show variation in pigment [3]. Up to 75 % of cases present with an overlying dark, coarse terminal hair [4]. They may be elevated, verrucous, papular, pebbly, or cerebriform, and they can change with age [3]. Approximately one in six lighten with age [4].

Workup

The different classes of nevi are distinguished from each other histopathologically [5]. A biopsy would confirm nevus type, as well as rule out malignancy. Dermatoscopic findings that would help distinguish congenital nevi from acquired nevi include small pigmented globules, prominent vessels, and perifollicular hypopigmentation [4].

Treatment

There is little consensus on how to manage small congenital nevi [3]. Dermatologists use the ABCDE rule of dermoscopy to assess risk of malignancy ([A] = asymmetry, [B] = borders, [C] = colors, [D] = diameter, [E] = evolution). Asymmetry in the outer structure or differential structures inside the lesion, irregular borders, three or more colors, diameter greater than 6 mm, and evolution over the last 3 months are all features of neoplasms that have been linked with a higher incidence of malignancy [3, 6]. Presence of more than one criterion increases that risk [6].

Treatment should take into account the various risk factors contributing to the likelihood of malignancy, including medical history, sun exposure, family history of skin cancer, and ABCDE criteria. If the lesion appears normal, lifelong observation with medical follow-up may be adequate. If abnormalities and risk factors are present, our practice routinely recommends biopsy to rule out cellular atypia.

Follow-Up

Following biopsy, patients with abnormal pathology results may need to have follow-up procedures to remove additional atypical tissue. The rate of recurrence of dysplasia in the same site following excision is low [7]; however, patients with abnormal biopsy results would be considered at risk to develop further atypical lesions.

Our practice advises all patients to wear sunscreen. We also recommend annual skin cancer screenings to all patients. This is especially prudent for patients with a history of risk factors mentioned above, who should also be advised to monitor their existing moles for any changes. Patients with history of melanoma and/or non-melanoma skin cancers should have screenings every 3–6 months.

Questions for the Dermatologist

– *Does a benign-appearing mole need to be biopsied even if it has been present since birth? What if it has been present since birth and is now changing?*

Change is a critical component of mole history. A mole that has only been present for 1 year but has not changed may be followed. A mole that has been present for the patient's whole life and has not changed can be followed. If either changes, it should be biopsied.

– *Does hair growth in the mole signify that it is benign? Is it okay to pluck hairs out of a mole?*

There is a myth that hair within a mole means there will be no malignant transformation. Hair in a mole has no predictive value on its behavior. Patients can laser, pluck, or wax the hair without risk.

– *If color variation is uniform, is it less concerning for malignancy?*

If there are 3 different colors throughout the mole, it should be biopsied. If there are two co-centric colors, which is referred to as a fried egg nevus, defer to patient history to determine the need for biopsy.

– *Which patients need yearly full body screening?*

There are no formal guidelines for yearly screenings. Generally, dermatologists recommend annual screenings for patients with history of extensive sun exposure, sunburns, fair skin, multiple nevi, giant nevi, or family history of melanoma. There are no formal guidelines for when to start this practice, but if any of the above factors are noted during a routine physical exam, a screening should be recommended. Patients should see a dermatologist if they have changing moles.

– *If a lesion looks suspicious, is it okay to only biopsy a portion of it?*

Taking a representative sample of the mole is fine. That minimizes the size of the scar, while giving a sense of what the mole is doing. If there is high suspicion of melanoma, removing the entire lesion in the same setting is recommended. While that is potentially fallible, it is well worth the increased risk of scar.

– *Can a congenital nevus become cancerous over time?*

The malignant transformation rate for small and medium-sized congenital nevi is very low (<1 %). There is a higher risk (up to 12 % has been reported) of transformation in giant congenital nevi. A patient with giant congenital nevus may be referred to dermatology for monitoring.

References

1. Moles: Who gets and types [Internet]. American Academy of Dermatology; 2014. Available from: http://www.aad.org/dermatology-a-to-z/diseases-and-treatments/m---p/moles/who-gets-types
2. Kane KS, Ryder JB, Johnson RA, Baden HP, Stratigos A. Chapter 7. Disorders of melanocytes. In: Kane KS, editor. Color atlas & synopsis of pediatric dermatology. New York: McGraw-Hill; 2002. p. 151.
3. Tannous ZS, Mihm MC, Sober AJ, Duncan LM. Congenital melanocytic nevi: clinical and histopathologic features, risk of melanoma, and clinical management. J Am Acad Dermatol. 2005;52(2):197–203.
4. Alikhan A, Ibrahimi OA, Eisen DB. Congenital melanocytic nevi: where are we now? J Am Acad Dermatol. 2012;67(4):495.e1–17.
5. Elewski BE, Hughey LC, Parsons ME. Differential diagnosis in dermatology. Philadelphia: Elsevier; 2005. p. 379.
6. Blum A, Rassner G, Garbe C. Modified ABC-point list of dermoscopy: a simplified and highly accurate dermoscopic algorithm for the diagnosis of cutaneous melanocytic lesions. J Am Acad Dermatol. 2003;48(5):672–8.
7. Goodson AG, Florell SR, Boucher KM, Grossman D. Low rates of clinical recurrence after biopsy of benign to moderately dysplastic melanocytic nevi. J Am Acad Dermatol. 2010;62(4):591–6.

Chapter 50
Dermatofibroma

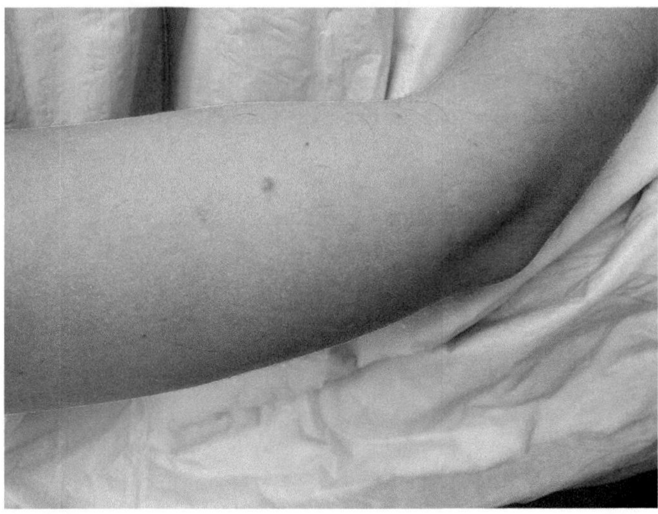

Fig. 50.1 Occasionally there is precursor nominal trauma (like a bug bite) described, but usually these dermal lesions appear spontaneously

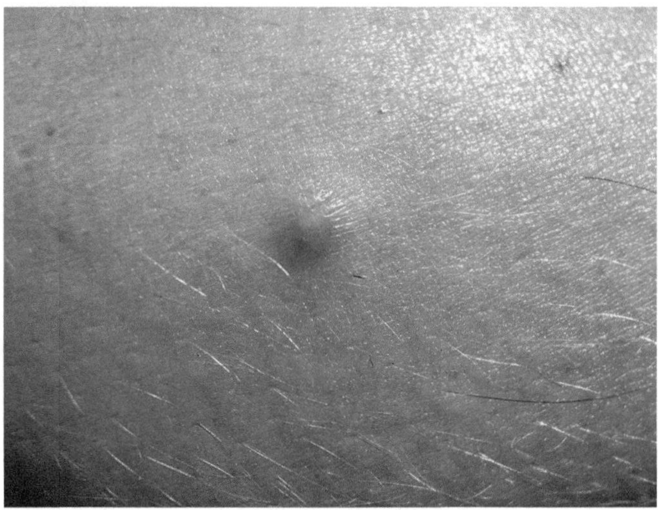

Fig. 50.2 Button-like firm dermal papule, asymptomatic

D. Reich et al., *Top 50 Dermatology Case Studies for Primary Care*,
DOI 10.1007/978-3-319-18627-6_50

Primary Care Visit Report

A 26-year-old female smoker presented with a "lump" on her right upper arm. She said it had been there for a few years and was unchanged until recently, when she noticed a "white thing on it." The patient wanted to have it removed.

Vitals were normal. On exam, there was a non-tender 4 mm hyperpigmented papule on her right upper arm with central white dome.

Unsure what this was, I referred the patient to dermatology. However, the patient did not want to pay the higher co-pay to go to a specialist and opted to leave the lesion alone.

Discussion from Dermatology Clinic

Differential Dx

- Dermatofibroma
- Prurigo nodularis
- Keloid
- Epidermal cyst
- Foreign body granuloma
- Common nevus
- Schwannoma

Favored Dx

The lesion has been present for a few years without change, which suggests it is benign. The growth is small, firm, and located on an extremity, all of which are features of dermatofibromas.

Overview

Dermatofibromas, also called histiocytomas, are benign dermal nodules that usually appear in the extremities. Dermatofibroma is a common skin lesion, accounting for 3 % of skin lesion specimens received by one laboratory [1]. Most cases occur in the third through fifth decades of life and show female predominance [2]. It represents a benign process with no malignant potential. Dermatofibroma may be associated with history of local trauma. Multiple eruptive dermatofibromas have been noted in patients with systemic lupus erythematosus and HIV [3]. It is unknown whether dermatofibromas are a true neoplasm versus an inflammatory response, and there are several histologic variants of the lesions [1, 2].

Presentation

Lesions present as hyperpigmented or flesh-colored firm nodules that are typically 0.3–1.0 cm in diameter. They are dome-shaped and have ill-defined borders. They may appear gradually over the course of months and persist unchanged for years [4]. Lesions most commonly occur on limbs but may also more rarely be seen on the trunk, face, and neck [1]. Patients may report arthropod bites, or minor injuries to the site preceding lesion appearance. Dermatofibromas tend to be asymptomatic but are sometimes accompanied by tenderness or pruritus.

Workup

Diagnosis is made on clinical and pathologic features. Dimpling can be noted when the lesion is pinched between two fingers, called the "dimple sign." Dermoscopy most often reveals a central white scar-like patch surrounded by a delicate pigment network [5].

Treatment

It is not necessary to treat dermatofibromas [4]. It is even possible (but rare) for lesions to regress spontaneously [4]. However, if patients are bothered by the cosmetic appearance, the primary treatment option is removal by excision. Removal by excision is the most definitive therapy but may leave a scar comparable in size to the original lesion, and there is a possibility of recurrence [6]. Cryotherapy improves cosmetic appearance by flattening raised dermatofibromas and reducing their pigmentation but may also leave a scar [7]. Pulsed dye lasers have been shown to reduce the size, volume, dyspigmentation, and symptoms (if present) [5, 8].

Follow-Up

Follow-up will only be required to monitor progress if any therapy is elected. If no treatment is elected, follow-up can be left open to the patient. They should be advised to return for evaluation if the dermatofibroma exhibits any change in size, color, or symptoms.

Questions for the Dermatologist

– *Which procedure is used to remove a dermatofibroma? Can a family physician do it?*

Dermatofibromas are removed by excision. There are currently no reliable injectable or laser removal options. A family physician who has been trained to do small excisions with a punch biopsy would be able to remove the lesion.

– *Is there any harm in leaving a dermatofibroma alone and not removing it?*

No there is not, as they are completely benign.

– *What causes them?*

The cause of dermatofibromas is not fully understood. They are sometimes accompanied by history of local trauma, even as innocuous as bug bites or scratches. Dermatofibromas are made up of collagen-producing cells called fibroblasts. The growths usually cluster on lower extremities, but the reason for that is not known.

References

1. Alves JV, Matos DM, Barreiros HF, Bártolo EA. Variants of dermatofibroma—a histopathological study. An Bras Dermatol. 2014;89(3):472–7.
2. Han TY, Chang HS, Lee JH, Lee WM, Son SJ. A clinical and histopathological study of 122 cases of dermatofibroma (benign fibrous histiocytoma). Ann Dermatol. 2011;23:185–92.
3. Winfield HL, Smoller BR. Fibrohistiocytic lesions. In: Grant-Kels JM, editor. Color atlas of dermatopathology. New York: Informa Healthcare; 2007.
4. Wolff K, Johnson R, Saavedra AP. Section 9. Benign neoplasms and hyperplasias. In: Wolff K, Johnson R, Saavedra AP, editors. Fitzpatrick's color atlas and synopsis of clinical dermatology. 7th ed. New York: McGraw-Hill; 2013. Available from: http://eresources.library.mssm.edu:5371/content.aspx?bookid=682&Sectionid=45130140. Accessed 5 Sept 2014.
5. Alonso-Castro L, Boixeda P, Segura-Palacios JM, de Daniel-Rodríguez C, Jiménez-Gómez N, Ballester-Martínez A. Dermatofibromas treated with pulsed dye laser: clinical and dermoscopic outcomes. J Cosmet Laser Ther. 2012;14(2):98–101.
6. Zelger B, Zelger BG, Burgdorf WH. Dermatofibroma—a critical evaluation. Int J Surg Pathol. 2004;12(4):333–44.
7. Andrews MD. Cryosurgery for common skin conditions. Am Fam Physician. 2004;69(10):2365–72.
8. Wang SQ, Lee PK. Treatment of dermatofibroma with a 600 nm pulsed dye laser. Dermatol Surg. 2006;32(4):532–5.

Appendix: General Guidance for Initial Topical Steroid Use in Adult Patients[1]

Body site	Steroid potency	Duration of treatment for flares
Scalp	Superpotent (Class I) or potent (Class II)	Up to 2 weeks
Face	Mild (Class V–VII)	Up to 7 days
Trunk	Medium (Class II–IV)	Up to 2 weeks
Arms and legs	Medium (Class II–IV)	Up to 2 weeks
Hands and feet	Superpotent (Class I) or potent (Class II)	Up to 2 weeks
Eyelids, intertriginous areas	Mild (Class VI or VII)	5–7 days
Genitals, mucosa	Mild (Class V–VII)	Up to 7 days

- BID dosing is appropriate for all body sites and steroid potencies.
- Children under 1 year should only be treated with mild (Class V-VII) corticosteroids. Children over 1 year may safely use short courses of medium (Class III, IV, or V) potency steroids. Patient or parent education about proper corticosteroid use (and cessation) is essential.
- If oral steroids are indicated due to rash severity, symptoms, large body surface area affected, or non-responsiveness to topical steroids, a 15-day prednisone taper starting at 1 mg/kg/day is appropriate for adults. Anything shorter could precipitate a rebound rash.

[1] These recommendations are intended as starting points, and should always take into account disease severity, impact on patient, and individual case history. The class chosen depends on anatomical location and severity of what is being treated.

D. Reich et al., *Top 50 Dermatology Case Studies for Primary Care*,
DOI 10.1007/978-3-319-18627-6

Glossary of Dermatological Terms

Acanthosis Diffuse epidermal thickening (hyperplasia) of the stratum spinosum (prickle cell layer) of the skin, which causes it to appear darker

Annular Used to describe the ring-like shape formed by certain skin lesions

Atrophy Thinning or depression of skin due to loss of epidermal layers and/or subcutaneous fat, as seen with overuse of corticosteroids

Burrow A linear or serpiginous tunnel formed by infesting mites

Comedo Accumulation of sebum and skin debris within hair follicles, described as open (whiteheads) or closed (blackheads) comedones

Confluence Describes the distribution of skin lesions that merge and run together

Desquamation Shedding or peeling of scales of the outer layers of the epidermis (stratum corneum)

Erosion Loss of superficial layers of skin, usually due to friction or pressure

Erythema Superficial redness of the skin caused by dilation of superficial blood vessels and capillaries

Eschar A hard, darkened plaque of dead skin that overlies injured tissue, usually from burns, ulcers, gangrene, or cutaneous anthrax

Excoriation A superficial skin abrasion caused by scratching or rubbing itchy skin

Hyperkeratosis Thickening of the stratum corneum of the epidermis, sometimes associated with an increased amount of keratin

Herpetiform A rash that resembles herpes, typically featuring a cluster of vesicles

Keloid A firm, hypertrophic scar that extends beyond the borders of the original injury

Koebnerized Describes a lesion that forms in the area of an injury or scar (also called the Koebner phenomenon)

Lichenification Diffuse thickening of epidermis due to chronic scratching or rubbing resulting in visible exaggeration of normal skin lines

Maceration Softening, disintegration, and peeling of skin that is subjected to prolonged wetting

Morbilliform Describes a confluent and erythematous macular rash, similar to the rash of measles

D. Reich et al., *Top 50 Dermatology Case Studies for Primary Care*,
DOI 10.1007/978-3-319-18627-6

Onycholysis Separation of the nail plate from the nail bed, usually beginning distally

Pruritus Itching; the sensation that produces an urge to scratch

Scale Dried shed flakes made up of fragments of the stratum corneum

Serpiginous Describes a pattern formed by certain lesions, which appear to be following the track of a snake

Telangiectasia A permanent dilation of small, superficial veins in the skin

Ulceration Localized loss of the outer layer of the epidermis resulting in a concave open sore; can extend to deeper skin layers

Umbilicated Describes the shape formed by raised lesions (eg. papules) that feature a central depression

Verrucous Meaning wart-like; describes raised firm, flesh-colored lesions with a rough cauliflower-like surface

Xerosis Pathological dryness of skin and/or mucous membranes

Index

D. Reich et al., *Top 50 Dermatology Case Studies for Primary Care*,
DOI 10.1007/978-3-319-18627-6